ond
ION

MW01106409

PARKLAND
TRAUMA
HANDBOOK

second
EDITION

PARKLAND
TRAUMA
HANDBOOK

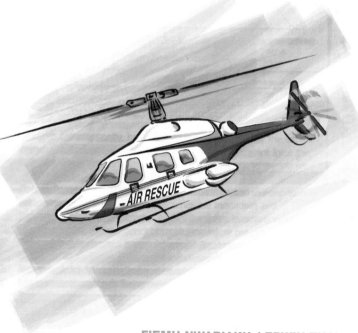

FIEMU NWARIAKU / ERWIN THAL

A *Harcourt Health Sciences Company*

Mosby
A *Harcourt Health Sciences Company*

Publisher	Laura DeYoung
Development Editor	Shelby McCoy
Project Manager	Steve Tromans
Designer	Pete Wilder
Layout	Christian Calisendorff
Illustration	Sandie Hill
	Mick Ruddy
	Susan Tyler
Cover design	Deborah Gyan
Copyeditor	Joanna Billing
Proofreader	Heather Russell
Production	Susan Walby
Index	Oliveira Potparic

Cataloging-in-Publication Data:
Catalogue records for this book are available from the US Library of Congress and the British Library

For full details of Mosby titles please write to:
Mosby International Ltd
Lynton House
7–12 Tavistock Square
London WC1H 9LB
UK

CONTENTS

ORTHOPEDIC TRAUMA

FOREWORD

It is rewarding to see the maturation in the Parkland Trauma Handbook in its second edition. In many ways, the changes appropriately match the changes in trauma care. The basic tenets have not changed. The care of the trauma patient is still based on an understanding of the pathophysiology of injuries, consistent application of established surgical principles, ongoing evaluation of clinical studies, knowledge of the surgical literature, extensive clinical experience and an organized team led by a surgeon with expertise in the field of trauma. At Parkland and most other teaching hospitals this team consists of residents and fellows who are under the guidance and careful supervision of experienced trauma-attending surgeons.

In contrast, the patterns of injury and many specific approaches have changed dramatically over the last several years. For a variety of reasons there is a notable increase in the relative proportion of blunt trauma This frequently requires more complex decision making, and non-operative care of visceral injuries continues to increase as a safe and rational approach. In addition, a number of new diagnostic and therapeutic modalities have become available. New diagnostic information can clarify or enhance the complexity of decision making and certainly increases the number of patients who can safely be considered for non-operative management.

These changes are reflected in the organization and content of many chapters of the second edition of the Parkland Trauma Handbook. There is much more emphasis on angiography and other imaging techniques in the decision-making regarding thoracic trauma. The evolution of ultrasonographic evaluation in the emergency department has significantly changed the diagnostic management of patients with torso trauma and this is reflected in the consolidation of several chapters into a single chapter on diagnostic tests and decision making. Changes in transfusion of blood and blood products, the management of head injuries and a variety of other advances are emphasized. The chapters are shortened and more concise in keeping with use of this as a handbook.

The revisions and rewriting has been led by one of our outstanding chief residents Fiemu Nwariaku and coordinated by the gentle but persistent hand of Dr. Thal. It continues to be a handbook for residents, written by residents and will be even more useful than the first edition. It is a pleasure to be associated with this fine piece of work.

James Carrico, MD
Professor and Chairman
Department of Surgery
UT Southwestern Medical Center
Dallas, Texas

FOREWORD FROM THE FIRST EDITION

Parkland Memorial Hospital is nationally recognized as a leader in the care of injured patients. Underpinning this recognition is a well established approach to the care of trauma patients. This approach is based on (1) an understanding of the pathophysiology of injury; (2) consistent application of established surgical principles; (3) ongoing evaluation of careful clinical studies; (4) knowledge of the surgical literature; and (5) decades of direct experience with the care of injured patients. This approach is carried out by a multidisciplinary team of surgeons led by general surgeons. The general surgery chief resident and the surgery specialty chief residents, under the careful supervision of experienced attending surgeons, play key roles in this system.

The Parkland surgical residents have developed formal and informal methods for transmitting this approach to each other. This handbook is the result of a suggestion by Miguel (Mike) Lopez-Viego that this information be codified into a handbook which could provide this information to surgical residents and students at Parkland and nationally. The result is a handbook written by residents for residents. Erwin Thal has played the role of an attending in a masterful fashion. He has made suggestions regarding organization, encouraged and occasionally cajoled the residents to meet deadlines. He has reviewed the manuscripts, made suggestions and provided a consistency in style and approach.

The result is this handbook which emphasizes a practical and consistent approach to the management of injured patients. It can be read from cover to cover or used as a pocket reference for immediate information on individual problems.

The handbook promises to be a major benefit to students, residents and to injured patients.

Drs Thal, Lopez and all the residents from the surgical specialties at Parkland are to be congratulated on this effort and the outstanding result.

James Carrico MD
Professor and Chairman
Department of Surgery
UT Southwestern Medical Center
Dallas, Texas

PREFACE FROM THE FIRST EDITION

This handbook is the result of the collaborative efforts of senior surgical residents and fellows from Parkland Memorial Hospital. The goal of this project was to construct a practical, portable, trauma reference source that would be of use to medical students, residents, and practicing physicians on a daily basis.

The material in this handbook is based solely on sound and established principles of trauma care. Where possible, we have included brief reviews of the historical, anatomic, and physiologic basis for the diagnostic and management regimens we recommend. The information in our book is tempered by the experiences and policies of the trauma services at Parkland Memorial Hospital. These, to a large extent, are based on decades of experience with the care of injured patients.

The authors of this text collectively dedicate this project to our teachers, past and present, senior residents and professors alike. For they provided us with the independence to manage complicated trauma patients and thus learn the art of trauma care through high volume personal experiences. These were always supported by an academic environment that was strict and demanding, but always constructive and supportive.

The support and guidance of Dr. C. James Carrico and Dr Erwin Thal during this project were critical to its completion and exemplify the dedication of the faculty at Southwestern Medical School to the field of trauma. We are also grateful for the support of Susie Baxter, Anne Gunter and Nancy at Mosby–Year Book.

The contributing authors also consider this handbook a salute to our professor and friend and our constant source of surgical wisdom, Robert N. McClelland, a man whose greatest interest has always been the education of surgeons and the advancement of surgical knowledge.

Miguel A. Lopez-Viego

CONTRIBUTORS

Farshid Araghizadeh MD
Resident, General Surgery

Aamer Ar'Rajab MD, PhD
Resident, General Surgery

Ernest Beecherl MD
Resident, General Surgery

Roger Blake MD
Resident, General Surgery

Juan M Castillo MD
Resident, General Surgery

Eric Coln MD
Chief Resident, General Surgery

Matthew H Conrad MD
Resident, Plastic Surgery

Kevin Crawford MD
Resident, Orthopedic Surgery

Jeffrey S Dean DDS, MD
Resident, Oral/Maxillofacial Surgery

Jeffrey DeCaprio MD
Resident, General Surgery

Teri DeCaprio MD
Resident, Obstetrics and
Gynecology

Brian J Eastridge MD
Trauma/Critical Care Fellow

Mark Eaton MD
Resident, General Surgery

Keith L Goldberg MD
Chief Resident, General Surgery

Lori L Gordon MD
Resident, General Surgery

Bryan Hambric MD
Resident, General Surgery

Anthony Hinz MD
Resident, Orthopedic Surgery

Jesus G Jimenez MD
Resident, General Surgery

Paul E Kaplan MD
Resident, Urologic Surgery

Anthony Macaluso MD
Chief Resident, General Surgery

Amy Macaluso MD
Resident, Anesthesia

Michael May MD
Resident, General Surgery

Kim Mezera MD
Fellow, Orthopedic and Hand
Surgery

Jennifer Moldovan MD
Resident, General Surgery

Oscar Molina MD
Resident, Emergency Medicine

Deborah L Mueller MD
Trauma/Critical Care Fellow

Fiemu E Nwariaku MD
Chief Resident, General Surgery

Nancy O'Neal MD
Chief Resident, General Surgery

Lyle H Pierce MD
Chief Resident, Urologic Surgery

Anant Praba MD
Chief Resident, General Surgery

John C Richier MD
Chief Resident, Urologic Surgery

Anneke Schroen MD
Resident, General Surgery

Daniel J Scott MD
Resident, General Surgery

Louis E Seade MD
Resident Orthopedic Surgery

Adam J Starr MD
Fellow Orthopedic Trauma Surgery

Patrick T Sweeney MD
Resident Ophthalmologic Surgery

Reggie Vaden MD
Chief Resident, General Surgery

Joseph Wells MD
Resident, General Surgery

Jonathan A White MD
Resident Neurologic Surgery

Keith J Wright MD
Resident, General Surgery

ACKNOWLEDGEMENTS

The Parkland Trauma Handbook has served as a useful, practical guide for physicians, medical students and other health care personnel since the first edition was published in 1994. There is usually little need for revision of a manual within a short period, however recent unprecedented changes in the care of the injured patient and tremendous increase in volume of surgical critical care knowledge has necessitated revision.

In spite of the large volume of new information, most chapters in the first edition were so well written that they rendered revision challenging. I thank our predecessors for such a thorough task. Although the chapters were reviewed by surgical faculty, all chapters were written by surgical residents at Parkland Memorial Hospital. Given the limited time that we possess as residents, I appreciate the effort involved and I am grateful to all the contributing authors.

My thanks to Lanette Strange, Diane Wynne and Judy Craig at the University of Texas Southwestern Medical Center for their secretarial assistance with manuscript preparation and mailing. I am also indebted to the staff at Mosby Inc. - Michael Brown, Laura DeYoung, Pui Szeto, Shelby McCoy and Simon Pritchard for their gentle reminders regarding manuscript deadlines.

In a project with so many authors, uniformity in style is difficult to maintain as is the verification of facts. For maintaining consistency, providing advice and keeping us honest I am thankful for the invaluable assistance of our teacher, advisor, mentor and friend- Dr. Erwin Thal. This book would definitely not be possible without his assistance.

I am thankful to Dr. C. J. Carrico for his encouragement, support and supervision and also for his vision for both editions of this handbook. Also I am grateful to all our teachers, and mentors for their tolerance and most of all to our patients who continue to challenge us and make the effort worthwhile.

For her patience, willingness to listen, and her support during the long and tedious editing process my deepest gratitude to my friend, Ruth Nwariaku.

Finally, to those whose contributions I have neglected to acknowledge here due to a feeble memory or weakness of character, please accept my apologies and my gratitude.

Fiemu E Nwariaku
September, 1998.

EPIDEMIOLOGY OF TRAUMA

I. OCCURRENCE

A. **INJURY** has prevailed as the leading public health problem in the United States since the early part of this century.

1. **Approximately 57 million Americans are injured each year.**
2. **Trauma remains the leading cause of death** up to the age of 44 years and accounts for more deaths than all other causes combined up to the age of 34 years.
3. **More than 150,000 people die annually from injuries.**
4. **Approximately one-third of the population** sustains an injury each year that is great enough to seek medical attention or to be unable to perform usual activities for at least a day or longer.

B. **HIGH-RISK GROUPS.**

1. **Children.**
2. **Minorities.**
3. **Elderly.**

C. **MOTOR VEHICLE COLLISIONS** (MVCs) are the leading cause of death secondary to injury from the age of 1 to 64 years.

1. **In 1995, 115 people died each day** in MVCs (one every 13 minutes) and 15 pedestrians were killed each day (one every 94 minutes).
2. **Two million traumatic brain injuries** and 10,000 traumatic spinal cord injuries occur each year.

II. ETIOLOGY

Unintentional injuries are the leading cause of death in the age group 1–44 years. Primary modes of injury include:

1. **Motor vehicle crashes.**
2. **Fires.**
3. **Burns.**
4. **Falls.**
5. **Drowning.**
6. **Poisoning.**

Drowning is the second leading cause of death due to unintentional injuries in ages 1–24 years. Homicide is the second leading cause of death in ages 15–24 years and the primary cause of death in African-American males aged 15–34 years. Burns result in about 60,000 hospitalizations and 7000 deaths annually. Falls account for about 10,000 deaths annually in people over age 65 years. Bicycle-related injuries result in almost 800 deaths and 50,000 injuries each year.

1

III. COST

1. **Annual costs secondary to injury** in the United States exceed $244 billion dollars when including death, disability, medical care, rehabilitation, and lost wages and taxes.
2. **For every death from trauma,** there are 18 patients hospitalized, 233 emergency department (ED) visits, and 450 physician office visits.
3. **Approximately 42% of all ED visits** (39.6 million annually) are related to injury.
4. **The federal government pays $12.6 billion in medical costs** and $18.4 billion in death and disability benefits annually.
5. **Traumatic brain injuries,** the leading cause of death and injury-related disability in children and young adults, cost $25 billion and spinal cord injuries more than $6 billion each year.
6. **Productive life years lost to injury** are greater than those attributed to heart disease, cancer, and stroke combined and are estimated to be >4 million annually.

IV. PREVENTION

Efforts at injury prevention focus on three major strategies:

1. **Persuasion,** which encourages persons at risk to alter their behavior voluntarily.
2. **Mandate,** which creates laws or rules to alter behavior.
3. **Protection,** which incorporates mechanisms or design alterations to protect people automatically.

From 1968 to 1991, for example, the national death rate from MVCs decreased by 21%, whereas deaths caused by firearms increased by 60%. This discrepancy is at least partially explained by systematic, national efforts to reduce fatalities by MVCs. In 1995, 46% of passenger car occupants and 53% of light truck occupants killed in car crashes were unrestrained. Similarly, 43% of motorcycle operators and 56% of passengers killed were not wearing helmets at the time of the crash. Alcohol and other drugs are implicated in approximately half of all deaths secondary to MVCs, 40% of deaths in residential fires, and 35% of all injuries seen in EDs.

TRAUMA SYSTEMS AND TRAUMA CENTER RESOURCES

I. HISTORICAL DEVELOPMENT

A. **MAJOR INNOVATIONS.** The major innovations in the development of organized trauma care stem from military conflict.

1. **The beginnings of a trauma system** within the United States are found during the Civil War when emphasis on the rapid treatment of injured soldiers dictated the organization of medical staff, transport crew, and field hospitals.

2. **This emphasis on rapid transport** and treatment was further refined in subsequent wars.

3. **A significant improvement occurred during the Korean War** with the introduction of helicopters delivering wounded soldiers directly to mobile army surgical hospitals located near the front lines.

B. **CIVILIAN TRAUMA.** Although civilian trauma care was evolving at specific centers in the United States by the 1950s, the notion of organized trauma systems came to the forefront with the publication of *Accidental Death and Disability: The Neglected Disease of Modern Society* in 1966.

C. **EMERGENCY MEDICAL SERVICES SYSTEM ACT.** The passage of the Emergency Medical Services System Act in 1973 provided financial incentives to states to coordinate regionalized EMS activities.

D. **REVIEW OF TRAUMA CARE.** Awareness of the staggering societal costs of trauma and of the widespread lack of organized care for trauma victims was further heightened by the publication of *Injury in America – A Continuing Public Health Problem* in 1985.

E. **TRAUMA CARE SYSTEMS PLANNING AND DEVELOPMENT ACT.** In 1990, Congress passed the Trauma Care Systems Planning and Development Act, marking the first time that the federal government specifically provided funding for the development of statewide trauma systems.

II. RATIONALE FOR REGIONALIZED CARE

Numerous studies have confirmed improved patient outcome and decreased mortality following trauma if medical care is provided by a specialized trauma center.

1. **Most notably, the comparison of the preventable death rates** in Orange County, California, where patients were delivered to the nearest hospital, and in San Francisco, California, where patients were delivered to the designated trauma center, by West and associates[1] illustrates the benefits of regionalized trauma care.

2. **The study also revealed** the preventable death rate in Orange County to be approximately 73%, in contrast to one preventable death in San Francisco.
3. **Following the implementation of trauma centers in Orange County,** the preventable death rate declined to 9% (Table 2.1).

III. STRUCTURE OF TRAUMA SYSTEMS

A. **PLANS AND PROTOCOLS.** The trauma system should provide well-organized plans and protocols to meet the following goals of regionalized care: access, prehospital care and triage, acute care at specialized centers, and rehabilitation.

B. **ESSENTIAL CHARACTERISTICS.** West and associates[1] have delineated eight essential characteristics of an inclusive, regional trauma system based on recommendations of the American College of Surgeons:

1. **Authority to designate trauma centers granted to a lead agency.**
2. **A formal process used for trauma center designation.**
3. **American College of Surgeons standards** applied to trauma centers.
4. **Trauma center reviews performed** by an out-of-area survey team.
5. **Designated centers limited in number** and based on community need.
6. **Written criteria established to determine hospital triage.**
7. **On-going evaluation and monitoring.**
8. **Trauma centers' availability structured on statewide basis.**

C. **RESOURCES AND CARE.** Hospitals included within a trauma system must provide care and resources commensurate with their designated level as suggested by the American College of Surgeons Committee on Trauma and local or state requirements. Table 2.2 delineates the characteristics of the various levels of trauma centers.

IV. DISASTER MANAGEMENT

Contending with disasters maximally stresses the resources and capabilities of a trauma system. Guidelines developed by the American College of Surgeons Committee on Trauma[2] provide basic recommendations for disaster management planning.

1. **Hospitals should designate a disaster committee** composed of representatives of all hospital departments.
a. Disaster plans should reflect the potential disasters for the region and differentiate between multiple and mass casualties with graded responses.
b. These plans should also integrate local or regional disaster agencies to ensure a coordinated response.
c. Lastly, the plan should reflect realistic response and care capabilities of the institution.

TABLE 2.1

COMPARISON OF NON-CNS TRAUMATIC DEATHS[a]

	San Fransisco 1974		Orange County, California						
			1974[b]		1978–1979		1980–1981		
							Trauma Center[b]		Nontrauma Center
Category	n	%	n	%	n	%	n	%	n	%
Preventable deaths	0/16	0	22/30	73	15/21	71	2/23	9	4/6	67
Appropriate operation performed	15/16	94	6/30	20	3/21	14	16/18	89	1/5	20
Hemorrhagic deaths (no surgery performed)	1/16	6	17/30	57	14/21	67	1/14	7	1/2	50

[a]From West JT, Cales R, Gazziniga A. Impact of regionalization: The Orange County Experience. *Arch Surg* 1983; 118:740–744.
[b]Region with an organized system of trauma care.

2. **Inventory of available and desired supplies**, including:
   a. Blood bank products.
   b. Local and regional blood suppliers.
   c. Space should be designated within the hospital and should include:
      1) Areas for triage, critical stabilization operations, and minor procedures.
      2) Hazardous chemical or radioactive material decontamination.
      3) Space for patients with nonsalvageable injuries and a morgue.
      4) Specified space should also be reserved for an administrative control center, a communications headquarters, and a counseling area.
3. **The disaster protocol should assign all personnel**, preferably working in teams of physicians, nurses, and administrators, to specific duties and work areas.
4. **A hospital disaster commander and a triage physician**, who is an experienced trauma surgeon, should be among the assigned personnel.
5. **A specified disaster site team** should be available if field triage and treatment is requested.
6. **Security staff and a public relations person** should be included in the personnel requirements.
7. **Disaster plan enactment** should ideally be practiced twice annually, followed by critical evaluation of system performance.

TABLE 2.2

TABULATION OF ESSENTIAL (E) AND DESIRABLE (D) CHARACTERISTICS OF TRAUMA CENTERS, BY LEVEL[a]

Characteristics	Levels		
	I	II	III
Hospital organization			
Trauma service	E	E	D
Surgery departments/divisions/services/			
(staffed by qualified specialists)			
Cardiothoracic surgery	E	D	—
General surgery	E	E	E
Neurologic surgery	E	E	—
Obstetrics and gynecologic surgery	D	D	—
Ophthalmic surgery	E	D	—
Oral surgery (dental)	D	D	—
Orthopedic surgery	E	E	—
Otorhinolaryngologic surgery	E	D	—
Pediatric surgery	E	D	—
Plastic and maxillofacial surgery	E	D	—
Urologic surgery	E	D	—
Emergency department			
(ED)/division/service/section			
(staffed by qualified specialists)[b]	E	E	E
Surgical specialties availability[c]			
In-house 24 hours a day			
General surgery[d]	E	E[d]	—
Neurologic surgery[e]	E[e]	E[e]	—
On-call and promptly available from			
inside or outside hospital			
Cardiac surgery	E	D	—
General surgery	—	—	E
Neurologic surgery	—	—	D
Microsurgery capabilities	E	D	—
Gynecologic surgery	E	D	—
Hand surgery	E	D	—
Ophthalmic surgery	E	E	D
Oral surgery (dental)	E	D	—
Orthopedic surgery	E	E	D
Otorhinolaryngologic surgery	E	E	D
Pediatric surgery	E	D	—
Plastic and maxillofacial surgery	E	E	D
Thoracic surgery	E	E	D
Urologic surgery	E	E	D

Characteristics	Levels		
	I	II	III
Nonsurgical specialties availability			
In-hospital 24 hours a day			
Emergency medicine	E[f]	E[f]	E
Anesthesiology[h]	E[g]	E[h]	E[i]
On-call and promptly available from			
inside or outside hospital			
Cardiology	E	E	D
Chest medicine	E	D	—
Gastroenterology	E	D	—
Hematology	E	E	D
Infectious diseases	E	D	—
Internal medicine	E	E	E
Nephrology	E	E	D
Neuroradiology	D	—	—
Pathology	E	E	E
Pediatrics	E	E	E
Psychiatry	E	D	—
Radiology	E	E	E
Special facilities, resources, capabilities			
ED personnel			
Designated physician director	E	E	E
Physician with special competence in care of the critically injured who is a designated member of the trauma team and physically present in the ED 24 hours a day	E	E	E
Nurses (RN and LPN) and nurses' aides in adequate numbers	E	E	E
Equipment for resuscitation and to provide life support for the critically or seriously injured shall include but not be limited to			
Airway control and ventilation equipment, including laryngoscopes and endotracheal tubes of all sizes, bag-mask resuscitator, sources of oxygen, and mechanical ventilator	E	E	E
Suction devices	E	E	E
Electrocardiograph, oscilloscope, and defibrillator	E	E	E
Apparatus to establish central venous pressure monitoring	E	E	E
All standard intravenous fluids and administration devices, including intravenous catheters	E	E	E

2

TRAUMA SYSTEMS AND TRAUMA CENTER RESOURCES

Characteristics	Levels		
	I	II	III
Sterile surgical sets for procedures standard for EDs, such as thoracostomy cut-down, etc.	E	E	E
Gastric lavage equipment	E	E	E
Drugs and supplies necessary for emergency care	E	E	E
Radiograph capability, 24-hour coverage by in-house technicians	E	E	E

aFrom American College of Surgeons Committee on Trauma. *Resources for optimal care of the injured patient.* Chicago: American College of Surgeons; 1990. Used by permission.

bThe ED staffing should ensure immediate and appropriate care for the trauma patient. The ED physician should function as a designated member of the trauma team, and the relationship between ED physicians and other participants of the trauma team must be established on a local level, consistent with resources but adhering to established standards and ensuring optimal care.

cRequirements may be fulfilled by senior residents capable of assessing emergent situations in their respective specialties. They must be capable of providing surgical treatment immediately and to provide the control and surgical leadership for the care of the trauma patient. When residents are used to fulfill availability requirements, staff specialists must be on call and promptly available.

dThe established trauma system should ideally ensure that the trauma surgeon will be present in the ED at the time of the patient's arrival. When sufficient prior notification has not been possible, a designated member of the trauma team will immediately initiate the evaluation and resuscitation. Definitive surgical care must be instituted by the trauma surgeon in a timely manner that is consistent with established standards.

eAn attending neurosurgeon must be promptly available and dedicated to that hospital's trauma service. The in-house requirement may be fulfilled by an in-house neurosurgeon or surgeon (or physician in level II facilities) who has special competence, as judged by the Chief of Neurosurgery, in the care of patients with neural trauma, and who is capable of initiating measures directed toward stabilizing the patient and initiating diagnostic procedures.

fIn level I and level II institutions, requirements may be fulfilled by senior level emergency medicine residents capable of assessing emergency situations in trauma patients and providing any indicated treatment. When residents are used to fulfill availability requirements, the staff specialist on call will be advised and be promptly available.

gRequirements may be fulfilled by residents capable of assessing emergent situations in trauma patients and of providing any indicated treatment. When residents are used to fulfill availability requirements, the staff anesthesiologist on call will be advised and be available promptly.

hMay be fulfilled when local conditions assure that the staff anesthesiologist will be in the hospital at the time of the patient's arrival in the hospital. During the interim period, prior to the arrival of the staff anesthesiologist, a certified registered nurse anesthetist (CRNA) capable of assessing emergent situations in trauma patients and of initiating and providing any indicated treatment will be available.

iRequirements may be fulfilled by CRNAs capable of assessing emergent situations in trauma patients and of providing an indicated treatment. When CRNAs are used to fulfill available requirements, the staff anesthesiologist on call will be advised immediately and will attend promptly.

V. REFERENCES

1. West JT, Cales R, Gazziniga A. Impact of regionalization: The Orange County Experience. *Arch Surg* 1983; 118:740–744.
2. American College of Surgeons Committee on Trauma. *Resources for optimal care of the injured patient*. Chicago: American College of Surgeons; 1993.

VI. FURTHER READING

Arroyo J, Crosby L. Basic rescue and resuscitation – trauma system concept in the United States. *Clin Orthop* 1995; Sept (318):11–16.

Bazzoli G, Madura K, Cooper G et al. Progress in the development of trauma systems in the United States. *JAMA* 1995; 273:395–401.

Eastman AB, Bishop G, Walsh J et al. The economic status of trauma centers on the eve of health care reform. *J Trauma* 1994; 36:6.

Moore E. Trauma systems, trauma centers, and trauma surgeons: Opportunity in managed competition. *J Trauma* 1995; 39:1–11.

West JT, Williams M, Trunkey D et al. Trauma systems: Current status – future challenges. *JAMA* 1988; 259:3597–3600.

TRAUMA SYSTEMS AND TRAUMA CENTER RESOURCES

2

ADVANCED TRAUMA LIFE SUPPORT

I. HISTORY

A. **ADVANCED TRAUMA LIFE SUPPORT COURSE.** Developed in 1978 by the Lincoln Medical Education Foundation, the Advanced Trauma Life Support course (ATLS) is a continuing medical education program which was adopted by the American College of Surgeons (ACS) Committee on Trauma in 1979.

1. **It was designed to educate** the first physician responder in the initial assessment and resuscitation of the multiply injured patient.

2. **The course**, which is taught to physicians from varying specialty backgrounds, standardizes the acute care of the multiply injured patient by training physicians to manage the resuscitation and stabilization, recognize potential problems, identify limitations of their facilities, and determine the need for early transfer.

B. **TRAUMA DEATHS.** The epidemiology of trauma deaths is triphasic.

1. **The first period, immediately after the incident,** can be impacted by effective prevention policy and is outside the realm of most acute care providers.

a. Most of these deaths are avoidable only through effective prevention programs, such as helmet and seat-belt legislation.

b. These early deaths usually involve severe injuries to multiple vital organs.

2. **The second mortality peak, during the hours after injury,** is usually due to preventable conditions such as cardiac tamponade, tension pneumothorax, and rapid exsanguination from intrathoracic or abdominal injuries.

a. This period is the primary focus of ATLS, the so-called golden hour, when rapid assessment and resuscitation improve survival dramatically.

b. Rapid intervention during this time can not only increase survival but may also greatly decrease patient morbidity.

3. **Prompt therapy during the initial period following injury** can affect mortality in the third phase of post-traumatic death which occurs days to weeks after injury, usually secondary to sepsis and multiple organ failure.

II. COURSE STRUCTURE

1. **The ATLS course is supervised by the Committee on Trauma of the ACS** both in the United States and several other countries.

2. **The ATLS student course** is conducted for physicians only.

a. Nonphysicians may participate only to audit the course and they require the written approval of a State or Provincial Committee on Trauma chairperson.

b. Senior medical students may be offered the course during the 3 months prior to graduation provided there is approval by the State or Provincial chairperson.

3. **The course has recently been revised** and consists of didactic lectures, interactive lectures and skills stations, wet lab exercises that teach invasive procedures, and moulaged patient assessments.

4. **We currently enroll** all prospective surgical interns in our training program in the ATLS course during the week prior to beginning their internship.

5. **All slides, manuals, skill station radiographs, and testing materials** are distributed by the ACS.

6. **Course participants must attend the entire 2-day course,** demonstrate knowledge in core content and skill stations, and have a written test score >80%.

7. **The written test includes 40 multiple choice items** and, if >8 incorrect answers are noted, the student is required to take a remedial written test within 3 months of the initial course.

8. **Reverification is required every 4 years** by successful completion of a refresher course.

9. **International requests for the ATLS program** are reviewed by the ATLS subcommittee of the ACS Committee on Trauma.

III. SKILLS REQUIRED

1. **ATLS focuses** on prompt, accurate initial assessment and immediate, appropriate maneuvers.

2. **The skills felt to be critical are as follows:**

a. Rapid initial assessment.

b. Resuscitation and stabilization in an organized fashion.

c. Preparation for definitive care or determination of need for transfer to a trauma center, and

d. Arrangement of interhospital transfer when indicated.

3. **Delivery of optimum care to the trauma patient** is the goal of the course.

4. **Successful completion of the initial assessment testing station** is required to complete the course successfully.

IV. OUTCOME

1. **The ATLS course has been widely successful** in improving outcome for of trauma patients.

2. **In one study, mortality was decreased** from 55.2% to 13.6% following institution of ATLS protocols[1].

V. REFERENCE

1. Adam R. Trauma outcome improves following ATLS. *J Trauma* 1993; 34(6):890–898.

VI. FURTHER READING

American College of Surgeons: Committee on Trauma. *Advanced Trauma life support course*. Chicago: ACS; 1997.

American College of Surgeons: Committee on Trauma. *Advanced Trauma life support course for physicians, instructor manual,* 5th edn. Chicago: ACS; 1993.

ADVANCED TRAUMA LIFE SUPPORT

3

I. OVERVIEW

1. **Triage of the trauma patient** attempts to assess multiply injured patients systematically in a reproducible and accurate way to prioritize care and assess injury.
2. **Appropriate triage is essential to minimize morbidity:** however, scoring systems are not fail-safe and thus there is an inherent bias toward overtriage in most scoring systems.
3. **Scoring systems** have the ability to identify high-risk patients requiring multidisciplinary care.
4. **These systems assess physiologic, anatomic, and biochemical measures** and correlate with morbidity and mortality to differing degrees.
5. **There is a general consensus** that a combination of physiologic and anatomic measures should be used to assess the trauma patient more accurately.

II. COMMON TRAUMA SCORING SYSTEMS

A. **GLASGOW COMA SCORE.** The GCS is a commonly used index for evaluating the level of consciousness and general status of the central nervous system (Table 4.1).

TABLE 4.1

GLASGOW COMA SCALE

Eye opening	
Spontaneous	4
To voice	3
To pain	2
None	1
Verbal response	
Oriented	5
Confused	4
Inappropriate words	3
Incomprehensible sounds	2
None	1
Motor response	
Obeys commands	6
Localizes pain	5
Withdraws from pain	4
Flexion to pain	3
Extension to pain	2
None	1

1. **Three physiologic categories** (eye opening, verbal response, and motor response) are assessed and the total score (3–15) is determined by the sum of the highest value the patient achieves in each category.
2. **The GCS correlates with mortality:** a conversion of the GCS is used to determine the Revised Trauma Score (RTS).
B. **REVISED TRAUMA SCORE.** The RTS evolved from the Triage Index and Trauma Score.
1. It utilizes the systolic blood pressure (SBP), respiratory rate (RR), and the converted GCS each on a scale from 0 to 4 (Table 4.2).
2. In the prehospital setting an RTS <11 is a strong indicator to transfer patients to a trauma center. As an in-hospital tool, the RTS score may be calculated using coded values to yield a score of 0–7.84 which correlates with in-hospital outcome (Figure 4.1):

$$\text{RTS score} = 0.9368(\text{coded GCS}) + 0.7326(\text{coded SBP}) + 0.2908(\text{coded RR})$$

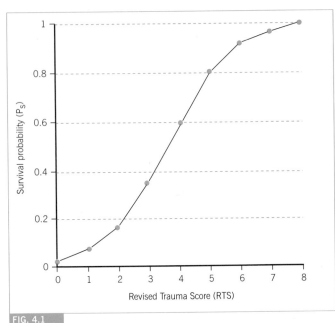

FIG. 4.1
Survival probability (P_s) vs Revised Trauma Score. (From Champion H, Sacco W, Copes W. Trauma scoring. In: Moore EE, Mattox KL, Feliciano DV, eds. *Trauma,* 3rd edn. Stamford, Connecticut: Appleton and Lange; 1996:53–67.)

TABLE 4.2

REVISED TRAUMA SCORE

Assessment	Method	Coding
Respiratory rate	Count total breaths in 15 seconds and multiply by 4	10–29 = 4
		>29 = 3
		6–9 = 2
		1–5 = 1
		0 = 0
Systolic blood pressure	Measure systolic cuff pressure on either arm by auscultation or palpation	>89 = 4
		76–89 = 3
		50–75 = 2
		1–49 = 1
		0 = 0

Glasgow Coma Scale
(see Table 4.1)
GCS conversion scale:
13–15 = 4
9–12 = 3
6–8 = 2
4–5 = 1
<4 = 0

C. **ABBREVIATED INJURY SCALE.** The AIS is a list of injuries which are assigned arbitrary values from 1 to 6, with 1 being minor and 6 nearly always fatal.
1. **Injuries are identified** in six major regions.
2. **The Injury Severity Score** (ISS) is a summary of AIS injuries and ranges from 1 to 75.
3. **A patient with an AIS** injury rated as 6 is given an ISS of 75.
4. **The ISS is calculated** as the sum of the squares of the three highest AIS scores of different body regions (Table 4.3). The ISS correlates well with mortality but is limited in that it uses only the three greatest AIS values and neglects other injuries.

TABLE 4.3

EXAMPLE CALCULATION OF INJURY SEVERITY SCORE

Body region	Injury	AIS score	ISS
Abdomen	Ruptured spleen	2	
Chest	Fractured ribs	2	$2^2 + 2^2 + 3^2 = 17$
Extremity	Fractured femur	3	

5. **The ISS does not consider** the relative importance of different body regions.
6. **ISS is one of the most commonly used scoring systems** and is useful as a clinical research tool when comparing patient groups. Figures 4.2 and 4.3 compare several rates with ISS for blunt and penetrating injuries.
D. **PEDIATRIC TRAUMA SCORE.** The PTS is a scoring system for pediatric patients which is similar to the RTS except for its use in children.
1. **It has six components:** weight, airway, systolic blood pressure, central nervous system (CNS), open wound, and skeletal injury.
2. **Each component is awarded a score** ranging from -1 to +2.
3. **Generally, patients with a PTS of <8 will benefit from transfer** to a pediatric trauma center.

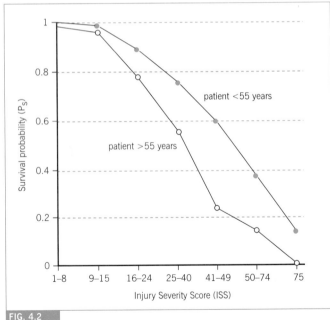

FIG. 4.2

Survival probability vs Injury Severity Score in patients with blunt injuries. (From Champion H, Sacco W, Copes W. Trauma scoring. In: Moore EE, Mattox KL, Feliciano DV, eds. *Trauma,* 3rd edn. Stamford, Connecticut: Appleton and Lange; 1996:53–67.)

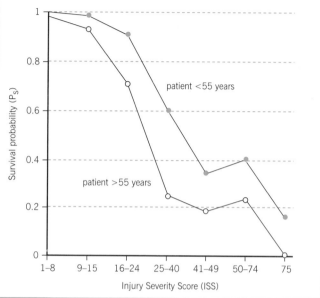

FIG. 4.3

Survival probability vs Injury Severity Score in patients with penetrating injuries. (From Champion H, Sacco W, Copes W. Trauma scoring. In: Moore EE, Mattox KL, Feliciano DV, eds. *Trauma,* 3rd edn. Stamford, Connecticut: Appleton and Lange; 1996:53–67.)

III. QUALITY IMPROVEMENT AND TRAUMA REGISTRY

1. **Data collection and frequent audit** of prehospital and in-hospital care will ensure that trauma patient outcomes are monitored and comparable to national norms. Availability of this information will also allow evaluation of the impact of instituting injury prevention programs.
2. **In keeping with the recommendations of the American College of Surgeons Committee on Trauma,** the trauma services at Parkland Memorial Hospital are part of a national trauma registry. Information from our local registry is being collated as part of the national repository.
3. **Trauma registries provide an extremely useful tool** in the hospital quality improvement program.
4. **Certain factors identify patients requiring in-depth audit.**
a. These audit filters include:
   1) Length of stay in the emergency department.

2) Excessive time to obtain a head CT scan in patients with altered mental status.

3) Time to operation in, for example, hemodynamically unstable patients.

b. Audit filters will identify patients with a delay or error in diagnosis, error in judgment, error in technique, or inappropriate care.

c. System problems and protocol procedures can be monitored as well.

d. All deaths are classified as nonpreventable, potentially preventable, or preventable.

e. This information can be used for trending of care and addressing special problems and is essential for the survey committees when reviewing trauma systems and hospitals for initial or repeat credentialing.

f. This activity is coordinated between the trauma medical director and the trauma nurse coordinator.

IV. FURTHER READING

Flint L, Richardson J. Organization for trauma care. In: Richardson J, Polk H, Flint L, eds. *Trauma: Clinical care and pathophysiology*. Chicago: Year Book; 8–9.

MECHANISMS OF INJURY AND BALLISTICS

I. GENERAL ASPECTS

A. **TRAUMA CHARACTERISTICS.** Trauma is a wound or injury characterized by a structural alteration or physiologic imbalance that results when energy is imparted during interaction with physical or chemical agents.

B. **MECHANISMS OF INJURY.** The mechanisms of injury can be generally broken down into penetrating, blunt, and miscellaneous forms of trauma.

1. **This separation is important** because the physiologic consequences of these differing forms of energy to the same organ system can vary considerably.

2. **Likewise, the treatment of these injuries is often very different.**

C. **INJURY SEVERITY.** Factors that determine injury severity, given the same mechanism of injury, include:

1. Age of the patient.
2. Anatomy.
3. Pre-existing disease.
4. Substance abuse.
5. Individual variations in response to the energy transfer of trauma.

II. BLUNT TRAUMA

Blunt trauma can be broken down into crushing or shearing mechanisms.

A. **CRUSHING MECHANISMS** involve three separate energy transfers.

1. **Primary collision initiating mass impacting the patient directly** (e.g. a car in a motor–pedestrian collision striking the patient).

2. **Patient's impact with objects in the surrounding environment** (e.g. the patient's chest striking the steering wheel in a motor vehicle collision).

3. **Internal organs contacting their supporting structures** (e.g. the brain contacting the cranial vault).

B. **SHEARING MECHANISMS** include those involving deceleration where the mobile portion of an organ shears against surrounding fixed structures (e.g. the descending thoracic aorta shears at the ligamentum arteriosum).

C. **MECHANISMS OF INJURY PRODUCING BLUNT TRAUMA** include:

1. **Motor vehicle collisions** (which account for 50% of all blunt traumatic injuries).
2. **Motor–pedestrian collisions.**
3. **Falls.**
4. **Aggravated assaults.**

D. THE LIVER AND SPLEEN are the organs most frequently injured by blunt trauma.

E. THE HISTORY taken from the patient, witnesses, and paramedics must be used to ascertain the mechanism of injury. Facts that should be gathered include:

1. Restraint devices and air bags.
2. Amount of vehicle damage.
3. Injuries or deaths of people in the same collision.
4. Ejection.
5. Location of the patient in the vehicle.

F. CERTAIN FRACTURES indicate a high-energy impact.

1. These include fractures of the scapula, first and second ribs, and femur.
2. These fractures are associated with a high likelihood of associated injuries.
3. Compression fractures (especially of the calcanei and lumbar spine) and deceleration injuries (e.g. shearing of the thoracic aorta) are common with falls over 15 feet.

G. AGGRAVATED ASSAULTS include injuries incurred from beatings, child abuse, and rape. The nature of the assaulting weapon is important in predicting the severity of the injury, and all body regions must be evaluated for occult injuries.

III. PENETRATING TRAUMA

A. PENETRATING TRAUMA refers to an injury produced when a foreign object dissipates energy to the tissue by passing through it. Although missiles do not always follow a straight path, injuries caused by penetrating trauma are often more predictable than those caused by blunt trauma.

B. ORGANS COMMONLY INJURED IN PENETRATING TRAUMA

1. Intestines.
2. Liver.
3. Vascular structures.
4. Spleen.

C. THE MOST COMMON MECHANISMS OF PENETRATING TRAUMA are knife and gunshot wounds.

1. Knife wounds cause a linear path of injury, the size of which can be deduced, to some degree, by examining the weapon.
2. Gunshot wounds, on the other hand, may result in injuries which deviate from the linear path from entrance to exit or point of rest.
   a. These injuries result from the missile's path being deflected by anatomic structures and by the blast effect.
   b. The physician with a basic knowledge of ballistics can better predict the extent of internal injuries caused by gunshot wounds.

D. BALLISTICS.

1. Most civilian gunshot wounds result from low-velocity impact (<1000 feet per second; 305m/s) and produce much less injury than the high-velocity (>3000 feet per second; 915m/s) injuries incurred in the military setting.

2. Tissue injury is proportional to the amount of kinetic energy dissipated to the tissues (which equals the product of the missile's mass and the square of the difference in entrance and exit velocities (mV^2)).

3. When a missile travels through tissue, the differential resistance it encounters causes its path to become unsteady. This instability results in yawing (deviation from the missile's longitudinal axis) and fragmentation (Figure 5.1). The amount of instability is directly proportional to the kinetic energy the missile imparts and the degree of tissue destruction (Figure 5.2).

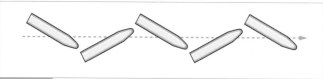

FIG. 5.1
The special ballistic property, yaw, associated with missiles of very high velocities (3000 feet per second) is depicted schematically. (From Swan KG, Swan RC. *Gunshot wound: pathophysiology and management,* 2nd edn. Chicago; 1989.)

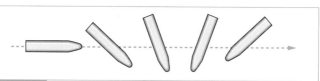

FIG. 5.2
The special ballistic property, tumble, associated with missiles of very high velocities (3000 feet per second) is depicted schematically. (From Swan KG, Swan RC. *Gunshot wound: pathophysiology and management,* 2nd edn. Chicago; 1989.)

4. **The recent development of ammunition** which is specifically designed to fragment upon entering tissue can increase tissue destruction.

5. **Cavitation** is the temporary lateral displacement of tissue as a missile travels through it. The displacement is proportional to the kinetic energy of the missile.

6. **Injury to the tissues lateral to the path of the missile** can also occur. This so-called blast effect is proportional to the kinetic energy dissipated by the missile.

7. Shotguns are short-range, low-velocity weapons (Figure 5.3). Shotgun shells contain 9–200 pellets.
8. Significant injuries, with massive tissue destruction, can occur at a range of 1–15 yards (0.9–13.5m).

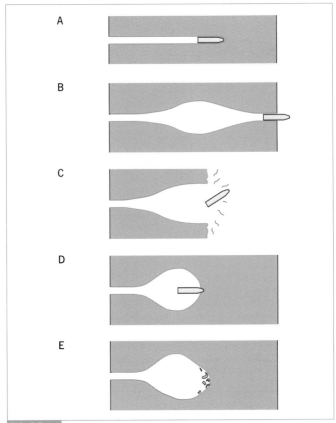

FIG. 5.3

(A) Low velocity; no cavitation; entrance and exit small. (B) Velocity, caliber, and thickness of tissue are such that cavitation occurs deep inside and entrance and exit are small. (C) Very high velocity; thin target; large and ragged exit. (D) Very high velocity; large cavity; small entrance. Exit may be small or nonexistent. (E) Asymmetric cavitation as bullet begins to deform, tumble, and fragment. (From Swan KG, Swan RC. *Gunshot wound: pathophysiology and management,* 2nd edn. Chicago; 1989.)

IV. MISCELLANEOUS FORMS OF TRAUMA

A. **EXPLOSIVE BLASTS** are the result of detonated explosives that have been converted into large volumes of gas. They can inflict damage by several mechanisms including:
1. **Fragments of casing**, causing high-velocity penetrating wounds.
2. **Shock waves with blast injury**, producing disruption of tissue.
3. **Evisceration and burns** from the explosion center.
4. **Traumatic amputations.**
B. **BURN TRAUMA** is the third most common cause of accidental death in the United States.
1. **This includes** thermal burns, scald burns, chemical burns, electrical burns, and frostbite injury.
2. **Burn patients frequently have other injuries** and the patients must be evaluated appropriately to rule out other injuries incurred.

V. FURTHER READING

Feliciano, DV. Patterns of Injury. In: Moore EE, Mattox KL, Feliciano DV, eds. *Trauma,* 3rd edn. Stamford: Appleton and Lange; 1996:85–103.

MECHANISMS OF INJURY AND BALLSITICS   5

INITIAL ASSESSMENT

I. PRIMARY SURVEY

1. **The purpose of the primary survey** is to rapidly identify life-threatening injuries rapidly in the first few minutes of evaluation.
2. **Strict adherence to the time-tested algorithms** of the primary survey minimizes the incidence of missed life-threatening injuries.

II. ABC OF TRAUMA CARE

A. AIRWAY AND CERVICAL SPINE.

1. **Injuries to the airway are rapidly fatal**, thus airway assessment is of the highest priority.
2. **Management objectives.**
   a. Maintain the intact airway.
   b. Protect the tenuous airway.
   c. Provide an airway if it is not patent.
3. **Asking the patient questions upon arriving in the emergency room** is a rapid way to ensure airway patency and to assess the mental status crudely.
4. **Look for chest wall expansion.**
5. **Listen and feel for air movement** at the patient's nose and mouth.
6. **The patient's mouth should be opened and examined** to make sure that a foreign body or flaccid tongue has not acutely occluded the airway. In the obtunded patient, an oral or nasal airway will facilitate ventilation if chin lift or jaw thrust maneuvers are successful.
7. **The cervical spine needs close attention** in all trauma patients.
   a. The cervical spine should be stabilized until it is proved to be normal, either by a cervical-spine radiologic series or by examination of an awake and oriented patient who is nontender to palpation.
   b. Stabilization of the spine is usually best accomplished with a cervical collar.
8. **Basic airway maneuvers.**
   a. Supplemental oxygen (Fio_2 >0.85) via non-rebreather mask.
   b. Chin lift and jaw thrust.
   c. Suction to evacuate secretions.
   d. Nasopharyngeal or oropharyngeal airway.
9. **Advanced airway maneuvers**. In the situation where the basic maneuvers are unsuccessful, advanced airway maneuvers will be necessary.
   a. Endotracheal intubation.
   b. Surgical airway (e.g. cricothyroidotomy, tracheostomy).

10. **Four groups of patients usually require advanced maneuvers**, namely those with:
a. Apnea.
b. Upper airway obstruction.
c. Altered mental status (Glasgow Coma Scale (GCS) <8).
d. Respiratory distress (respiratory rate >40, Pao_2 <60torr with Fio_2 0.4, $Paco_2$ >50).

11. **Oral or nasotracheal intubation** with inline cervical spine stabilization is our preferred method of obtaining a definitive airway.
a. Nasotracheal intubation requires that the patient be spontaneously breathing.
b. Also pre-oxygenation, to maintain oxygen saturation close to 100%, is required prior to intubation by any method.

12. **Open cricothyroidotomy**. The most difficult aspect of cricothyroidotomy is identifying and maintaining the surgical landmarks. The following technique reduces this difficulty:
a. The surgeon first identifies the cricothyroid membrane (Figure 6.1A) and immobilizes it between the thumb and index finger of his or her left hand (Figure 6.1B).
b. Throughout the procedure the surgeon never moves this hand, thus the cricothyroid membrane is always localized.
c. With the right hand a vertical midline incision is made down to the cricothyroid membrane (Figure 6.1C). A midline incision greatly minimizes bleeding.
d. An assistant grasps the lateral tissues with forceps to provide exposure. The cricothyroid membrane is then opened transversely with the scalpel, and a no. 4 or no. 6 tracheostomy tube is inserted (Figure 6.1D).
e. A hemostat can be inserted prior to tube placement to dilate the membrane and confirm location.
f. This procedure sounds simple but is often very difficult in the unstable patient who may be agitated or combative secondary to hypoxia and in whom one does not have the luxury of extending the neck.

13. **Needle cricothyroidotomy.**
a. This procedure is performed by placing a large intravenous (i.v.) cannula in the trachea and connecting it to oxygen flowing at 15L per minute.
b. A Y connector makes the exhalation step easier.
c. The patient is then ventilated for 1 second and allowed to exhale for 4 seconds.
d. Hypercarbia limits this technique to 30–45 minutes of ventilation.
e. Surgical cricothyroidotomy is contraindicated in children younger than 13 years.
f. Needle cricothyroidotomy may be the only option available until a formal tracheostomy can be performed.

g. Because cricothyroidotomy can be so difficult, oral intubation with
    inline stabilization is usually our preference when status of the cervical
    spine is in question.

    1) The assistant reaches over the patient's chest to hold the head in
        the midline and stable position while the intubation is performed.
    2) Most of these patients can be intubated with sedation alone.
    3) If a patient has laryngeal crepitance, significant stridor, or other signs
        of laryngeal fracture or edema, special caution must be used.

6

INITIAL ASSESSMENT

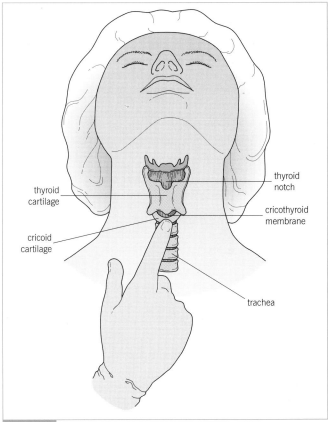

thyroid
notch

thyroid
cartilage

cricothyroid
membrane

cricoid
cartilage

trachea

FIG. 6.1A

Surgical cricothyroidotomy. A–D, see text for details.

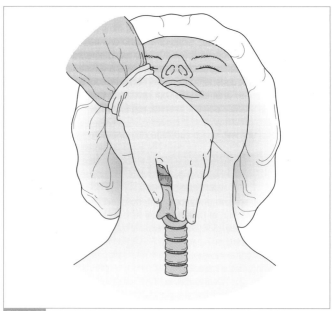

FIG. 6.1B

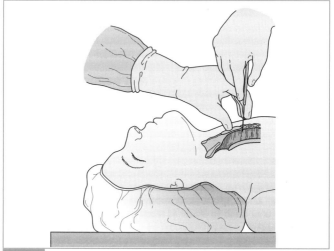

FIG. 6.1C

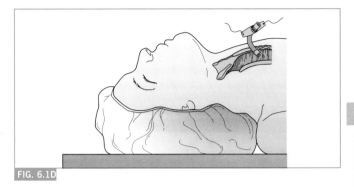

FIG. 6.1D

    4) These patients are best served by being placed in a very sterile, controlled setting (such as in the operating room) with the neck prepared, and the surgeon gowned and ready, while the anesthesiologist evaluates the airway for oral intubation.

    5) If this is unsuccessful, the surgeon can then proceed with tracheostomy or cricothyroidotomy under local anesthesia.

h. A needle cricothyroidotomy can be performed in the emergency department until a definitive airway can be obtained.

B. BREATHING.

1. **Look for chest movement and listen to breath sounds.**
2. **If breath sounds are unequal,** assessment of the tracheal position will determine if there is mediastinal shift which indicates tension pneumothorax or massive hemothorax.
3. **These should be treated immediately** by needle thoracostomy and chest-tube placement, respectively, prior to proceeding with the remainder of the evaluation.

C. CIRCULATION.

1. **Assessment of circulation** begins by observing the color and feeling the temperature of the skin.
2. **Hypovolemic shock** is characterized by cool clammy skin, pallor, and a weak pulse.
3. **Septic shock** is characterized by warm and dry extremities.
4. **Evaluation should also include** listening for heart sounds, palpation of peripheral pulses, and blood pressure measurement.
5. **Management of circulatory deficits** is begun by immediate vascular access with large bore i.v. catheters and administration of 2L of crystalloid solution (see Chapter 7).
6. **At Parkland Memorial Hospital** we do not routinely obtain central venous access as first choice except for patients with no upper-extremity access and massive intra-abdominal bleeding.

D. **DISABILITY.**
1. **A minineurologic examination** will rapidly evaluate the presence of significant intracranial injuries that will require operation.
2. **Assessment of gross neurologic function** is carried out at Parkland Memorial Hospital using the mnemonic AVPU: A – Alert patient; V – responds only to verbal stimulus; P – responds only to painful stimulus; and U – unresponsive.
3. **A rapid examination of the pupils and documentation of gross motor function** in all extremities is also performed.
E. **EXPOSURE.**
1. **The incidence of late diagnosis of significant injuries** in the trauma patient can be minimized by exposure and a careful examination of the patient's body.
2. **Hair-bearing areas,** such as the axilla, perineum, and head, have been identified by Parkland Memorial Hospital as high-risk areas for missed penetrating injuries.
3. **Maintaining comfortable ambient temperature** is a concurrent goal, especially in burn patients, since they do not possess normal skin homeostasis.
4. **Warming** is achieved by warm blankets, warm air devices, and reflective shields at our hospital.
F. **OTHER ASPECTS OF INITIAL ASSESSMENT.**
1. Resuscitation.
2. Insertion of a nasogastric tube.
3. Use of a Foley catheter.

III. SECONDARY SURVEY

The secondary survey, or complete history and physical examination, of the injured patient does not begin until the primary survey has been completed and the resuscitation phase has begun.
1. **A minority of patients will continue to remain unstable after resuscitation** and will require emergent operative intervention to control hemorrhage or evacuate lesions that are creating a mass effect within the cranial vault.
2. **The majority of patients are hemodynamically stable**.
3. **Stable patients should undergo** a complete history and head-to-toe physical examination.
4. **The secondary survey has been described**, by some, as tubes and fingers in every orifice.
5. **The survey includes special procedures** such as radiography, laboratory tests, ultrasound, CT scans, and peritoneal lavage. Chest, cervical spine, and pelvic radiographs take precedence over other studies.

6. **A nasogastric tube should be inserted**, if not contraindicated, prior to obtaining chest radiographs.
7. **The ABC should be constantly reassessed** during the secondary survey and interventions made as indicated.

A. HISTORY AND MECHANISM OF INJURY.
1. **A pertinent past medical history** should be obtained.
2. **AMPLE**: A – allergies; M – medications; P – past illnesses; L – last meal; and E – events of injury.
3. **Historical events details** should be obtained from the emergency medical technicians.

B. VITAL SIGNS.
1. **Blood pressure**: narrow pulse pressure is the earliest sign of hypovolemia.
2. **Pulse**: look for orthostatic changes, tachycardia, and arrhythmias.
3. **Respiration**: look for apnea or tachypnea.
4. **Temperature**: look for hypothermia or hyperthermia.

C. HEAD.
1. **Skull**: inspect and palpate for skull fractures and perform repeated neurologic examinations.
2. **Eyes**: check pupillary size, conjunctival or fundal hemorrhages, lens dislocation, hyphema, contact lenses, Raccoon sign, globe entrapment, and nystagmus. For a quick visual check, ask the patient to read the print on the side of an i.v. bag with each eye.
3. **Ears**: check for hemotympanum, perforation, cerebrospinal fluid (CSF) leak, and Battle's sign.
4. **Nose**: check for CSF leak, septal deviation, septal hematoma, and fracture.
5. **Mouth**: check for aspiration, hemorrhage, laceration, dental injuries, and foreign bodies.

D. MAXILLOFACIAL.
1. **Maxillofacial trauma is associated with two life-threatening conditions**: airway obstruction and hemorrhage.
2. **Patients with midface fractures** may also have fractures of the cribriform plate, and should have gastric intubation performed by the oral route, rather than nasally.

E. CERVICAL SPINE AND NECK.
1. **Principles**. All patients with maxillofacial trauma caused by blunt force should be presumed to have a cervical spine injury.
a. The neck must be protected until a fracture can be excluded, either by nontender examination of an alert, oriented, nonintoxicated patient, or by radiographic evaluation (plain films, CT, magnetic resonance imaging (MRI)) of the obtunded patient.
b. However, following manual stabilization of the neck, the cervical collar should be unfastened temporarily to allow adequate examination of the neck.

    c. The absence of a neurologic deficit or pain does not rule out injury to the cervical spine.

2. Assessment.

a. Inspection for jugular venous distention, tracheal deviation, hemorrhage, penetrating wounds, and hematoma.

b. Palpation for deformity, fracture, crepitance, masses, and thrill.

c. Auscultation for stridor and bruit.

3. Diagnostic radiography. An adequate cervical spine radiogram must show the C7–T1 junction.

4. Management. Maintain adequate immobilization of the cervical spine.

F. CHEST.

1. Assessment.

a. Visually check for symmetrical excursions, deformity, flail chest, retraction, penetrating wound, sucking chest wound, contusions, and hematomas.

b. Feel each rib and clavicle individually for crepitance or fracture.

c. Listen high on the anterior chest for pneumothorax; listen low on the posterior chest for hemothorax, decreased breath sounds, and distant heart tone.

2. Therapeutic and diagnostic techniques.

a. Chest radiograph.

b. Pleural decompression (chest-tube thoracostomy).

c. Needle thoracentesis.

d. Pericardiocentesis.

G. ABDOMEN.

1. Principles.

a. Nearly 40% of patients with significant hemoperitoneum will have no clinical manifestations.

b. Distention is a late sign.

c. A 1cm change in abdominal girth may account for as much as 3L of blood loss.

d. Initial examination and frequent re-evaluation are paramount to the management of abdominal trauma.

2. Assessment.

a. Look for a penetrating wound, hemorrhage, hematoma, contusion, and distention.

b. Listen for bowel sounds and bruit.

c. Feel for tenderness, rebound, crepitance, masses, and thrill.

3. Diagnostic studies.

a. Trauma ultrasound:

    1) This technique is emerging as the initial diagnostic study of choice in blunt abdominal trauma.

    2) Utility lies in the ability to detect free intraperitoneal fluid (i.e. blood) with up to 98% sensitivity.

3) Ability to diagnose solid-organ injury is poor.
b. Peritoneal lavage:
   1) Must be considered in patients with altered sensorium from trauma, alcohol, or drugs.
   2) Should be considered for patients undergoing anesthesia for other procedures (orthopedic or neurosurgical), because the abdominal examination is unreliable.
c. Local wound exploration for stab wounds to anterior abdominal wall.
d. CT scanning.
e. Exploratory laparotomy, if indicated.

H. RECTUM AND PERINEUM.
1. **Assessment.**
a. Anal sphincter tone.
b. Rectal blood.
c. Bowel wall integrity.
d. Prostate position.
e. Blood at the urinary meatus.
f. Scrotal or perineal hematoma.
g. Vaginal wall integrity.
2. **Management.**
a. Foley catheter, if there is no blood at meatus, no high-riding prostate gland, and no scrotal or perineal hematoma.
b. If any of these are present, a retrograde urethrogram should be obtained prior to inserting the Foley catheter.

I. BACK.
1. **Palpate each spinous process** for bony deformity.
2. **Look for evidence of** blunt or penetrating trauma.

J. EXTREMITIES AND FRACTURES.
1. **Assessment.**
a. Inspection for deformities, expanding hematoma, and open wound.
b. Palpation for tenderness, crepitance, abnormal movement, fracture, and pulses.
2. **Management.**
a. Appropriate use of splints.
b. Tetanus prophylaxis as indicated.
c. Pain relief, only if there are no other associated intra-abdominal concerns.

K. NEUROLOGIC.
1. **Assessment.**
a. Glasgow coma scale.
b. Sensory and motor evaluation.
c. Paralysis or paresis.
2. **Management.** Adequate immobilization of the entire patient with neurosurgical consultation, if indicated.

L. VASCULAR.

1. **Assessment.**

a. Palpate or Doppler test all extremity pulses; however, the presence of these does not rule out an arterial injury.

b. Record details of vascular examination.

c. Capillary refill.

d. Signs of a vascular injury.

e. Bleeding.

f. Expanding hematoma.

g. Bruit.

h. Abnormal pulses.

I. Impaired distal circulation.

j. Decreased sensation.

k. With increasing pain compartment syndrome should be ruled out.

l. Continued re-evaluation.

2. **Management.**

a. Angiogram, if arterial injury is suspected.

b. Fasciotomies, if indicated.

c. Amputation, if indicated.

V. FURTHER READING

American College of Surgeons: Committee on Trauma. *Advanced trauma life support program for physicians,* 5th edn. Chicago; 1993.

7

A. **DEFINITION.** Shock may be defined as the clinical state characterized by inadequate tissue perfusion. Untreated, this hypoperfusion leads to organ failure and patient death. The ability to recognize and treat shock and its underlying causes, is essential in trauma care. Classification of the types of shock allows better understanding of the pathophysiology and treatment of inadequate tissue perfusion (Table 7.1).

B. **TYPES OF SHOCK.**

1. **Hypovolemic (hemorrhagic) shock** is the result of acute blood loss, or the loss of plasma and extracellular fluid, with a reduction in the circulating intravascular volume. This is the most common form of shock in the injured patient.

2. **Cardiogenic shock** is diminished cardiac output resulting from failure of the heart as a pump or mechanical restriction of cardiac function by impaired venous return, as with cardiac tamponade or tension pneumothorax.

3. **Neurogenic shock** is caused by relative hypoperfusion due to the loss of vascular tone following spinal cord injury. Neurogenic shock is rarely the result of an isolated head injury and this form of shock signals the surgeon to search for another cause of hypotension in the head-injured patient.

4. **Septic shock** is characterized by decreased systemic vascular resistance with increased venous capacitance and arteriovenous shunting secondary to infection. Septic shock is uncommon immediately after injury but may occur with a delay in presentation, especially following penetrating abdominal trauma.

C. **INITIAL ASSESSMENT.** Following the establishment of an adequate airway and ventilation with supplemental oxygen, the circulatory system is evaluated.

D. **DIAGNOSIS.** Vital signs and physical examination, combined with a simultaneously obtained pertinent history, are essential in the diagnosis and proper treatment of shock.

E. **FURTHER ACTION.** The following initial steps in the treatment of shock in the trauma patient are appropriate regardless of its cause.

TABLE 7.1

CHARACTERISTICS OF SHOCK STATES

Physiologic sign	Hypovolemic	Cardiogenic Myocardial	Cardiogenic Mechanical	Neurogenic	Septic
Pulse	+	+	+	nl or −	+
Blood pressure	−	− to nl	−	−	−
Respiratory rate	+	+	+ +	nl/+	+ +
Urine output	−	−	−	−	−
Neck veins	Flat	Distended	Distended	Flat	Flat
Skin temperature	Cold	Cold	Cold	Warm	Warm
Skin sensation	Clammy	Clammy	Clammy	Dry	Moist/dry
Cardiac index	+/−	−	−	+/−	+ +
Central venous pressure	−	+	+ +	−	nl/+
Pulmonary capillary wedge pressure	−	+ +	+	−	−/nl
Systemic vascular resistance	+ +	+ +	+ +	−	−
Response to volume	+ + +	−	+	+	+

− = decreased; + = increased; nl = normal

II. VASCULAR ACCESS

A. **OBTAIN ACCESS.** Prompt access to the vascular system is rapidly obtained by insertion of two large-bore (≥ 16 gauge) intravenous (i.v.) catheters into the patient's arms.

1. **Blood is obtained** for type and cross-matching during insertion of the catheters.
2. **Saphenous vein cutdowns** are employed if upper-extremity peripheral access is unobtainable.
3. **Large-bore catheters** allow rapid instillation of fluid.
4. **The limiting factors** in fluid administration include catheter length and diameter.
5. **Vein size** has no clinical effect on the rate of fluid administration.
6. **The use of pressure devices,** such as on the 'Level One' warming unit, allows the administration of up to 1–2L of fluid per minute.
7. **Percutaneous femoral venous catheters** provide a readily available alternative when peripheral access is unobtainable.
8. **Catheters should be of sufficient length** to prevent dislodgment associated with the activity in the emergency department or during transport.
9. **Potential abdominal injury** is not a contraindication to lower extremity access and infusion.

B. **RISKS DURING INITIAL RESUSCITATION.** Central venous catheters should be avoided during the initial resuscitation, whenever possible, because of the risk of pneumothorax and the difficulty of rapid infusion of large volumes of fluid through the long catheters.

1. **Complications** are more common under emergency conditions and hemodynamic monitoring is generally not a high priority during the initial resuscitation.
2. **Introducer sheaths,** normally used during the insertion of pulmonary artery catheters, will allow rapid volume infusion through the subclavian or jugular veins when these routes must be used.

C. **FLUID CHALLENGE.**

1. **A bolus infusion** of up to 2L of lactated Ringer's solution may stabilize the tachycardic or hypotensive patient and identify those patients who require immediate therapy.
2. **Therapeutic decisions** are based on the trauma patient's response to fluid challenge in combination with findings or changes in physical examination or diagnostic tests.
3. **Patients who have ceased bleeding** tend to respond permanently to the fluid challenge, but patients who respond transiently usually have ongoing blood loss.

III. HYPOVOLEMIC SHOCK

A. **HEMORRHAGIC OR HYPOVOLEMIC SHOCK.** This is the most common form of shock encountered in the care of the injured patient.

1. **It may result from the loss** of whole blood, or of plasma and extracellular fluid, as is seen in the burn or crush injury patient.

2. **The loss of intravascular volume** causes the sympathetic and adrenal responses to increase peripheral vascular resistance and heart rate rapidly in an attempt to maintain blood pressure.

3. **Vasoconstriction** in the skin, muscle, kidney, and splanchnic vascular beds results in a redistribution of blood flow to the heart and brain.

4. **Simultaneous venoconstriction** prevents blood from pooling in the venous capacitance vessels.

5. **As the volume deficit grows**, the pulse pressure narrows with the rise in diastolic pressure secondary to sympathetic discharge.

6. **Continued hemorrhage** leads to a fall in systolic pressure and progressive hypotension as the compensatory mechanisms are overwhelmed.

7. **A rise in the precapillary:postcapillary resistance ratio** leads to a decrease in capillary hydrostatic pressure and the movement of fluid from the extracellular to the intravascular space.

8. **The decreased organ blood flow** leads to decreased oxygen delivery and waste removal.

9. **Cells shift from aerobic to anaerobic metabolism**, with a resultant increase in lactic acid production and a fall in pH.

10. **Altered cell membrane permeability** and the inability to maintain electrolyte gradients leads to sodium and water shifts into the cell, with further depletion of the extracellular fluid volume.

11. **Without correction of these shock-induced abnormalities**, depletion of high-energy phosphate stores, further loss of membrane integrity, cellular swelling, and organelle breakdown lead to cell death.

12. **Advanced Trauma Life Support guidelines** describe four classes of hemorrhage based on the percent of acute blood volume loss (Table 7.2).

13. **Adult blood volume** is approximately 7% of normal body weight.

B. **CLASSIFICATION OF HEMORRHAGIC SHOCK.**

1. **Class I hemorrhage:** loss of up to 15% of blood volume.

2. **Class II hemorrhage:** 15–30% blood loss or 800–1500mL of blood in a 70kg man.

3. **Class III hemorrhage:** 30–40% blood loss, approximately 2000mL in an adult.

4. **Class IV hemorrhage:** >40% blood loss.

While these classifications are important in understanding the pathophysiology of shock, they are not extremely useful clinically.

TABLE 7.2

HEMORRHAGIC SHOCK[a]

Physiologic sign	Class I	Class II	Class III	Class IV
Blood loss (% blood volume)	>15	15–30	30–40	≥40
Pulse rate (b.p.m.)	<100	>100	>120	>140
Blood pressure	Normal	Normal	Decreased	Decreased
Pulse pressure (diastolic)	Normal or widened	Narrowed	Narrowed	Very narrow or absent
Capillary refill	Normal	Delayed	Delayed	Delayed
Skin	Normal	Cool, pale	Cool, pale	Cold, ashen with mottling
Respiratory rate	14–20	20–30	30–40	>35
Urine output (mL/h)	>30	20–30	5–15	Negligible
Mental status	Slightly anxious	Mildly anxious, thirsty	Anxious and confused, or apathetic	Lethargy progressing to coma

[a] Modified from American College of Surgeons. *Advanced trauma life support program.* Chicago; 1988:72.

7

SHOCK

C. **TREATMENT OF HEMORRHAGIC SHOCK.**

1. **Control of external hemorrhage** is accomplished by direct digital pressure.

2. **Initial fluid challenge** of 1–2L of lactated Ringer's solution allows rapid, inexpensive replacement of intravascular and aforementioned extracellular fluid losses during the initial resuscitative period.

3. **Crystalloid resuscitation** reduces the necessity for blood transfusion in many patients with mild to moderate shock.

4. **The majority of patients will respond to the initial volume challenge**. However, deterioration will occur following slowing of the infusion in patients experiencing continued fluid losses or ongoing hemorrhage.

5. **Trauma patients with continued signs of hypoperfusion** following lactated Ringer's infusion require whole blood or packed red blood cell replacement when hypovolemia results from blood loss.

a. Fresh whole blood is the primary therapy for hemorrhagic shock.

b. When typed and cross-matched blood is not available, universal donor type O, Rh negative blood, or preferably type-specific blood is administered.

c. Packed red blood cells may be transfused when whole blood is not available.

6. **During the initial resuscitation phase**, diagnostic tests and repeated physical examinations are performed to identify sites of continued hemorrhage.

D. **EXSANGUINATING HEMORRHAGE.** Failure to respond to adequate crystalloid and blood administration indicates exsanguinating hemorrhage and the need for immediate surgical intervention or search for other causes of shock, such as:

1. Spinal cord injury (neurogenic).

2. Myocardial infarction.

3. Cardiac tamponade or tension pneumothorax (cardiogenic).

E. **COLLOID RESUSCITATION.**

1. **Initial treatment** with colloid volume expanders (albumin, dextran, hydroxyethyl starch) has the hypothetical advantages of greater residence time in the intravascular space and less total fluid administration when compared with crystalloid resuscitation.

2. **When titrated to similar therapeutic end points**, colloid resuscitation offers no improvement over crystalloid resuscitation in mortality, morbidity, or length of hospital stay.

3. **Colloid volume expanders** are considerably more expensive than crystalloid solutions and, by remaining in the intravascular space, do not allow replenishment of the depleted interstitial space.

4. **The use of colloid resuscitation is avoided** in the acute setting at Parkland Memorial Hospital, with the exception of blood.

F. **HYPERTONIC RESUSCITATION.**

1. **Hypertonic saline solution** (with or without dextran) has been advocated for the initial resuscitation of shock, especially during prehospital transportation.

2. **Small boluses of hypertonic fluid** allow more rapid restoration of hemodynamic parameters in the injured hypovolemic patient, presumably by the osmotic transfer of interstitial and intracellular fluid into the intravascular space (Figure 7.1).

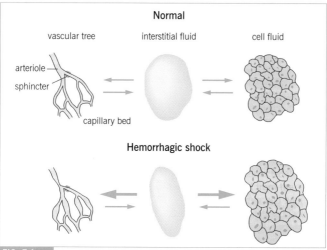

FIG. 7.1
Response of interstitial fluid to hemorrhagic shock. (From Shires GT III et al. Shock. In: Schwartz SI, ed. *Principles of surgery,* 5th edn. New York: McGraw-Hill; 1989.)

3. **The use of hypertonic resuscitation fluids** has not been shown to influence morbidity or mortality in trauma patients.
4. **No lasting hemodynamic benefit of hypertonic saline resuscitation** over routine crystalloid administration was demonstrated during a study at Parkland Memorial Hospital. These solutions are not used in our institution.

G. PNEUMATIC ANTISHOCK GARMENTS (MAST TROUSERS).

1. **Inflated MAST trousers** cause an increase in peripheral vascular resistance and may rapidly improve hemodynamic parameters.
2. **Because of the increased peripheral resistance** the cardiac output may fall, resulting in decreased tissue perfusion despite elevation of the blood pressure.
3. **MAST garments do not improve survival**, in the urban setting, and their application must not delay transport or fluid resuscitation.
4. **Application has been associated with** the development of compartment syndromes following prolonged inflation of the leg segments.

5. **Inflation of the abdominal compartment** may increase respiratory distress, especially in blunt trauma victims with rupture of the diaphragm.

6. **MAST trousers may have a benefit** in providing temporary stabilization of pelvic fractures associated with hemorrhage during transport of patients over long distances.

7. **Deflation of the trousers should be gradual and sequential**, one compartment at a time, and should be stopped if the patient exhibits a blood pressure drop ≥ 10–15mmHg.

H. AORTIC CROSSCLAMPING.

1. **Crossclamping of the aorta** has been recommended in the patient with intra-abdominal injuries and persistent hypotension despite aggressive resuscitation.

2. **The efficacy of this procedure** has no consensus among many authors.

3. **Resuscitative emergency department thoracotomy,** with occlusion of the descending thoracic aorta and open cardiac massage, may be useful for the patient in refractory shock to allow effective resuscitation en route to the operating room for definitive control of intra-abdominal bleeding.

4. **This procedure is used infrequently at Parkland** and, if the patient decompensates in the operating room, we prefer rapid entry celiotomy and intra-abdominal control of the aorta at the diaphragm.

I. VASOPRESSORS.

1. **The use of vasopressors in hypovolemic shock is contraindicated**.

2. **These agents act by elevating blood pressure** through increasing peripheral vascular resistance and, as a result, they decrease tissue perfusion and aggravate the cellular derangements of hypoperfusion.

J. END POINTS OF RESUSCITATION.

1. **Frequent re-evaluation** of the injured patient during the resuscitation period is necessary to determine the adequacy of treatment.

2. **Improvement of the volume deficit** is signaled by the improvement in the following parameters:

a. Resolution of tachycardia.

b. Pulse pressure.

c. Blood pressure.

d. Improvement in mentation.

e. Skin perfusion.

f. Urine output.

3. **The base deficit and serum lactate** are sensitive indicators of the degree of anaerobic metabolism during shock.

a. The initial base deficit predicts the magnitude of volume deficit.

b. A persistent or worsening base deficit, despite efforts at resuscitation, signals ongoing bleeding and should provoke both a search for the cause and therapeutic intervention.

c. Serum lactate may be utilized in a similar fashion.

4. **The gastric mucosal pH**, or pH$_i$, has recently been proposed as an even more sensitive guide to adequate tissue perfusion and is utilized in our intensive care unit (ICU) to monitor adequacy of resuscitation in patients who do not respond appropriately to routine interventions.
a. The splanchnic bed is among the first to be affected in shock and the last to be restored to normal after resuscitation.
b. The pHi is readily measured in the ICU using a gastric tonometer and may provide not only a measure of the adequacy of resuscitation but also an early warning system for systemic complications following initial stabilization.
5. **Hemodynamic monitoring,** with a central venous pressure or pulmonary artery catheter, may assist in following volume status and managing superimposed cardiac dysfunction or septic shock. We routinely resuscitate our geriatric patients in the ICU, within 2 hours of admission, with invasive monitoring since these patients do not manifest normal signs of under-resuscitation.

IV. CARDIOGENIC SHOCK

A. **CARDIOGENIC SHOCK.** This type of shock is a manifestation of failure of the heart as a pump secondary to myocardial dysfunction, arrhythmias, or mechanical factors restricting cardiac output or venous return.
B. **DIAGNOSIS.** History, physical examination, selective hemodynamic monitoring, diagnostic tests, and a high index of clinical suspicion all play a vital role in determining the cause of cardiogenic shock.
C. **MYOCARDIAL DAMAGE.** Shock resulting from direct myocardial damage may occur following a rapid deceleration injury to the thorax.
1. **Myocardial infarction** will, occasionally, be the cause of a crash, especially in the elderly population with atherosclerosis. These patients may benefit from inotropic support, after first eliminating hypovolemia or mechanical causes of decreased perfusion.
2. **Hemodynamic monitoring** simplifies the diagnosis of myocardial dysfunction.
3. **The pulmonary capillary wedge pressure** or CWP is typically elevated, or rises sharply following a fluid challenge, with depression of the cardiac output.
4. **A positive response to fluid challenge** signals continued hypovolemia and an unrecognized cardiac tamponade or tension pneumothorax.
5. **Constant electrocardiographic monitoring** is necessary to detect dysrrhythmias accompanying myocardial contusion or infarction. These must be treated promptly.
D. **MECHANICAL FACTORS.** Mechanical obstruction of cardiac output following trauma most frequently results from cardiac tamponade or tension pneumothorax.
1. **Rapid diagnosis and treatment** are needed for these life-threatening conditions.

2. **Cardiac tamponade** occurs most commonly following penetrating thoracic trauma, although it is occasionally encountered in the patient with blunt chest injuries.

3. **Hypotension, muffled heart tones, narrow pulse pressure, and distended neck veins** accompanied by tachycardia, a paradoxical pulse, and central cyanosis suggest a diagnosis of tamponade.

4. **Abnormalities seen on the chest radiograph or an elevated CVP reading** following fluid administration, with transient improvements in blood pressure or cardiac output, may help confirm the diagnosis in the patient who is relatively stable.

5. **Therapeutic pericardiocentesis** in the unstable patient may be lifesaving but is only a temporizing maneuver.

6. **Emergent thoracotomy or sternotomy** is required for definitive treatment and repair of cardiac injuries.

7. **Emergency department thoracotomy** is indicated in the patient with suspected tamponade following penetrating thoracic trauma and who presents following a witnessed cardiac arrest.

E. **TENSION PNEUMOTHORAX.** This condition may mimic cardiac tamponade in presentation, with hypotension, tachycardia, and evidence of elevated CVP.

1. **Decreased breath sounds,** with hyper-resonance to percussion on the affected side and tracheal deviation to the opposite side, strongly suggest this diagnosis.

2. **Needle aspiration of the involved pleural cavity** is diagnostic and therapeutic and should be followed rapidly by tube thoracostomy when the diagnosis is confirmed.

V. NEUROGENIC SHOCK

Neurogenic shock, caused by a loss of sympathetic tone or an imbalance of vasodilator and vasoconstrictor influences on vascular tone, most frequently follows spinal cord injury.

1. **Sympathetic denervation** causes a relative hypovolemia with hypotension.

2. **Unlike the situation in hypovolemic shock**, the pulse pressure is wide and the skin is dry and warm in neurogenic shock.

3. **Mentation and urine output** may be normal despite the low blood pressure.

A. **TREATMENT.** The initial treatment should be as for hypovolemia, with fluid administration.

1. **If symptomatic hypotension persists** after restoration of intravascular volume, small doses of vasopressors may be necessary to support arterial pressure.

2. **Hemodynamic monitoring** may be helpful, and demonstrates a low-to-normal CVP with a normal-to-elevated cardiac output.

3. **Injudicious use of fluids** in an attempt to elevate blood pressure can result in volume overload. However, vasopressors should not be used until fluid replacement is adequate.
4. **Vasopressors are withheld in the asymptomatic patient** in spite of a low (80–90mmHg) blood pressure.

B. **ACCOMPANYING CONDITIONS.** Neurogenic shock may be accompanied by hemorrhagic shock in the patient with multiple injuries.
1. **Hemorrhage at the site of spinal cord injury** may also produce hypovolemia in the patient with an isolated injury.
2. **Hemodynamic measurements** will show a decreased CVP with a depressed, or falling, cardiac output, indicating increased volume requirements.

C. **OTHER CAUSES.** Neurogenic shock may also be caused by high spinal anesthesia with loss of vasomotor tone and acute gastric dilatation.

D. **HEAD-INJURED PATIENT.** Isolated head injuries do not cause hypotension or shock except as a preterminal event. The presence of shock in the head-injured patient requires the search for another cause of hypotension, which is generally blood loss in the chest or abdomen, or blood loss associated with pelvic and long bone fractures.

VI. VASOGENIC SHOCK

A. **SEPTIC SHOCK.** This is uncommon immediately following injury, although it is the most common cause of death in ICU patients.

B. **PRESENTATION.** The trauma victim may present in septic shock following a delay in arrival, especially after penetrating abdominal trauma or other causes of intestinal perforation.

C. **DIAGNOSIS.** The presence in the bloodstream of microorganisms, or their toxins, leads to a systemic response characterized by cardiovascular insufficiency.

D. **MANIFESTATION.** Early septic shock manifests as a hyperdynamic state with decreased systemic vascular resistance, increased cardiac output, and increased oxygen consumption.
1. **Relative hypovolemia exists,** leading to hypotension and oliguria.
2. **Progression to multiple organ failure** and death over a period of hours to weeks is not uncommon.

E. **TREATMENT.** Identification and elimination of the infectious focus form the mainstay of the treatment of septic shock.
1. **Antibiotic administration** and, more importantly, surgical drainage or débridement when appropriate, are crucial for patient survival.
2. **Adjunctive therapy** is useful to prepare the patient for operation or support the patient until the infectious process is eliminated.
3. **Correction of intravascular and extravascular volume deficits** is essential to restore tissue perfusion.

4. **Crystalloid-balanced salt solutions** are used to replace third-space volume losses.
5. **Blood may be necessary** to maximize oxygen delivery, depending on the hemoglobin level.
6. **Pulmonary artery catheter monitoring** is beneficial in assessing the adequacy of volume replacement and the response to fluid challenge in the septic patient.
7. **The persistence of hypotension,** despite adequate volume replacement and appropriate treatment of infection, often indicates myocardial depression or very low systemic vascular resistance. In these instances, hemodynamic support with an inotropic agent with α-adrenergic activity, such as dopamine, is necessary.
8. **Invasive monitoring** is essential when using vasoactive drugs.
9. **Steroids do not improve survival** when given to patients in septic shock.

VII. FURTHER READING

American College of Surgeons Committee on Trauma. *Advanced trauma life support courses*. Chicago: American College of Surgeons; 1997.

Carrico CJ, Canizaro PC, Shires GT. Fluid resuscitation following injury: rationale for the use of balanced salt solutions. *Crit Care Med* 1976; 4:46–54.

Davis JW, Shackford SR, Holbrook TL. Base deficit as a sensitive indicator of compensated shock and tissue oxygen utilization. *Surg Gynecol Obstet* 1991; 173(6):473–476.

Eddy AC, Rice CL. The right ventricle: an emerging concern in the multiply injured patient. *J Crit Care* 1989; 4:58–66.

Edwards JD. Practical application of oxygen transport principles. *Crit Care Med* 1990; 18:45–48.

Fortune JB, Feustel PJ, Saifi J et al. Influence of hematocrit on cardiopulmonary function after acute hemorrhage. *J Trauma* 1987; 27(3):243–249.

Ivatury RR, Simon RJ, Havriliak D et al. Gastric mucosal pH and oxygen delivery and oxygen consumption indices in the assessment of adequacy of resuscitation after trauma: a prospective randomized study. *J Trauma* 1995; 39(1):128–134.

Lollgen H, Drexler H. Use of inotropes in the critical care setting. *Crit Care Med* 1990; 18:56–60.

Luce JM. Pathogenesis and management of septic shock. *Chest* 1987; 91:3–10.

Mueller HS. Inotropic agents in the treatment of cardiogenic shock. *World J Surg* 1985; 9:3–10.

Mullins RJ. Management of shock. In: Moore EE, Mattox KL, Feliciano DV, eds. *Trauma*. Stamford: Appleton and Lange; 1996:159–180.

Nathanson C, Parrillo JE. Septic shock. *Anesth Clin North Am* 1988; 6:73–85.

Provost DA, Weigelt JA, Lewis FR Jr. Cardiorespiratory physiology and oxygen delivery. In: Weigelt JA, Lewis Jr FR, eds. *Surgical critical care*. Philadelphia: WB Saunders Co.; 1996:49–65.

Putterman C. The Swan–Ganz catheter: a decade of hemodynamic monitoring. *J Crit Care* 1989; 4:127–146.

Shires GT. Principles in the management of shock. In: Shires GT, ed. *Principles of trauma care,* 3rd edn. New York: McGraw-Hill; 1985: 3–43.

Wiencek RG, Wilson RF. Injuries to the abdominal vascular system: how much does aggressive resuscitation and prelaparotomy thoracotomy really help? *Surgery* 1987; 102:731–736.

7

SHOCK

TRANSFUSION THERAPY

I. INTRODUCTION

Blood and blood component transfusions are useful supportive therapy when indicated throughout the entire management period. Indications for transfusion of blood products are generally more liberal in trauma patients than in nontrauma patients.

II. INDICATIONS

A. RESTORATION OF INTRAVASCULAR VOLUME.

1. **This is the most common indication for red blood cell transfusion**. Empirical transfusion with packed red blood cells (PRBC) is indicated in the emergency department when the patient remains hypotensive [systolic blood pressure (SBP) <90] after sufficient crystalloid administration (usually 2000mL) and no other source of hypotension is identified.
2. **Type specific and, if necessary, type O negative blood** is administered in this situation en route to the operating room or intensive care unit. Patients with a class II hemorrhage (15–30% blood volume loss) usually do not require transfusion if their source of hemorrhage is controlled.
3. **Blood transfusion is always necessary** for those patients with obvious evidence of hypoperfusion (class III and IV shock).
4. **Most patients who are hypotensive** from a hemorrhagic source have lost about 2000mL of blood.

B. RESTORATION OF OXYGEN-CARRYING CAPACITY.

1. **A hemoglobin of 7mg/dL** (Hct 20–21) is well tolerated in most trauma patients and is an acceptable end point once surgical lesions are corrected and hemostasis is achieved.
2. **A hemoglobin of 10mg/dL** (Hct 30) may be optimal in the elderly and in patients with evidence of cardiovascular compromise.
3. **This 'transfusion trigger'** should be individualized based on multiple factors including:
   a. Mental status changes.
   b. Tachycardia.
   c. Respiratory rate.
   d. Cardiac output and index.
   e. Arterial pH.
   f. Base deficit.
   g. Urine output.
   h. Gastric tonometry.

C. CORRECTION OF COAGULOPATHY.

1. **Coagulopathy is often seen in patients** with massive transfusions (>12 units), hypothermia, crystalloid over-resuscitation, and prolonged shock.
2. **Significant platelet dysfunction** may develop in these patients.
3. **The platelet 'transfusion trigger'**, in this setting, should be 100,000/μL.
4. **When the patient is fully resuscitated**, platelet counts of 20,000–40,000/μL are acceptable.
5. **Normal values for prothrombin (PT) and partial thromboplastin times (PTT)** are not accurate in the hypothermic patient as this study is performed at normal body temperature. Achieving normothermia is a critical step when correcting coagulopathy in the trauma patient.

III. BLOOD PRODUCTS
A. PACKED RED BLOOD CELLS.

1. **This product is obtained after centrifugation of whole blood** (Table 8.1).
2. **PRBCs are usually stored in sodium citrate anticoagulant solution,** which functions by binding calcium, thus depleting calcium levels.
3. **PRBCs are used** to replenish volume and oxygen-carrying capacity.
4. **Each unit is 200–300mL in volume.**
5. **Citrate is converted to lactate** and then bicarbonate in the patient, which provides an alkaline load.
6. **Although PRBCs are prepared by centrifugation,** up to 40% of a unit may consist of leukocytes, plasma, and platelets.
7. **Washed red blood cells are available,** which are further depleted of leukocytes, platelets, and plasma.
8. **Washed red blood cells may be useful** in preventing a nonhemolytic febrile reaction that is caused by host antibodies to foreign leukocytes.

B. WHOLE BLOOD.

1. **Theoretically, this is the ideal transfusion product** because it contains a full complement of red blood cells, platelets, and coagulation proteins.
2. **With storage over 24–48 hours** there is significant platelet dysfunction and decrease in clotting factor activity.
3. **This product has limited utility** in the trauma patient.

C. PLATELETS.

1. **Patients with thrombocytopenia and hemorrhage** require platelet transfusions.
2. **Platelets are obtained** from the buffy coat layer seen after centrifugation of whole blood.
3. **Platelets can be stored frozen** for up to five days.
4. **Each unit will increase platelet count** by approximately 10,000/μL and contains coagulation factors.
5. **Platelet transfusions are usually administered** in six-unit increments.

TABLE 8.1

BLOOD PRODUCTS

Blood product	Characteristics
Whole blood	(500mL); 35–40% hematocrit (Hct); no platelets or coagulation factors active; frequently unavailable
Packed red blood cells	(300mL); 65–80% Hct; no platelets, white blood cells, or plasma. Each unit should raise Hct 3% and hemoglobin by 1g/dL. Children are frequently transfused in 10mL/kg volumes
Leukocyte-poor red blood cells	(300mL); 65–80 Hct; 70% leukocytes removed; for patients with frequent febrile reactions
Washed red blood cells	(300mL); 65–80% Hct; 85% leukocytes and 99% plasma removed; for patients with allergic reaction to plasma protein in donor blood
Frozen red blood cells	(250mL); 65–80% Hct; 3-year shelf-life storage of rare blood or autologous donor cells
Platelets	(40–70mL); 5.5×10^3 platelets per unit. Each unit should raise platelet count 5000–10,000; 6–10 units are usually given at a time
Fresh frozen plasma	(180–300mL); 200 units factor VIII and 200–400mg fibrinogen per unit. Must be used within 6 hours of thawing. Requires ABO typing. Adequate source of all coagulation proteins
Cryoprecipitate	>80 units factor VIII (VIII:C); good source of factor VIII:vWF and fibrinogen in <15mL plasma

8

TRANSFUSION THERAPY

D. **FRESH-FROZEN PLASMA.**
1. **Immediate freezing of the supernatant,** left after removal of red blood cells and buffy coat, results in fresh-frozen plasma.
2. **It contains high levels of coagulation factors** including II, V, VII, IX, and XI but may require up to 45 minutes to thaw and should be used promptly.
3. **Fresh-frozen plasma is used liberally** at the Parkland Memorial Hospital in coagulopathic patients with solid-organ injuries (liver or spleen) or intracranial hemorrhage.
E. **CRYOPRECIPITATE.**
1. **Cryoprecipitate is used infrequently in patients with acute trauma.**
2. **It contains concentrated factor VIII, von Willebrand factor, and fibrinogen.** It is most useful in specific conditions such as:
a. von Willebrand's disease.
b. Hemophilia A.
c. Hypofibrinogenemia.
d. Factor XIII deficiency.

F. **FACTOR CONCENTRATES.**

1. **Specific factor concentrates,** such as factor VIII, are produced by isolation and concentration techniques that are expensive and labor intensive.

2. **They are of limited use in the absence of specific factor deficiencies** and should be reserved for patients with known pre-existing deficiencies.

IV. COMPLICATIONS OF BLOOD TRANSFUSION

A. **IATROGENIC.**

1. **Administration of incompatible blood** or use of an incompatible carrier can lead to transfusion complications.

2. **When hypotonic or calcium-containing solutions are used** (e.g. 5% dextrose or lactated Ringer's solution), red blood cell clumping, hemolysis, and clot formation will occur.

3. **Blood should be infused through lines carrying isotonic fluid,** such as normal saline or Plasmalyte.

B. **IMMUNOLOGIC.** The incidence of hemolytic reactions is 0.03–2% per unit: it is fatal in 1/100,000.

1. **Acute hemolytic reaction** is the result of transfusion of ABO incompatible blood.

a. Hypotension, fever, chills, hemoglobinuria, confusion, chest pain, back pain, dyspnea, and bleeding diathesis mark this reaction.

b. The transfusion should be stopped and the patient's blood sent for free hemoglobin, haptoglobin levels, and a Coombs' test.

c. Treatment is supportive with maintenance of good urine output.

2. **Delayed hemolytic reaction** is due to prior sensitization in a patient who has a nondetectable level of antibody at the time of typing.

a. These patients present with indirect hyperbilirubinemia and hemoglobinuria several days after transfusion.

b. This reaction is generally well tolerated and milder than the former.

3. **Febrile reactions** are probably due to antileukocyte antibodies and are seen in patients who have had prior transfusion. Even though this is a mild reaction the patient must be evaluated to exclude an acute hemolytic reaction before transfusion is continued.

4. **Nonhemolytic allergic reactions** are encountered in 1–4% per unit transfusion.

a. These reactions generally occur in patients who have not had previous transfusions and may be caused by a reaction to leukocytes or plasma proteins.

b. The reaction is usually mild with urticaria, fever, hives, and bronchospasm but may be severe and even present with anaphylaxis.

c. Treatment is supportive: antihistamine (diphenhydramine 25mg i.v.), epinephrine (1:1000) 0.1–0.5mg i.m. or s.c. every 10–15 minutes , and i.v. steroids (hydrocortisone 40–100mg) may be indicated.

5. **Immunosuppression**

a. Controversial data from colon cancer and renal transplant studies show decreased T-lymphocyte proliferation, reversed CD4:CD8 ratio, depression of natural killer cells, decreased B-lymphocyte reactivity against antigens, and decreased macrophage phagocytosis.

b. These are not just theoretical concerns because sepsis is the major non-neurologic cause of death associated with trauma.

c. However, fear of immunosuppression should not override the need for appropriate blood replacement in the acute setting.

C. INFECTIONS.

1. **Viral contamination per unit transfusion** is reported as:

a. HIV – 1/225,000.

b. Hepatitis B – 1/200,000.

c. Hepatitis C – 1/3300.

d. Human T-cell lymphocytotrophic virus (HTLV) types I and II – 1/50,000.

2. **Cytomegalovirus** (CMV) is the most common virus transmitted with transfusions in the United States.

a. Because it is endemic, routine screening for CMV is not performed.

b. Immunocompromised patients should receive CMV-tested blood products.

c. Transfusions of products with bacterial contaminants may occur (e.g. syphilis, malaria, *Yersinia enterocolitica*, *Babesia microti*, and *Trypanosoma cruzi*).

3. **The onset of fever, chills, and hypotension shortly after transfusion** make the distinction between acute allergic and hemolytic reaction difficult.

4. **These patients may become very ill** and may need to be treated with broad-spectrum antimicrobial agents and supportive care.

D. METABOLIC COMPLICATIONS.

1. **Potassium.**

a. Packed red blood cells contain 30–40mEq per unit after 3 weeks of storage secondary to cell lysis.

b. At infusion rates over 150mL per minute, hyperkalemia can be seen, especially if the patient is oliguric or in renal failure.

c. Hypokalemia is seen in the shock state secondary to increased aldosterone secretion.

d. Symptoms are predominantly cardiac arrhythmias. Treatment is potassium chloride 40–80mEq by slow infusion.

2. **Calcium**

a. Citrate binds calcium to prevent clotting during storage.

b. At infusion rates >1 unit per 5 minutes, hypocalcemia may occur.
c. Calcium is normally metabolized by the liver; hence a decreased clearance in liver disease and in the shock state can cause hypotension, myocardial depression, arrhythmias, and coagulopathy.
d. Treatment is slow i.v. calcium gluconate (0.45mEq elemental calcium) per 100mL of citrated blood transfused.

3. **Acid–base**
a. Stored PRBCs contain citrate which is converted by the liver to bicarbonate, thus perpetuating an alkalotic effect causing increased oxygen affinity and decreased myocardial contractility.
b. However, in shock or liver failure, acidosis is more common following anaerobic glycolysis after ischemia.
c. Treatment of acidosis is necessary when the serum pH falls below 7.25: a sodium bicarbonate drip is administered.
d. The dose of HCO_3 is calculated as:
    HCO_3 = base deficit (meq/L) $\times$ (0.25 $\times$ patient weight in kg).
e. Half of the total dose of sodium bicarbonate is given over 3 hours and the remainder over 12 hours.

4. **Hypothermia**
a. Defined as temperature <34ºC. (PRBCs are stored at 1–6˚C and have a shelf life of 35 days.)
b. Elderly patients are especially vulnerable to hypothermia, owing to impaired ability to increase heat production and to decrease heat loss by vasoconstriction.
c. Infusion of cold blood products augments heat loss caused by exposure and has several detrimental effects including:
    1) Acidosis.
    2) Leftward shift of the oxygen dissociation curve.
    3) Increased oxygen affinity.
    4) Impaired platelet function.
    5) Myocardial depression.
    6) Arrhythmias.
    7) Respiratory depression.
d. Treatment consists of:
    1) Initial passive rewarming with warming blankets, warm i.v. fluid, warm inspired gasses, and increased ambient environmental temperature.
    2) Active rewarming with peritoneal lavage, chest tube lavage, enemas, and cardiopulmonary bypass.

E. **COAGULOPATHY**
1. **Microvascular nonmechanical bleeding (MVB)**
a. This is defined as onset of oozing from mucosal surfaces, raw wounds, or puncture sites, or as reappearance of bleeding at sites of previous hemostasis.

b.   It is usually refractory to cautery and suture ligation.
c.   The incidence is 18–30% in patients receiving massive transfusion [>1 blood volume (10 units) in 24 hours].
d.   The etiology is multifactorial and implicating factors include hypothermia-induced platelet dysfunction, dilutional thrombocytopenia, and dilution of clotting factors.
e.   Studies have documented diminished platelet metabolism including thromboxane production at temperatures <34ºC. Clotting factor and platelet dilution have also been described.
f.   Appropriate treatment has to address these components individually:
   1)   Initial therapy involves rapid rewarming of the patient to maintain core temperatures >35ºC.
   2)   If coagulopathy is persistent in the setting of a normal platelet count, then replenishment of clotting factors is undertaken with fresh-frozen plasma (2–4 units every 2 hours) until clotting times return to normal.
   3)   Platelet transfusion is reserved for microvascular bleeding in the face of documented thrombocytopenia after correction of hypothermia and acidosis.
   4)   It has not been our practice to routinely administer platelets prophylactically after a threshold number of blood transfusions, since infusions of cold platelets and fresh-frozen plasma in an effort to stop microvascular bleeding can aggravate the coagulopathy.
   5)   Prophylactic administration of fresh-frozen plasma is also unnecessary and potentially harmful since there is no difference in bleeding rates between patients receiving prophylactic fresh-frozen plasma (25%) and those not receiving the product (30%).

2.   **Disseminated intravascular coagulation (DIC)**. Red blood cell adenosine diphosphate (ADP) and membrane phospholipoprotein activate the procoagulant system via factor XII and complement. Diffuse microvascular thrombosis, consuming platelets and coagulation factors, occurs. Simultaneous fibrinolysis releases fibrin split products into the circulation.
a.   The etiology of DIC includes:
   1)   Massive transfusion.
   2)   Sepsis.
   3)   Crush injury.
   4)   Multiple injuries.
b.   Clinical features include:
   1)   Fever.
   2)   Hypotension.
   3)   Acidosis.
   4)   Proteinuria.
   5)   Hypoxia.

c. Laboratory features include:
   1) Thrombocytopenia ($<80,000/mm^3$).
   2) Decreased fibrinogen (0.8g/L).
   3) Prolonged PT and PTT.
   4) Elevated fibrin-degradation products or D-dimers.
   5) Fragmented red blood cells on smear.
d. Treatment involves aggressive hemodynamic support, removal of underlying cause (transfusion of compatible washed PRBCs). If these measures fail we have used i.v. heparin infusion (titrated to maintain international normalized ratio (INR) between 1.1 and 1.5), antithrombin III, or ε-aminocaproic acid (Amicar) with variable success. The onset of DIC portends a poor prognosis. Mortality is high, mainly owing to end organ damage and failure.

3. Acute respiratory distress syndrome (ARDS).
a. This syndrome occurs in patients with an average incidence of 0.02% per unit blood transfused.
b. It can occur with any blood product containing plasma and signs usually appear during transfusion or within 3–4 hours.
c. The clinical features include fever, chills, hypotension, and progressive respiratory insufficiency.
d. Hypoxemia is refractory to supplemental oxygen and ARDS can be avoided by transfusing washed PRBCs in symptomatic patients.
e. Treatment consists of aggressive pulmonary support and possible mechanical ventilation.
f. The syndrome follows a milder course when caused by transfusion, usually resolving within 48–96 hours.
g. The mortality rate is significantly lower than the mortality of ARDS associated with other etiologies (10% vs 60%).

V. PEARLS AND PITFALLS

A. **HYPOTHERMIA.** Prevention and treatment of hypothermia is essential to achieving hemostasis and avoiding physiologic impairments.
B. **INFECTIOUS RISK.** Prophylactic platelet and fresh-frozen plasma transfusions carry infectious risk and are not warranted unless there is thrombocytopenia and acidosis is corrected.
C. **FACTOR DEPLETION.** PT, PTT, and fibrinogen are reliable predictors of factor depletion and should be used to assess the need for replacement of clotting factors.

VI. FURTHER READING

Carrico CJ, Mileski WJ, Kaplan HS. In: Moore EE, Mattox KL, Feliciano DV, eds. *Trauma*. Stamford: Appleton and Lange; 1996:181–191.

Fakhry SM, Sheldon GF. Blood transfusions and disorders of surgical bleeding. In: Sabiston DC, ed. *Textbook of surgery,* 15th edn. Philadelphia: WB Saunders; 1997:119–136.

Per Lundsgaard-Hansen, MD. Safe hemoglobin or hematocrit levels in surgical patients. *World J Surg* 1996; 20:1182–1188.

Phillips GR III, Rotondo MF, Schwab CW. Transfusion therapy. In: Maull KI, Rodriquez A, Wiles CE III, eds. *Complications in trauma and critical care*. Philadelphia: WB Saunders; 1996:73–80.

Dennis RC, Clas D, Niehoff JM, Yeston NS. Transfusion therapy. In: Civetta JM, Taylor RW, Kirby RR, eds. *Critical care,* 3rd edn. Philadelphia: Lippincott–Raven; 1992:639–659.

DIAGNOSTIC MODALITIES IN THE EMERGENCY DEPARTMENT

I. INTRODUCTION

A. **PRINCIPLES.** The most important aspect of obtaining an accurate diagnosis is an accurate history and a careful physical examination.

1. **The mechanism of injury** coupled with the physical findings will facilitate the selection of diagnostic procedures.

a. The patient in extremis will often require simultaneous evaluation and treatment, with the response to treatment modifying the priority of subsequent diagnostic procedures.

b. At times, a minimum number of diagnostic studies should be performed initially in order to expedite life-saving measures.

2. **Advanced Trauma Life Support procedures** are always followed and, while diagnostic procedures are important, they should never delay resuscitative efforts.

II. INITIAL DIAGNOSTIC STUDIES

These are immediately available at the bedside.

A. **SCREENING RADIOGRAPHS.** Screening radiographs consist of chest (inspiratory and expiratory), cervical spine, and pelvic films obtained early in most cases of blunt trauma. Additional radiographs should be obtained as indicated by history, mechanism of injury, physical examination, and stability of the patient (Table 9.1).

B. **CHEST RADIOGRAPHS.**

1. **Important screening study** for all multisystem trauma patients.

2. **Establishes baseline** for comparison of subsequent studies during hospitalization and follow-up.

3. **Essential for diagnosis** of pneumothorax, pulmonary contusion, hemothorax, and great vessel injury (Table 9.2).

4. **Inspiratory and expiratory films** are ordered to rule out pneumothorax.

5. **It is not very reliable** in the diagnosis of diaphragmatic injury.

C. **CERVICAL SPINE RADIOGRAPHS.**

1. **Lateral radiographs** demonstrating all cervical vertebrae and the C7–T1 junction will enable detection of up to 90% of all significant injuries (Table 9.3).

2. **An anteroposterior (AP) view** is useful in evaluating transverse processes and rotary injuries (spinous processes should all be in the midline). Increased distance between spinous processes suggests flexion injury.

3. **Oblique views** are useful to evaluate pedicles, intervertebral foramina, facet joints, and lamina. These are generally ordered when abnormalities are detected on the AP or lateral views.

9

TABLE 9.1

RADIOGRAPHS FREQUENTLY REQUESTED FOR EVALUATION OF TRAUMA PATIENTS

Examination	Indication
Cervical spine[a]	All blunt trauma and injuries above the clavicles
Chest[a]	All patients
Pelvis [a]	All blunt trauma
Excretory urogram (IVP)	Gross hematuria or microscopic hematuria depending on mechanism and physical findings
Retrograde cystogram	Fractured pelvis (anterior); gross hematuria
Retrograde urethrogram	Blood in penile meatus; scrotal or perineal hematoma; high-riding prostate
Face and mandible	Clinical evidence of facial fracture; diplopia; malocclusion
Spine	Pain and tenderness; hematoma; crepitance; deformity; neurologic deficit
Extremities	Pain and tenderness; deformity; crepitance
CT scan of head	Head injury; history of loss of consciousness; altered mental status; GCS <8; neurologic deficit
Abdomen	Suspected perforated viscus; localization of foreign body; penetrating wounds to abdomen and back
Ultrasound of abdomen	Screening study of intra-abdominal injury
CT scan of abdomen	Unreliable or equivocal abdominal examination; possible nonoperative management of intra-abdominal injury
Esophagram subcutaneous mediastinum	Penetrating neck injury; air in neck

[a]For most blunt trauma

TABLE 9.2

CRITERIA FOR SUSPECTED RUPTURED AORTA ON CHEST RADIOGRAPHS

Widening of the superior mediastinum >8cm[a]

Depression of the left mainstem bronchus >140°

Obliteration of the aortic knob[a]

Deviation of the nasogastric tube, endotracheal tube, or trachea to the right

Fracture of the first or second rib, scapula, or sternum

Left apical hematoma and capping

Obliteration of the aortopulmonary window on the lateral chest radiograph

Anterior displacement of the trachea on lateral chest radiograph

Fracture or dislocation of the thoracic spine

Calcium-layering in the aortic knob area

Obvious double contour of the aorta

Multiple left rib fractures

Massive hematoma

[a]Most reliable signs

TABLE 9.3

EVALUATION OF LATERAL VIEW OF CERVICAL SPINE

Upper cervical spine (C1–C2)

Distance from anterior ring of C1 to odontoid

  Adults ≤ 2.5mm

  Children ≤ 4.5mm

Prevertebral soft tissue

  Airway to anterior–inferior margin of C2

  Adults and children ≤ 7mm

Lower cervical spine (C3–C7)

Soft tissues

  Airway to anterior–inferior margin of C6

    Adults ≤ 22mm

    Children ≤ 14mm

Alignment

  Subluxation (<3mm) may be seen C2 on C3 and C3 on C4 in children up to

  late teens (rarely in the early 20s)

  Subluxation in adults is abnormal (usually C4–C7)

Disk space

  Uniform normal

  Compressed–inflexion injury

  Widened anterior–extension injury

Interspinous distance should decrease from C3 to C7

4. **The odontoid (open mouth) view** is used to evaluate odontoid and lateral processes of C1.

5. **Tomography (plain or computed)** is useful to define injuries further and to provide information when the plain film studies do not provide adequate visualization of the entire cervical spine.

6. **A Davis series (flexion–extension views)** will help evaluate ligamentous stability in the awake, alert, and oriented patient. A delay of 48 hours is generally required for resolution of muscle spasms. Patient co-operation is essential during this examination.

D. **PELVIC RADIOGRAPHS.**

1. **Pelvic films** should be obtained in patients with blunt trauma to the torso.

2. **Fractures that are detected** frequently require genitourinary evaluation.

3. **Pelvic fractures** may require an alternative approach to peritoneal lavage. Supra-umbilical incisions are required. Obtain inlet, outlet, and Judet views as well as a CT scan for definitive treatment of significant pelvic fractures.

E. AXIAL SKELETAL RADIOGRAPHS. Views of the cervical, thoracic, lumbar, and sacral spine are ordered in symptomatic patients and in those patients with altered mental status and significant blunt injury.

F. EXTREMITY RADIOGRAPHS.

1. **Radiographs of the hands and feet** are selectively ordered, when indicated, following the physical examination.

2. **It is important to define fractures** as soon as possible so splints can be applied and fractures can be reduced in a timely matter. This becomes an urgent matter if distal pulses are decreased or absent.

G. ULTRASOUND.

1. **Abdominal ultrasonography** has been shown to be accurate in identifying free intraperitoneal fluid in the trauma patient.

2. **The technique is portable, rapid, noninvasive,** and can be performed by any trained personnel.

3. **This is a focused, limited examination** for detection of fluid in dependent regions:

a. Pericardial area for pericardial fluid.

b. Right upper quadrant to examine liver, kidney, diaphragm, and Morrison's pouch.

c. Left upper quadrant to examine the spleen, kidney, and surrounding area.

d. Suprapubic – pouch of Douglas, and bladder.

e. May also be used to examine pleural spaces for effusions, major blood vessels, and the pericolic gutters.

4. **Sensitivity is 85–95% (operator dependent), specificity is 96–100%, and accuracy is 94–99%.**

5. **There is a direct correlation between operator experience and training and the quality of the study**.

6. **Results** are not as good in patients who are obese, or those with subcutaneous emphysema, significant bowel distention, empty bladder, retroperitoneal injury, or penetrating injury.

7. **Sonography** should be followed by diagnostic peritoneal lavage (DPL), CT, or exploratory celiotomy if the patient becomes transiently hypotensive, continues to have significant abdominal pain or tenderness, or becomes hemodynamically unstable.

8. **The study can be used** for serial examinations and short- or long-term follow-up.

H. PERITONEAL LAVAGE.

1. **Diagnostic peritoneal lavage** is relatively fast, safe, and reliable for patients with blunt injury and stab wounds to the anterior abdomen (98% accurate with 2% false-positive and 1–2% false-negative rates).

2. **Common clinical indications** are described below:

a. If the patient is hemodynamically unstable and capabilities for sonography are unavailable.

b. Used for penetrating abdominal stab wounds after positive local wound exploration (see below) or suspected hollow viscus injury (seat-belt injury).

c. DPL may also be used following an abnormal ultrasound exam or when a patient has a normal ultrasound but exhibits signs and symptoms suggestive of intra-abdominal injury.

d. Lavage is considered positive if 10mL of gross blood is aspirated or if 1L of lactated Ringer's is infused into the peritoneal cavity and microscopic evaluation reveals red blood cells >100,000/mm^3, white blood cells >500/mm^3, or the presence of bile, particulate matter, or amylase greater than the normal serum value.

I. LOCAL WOUND EXPLORATION.

1. This exploration is used to determine whether a nonthoracic stab wound is superficial.

2. Wounds located above the costal margin have been excluded from exploration mainly to avoid the complication of a pneumothorax.

3. Technique:

a. Extend wound margins with a scalpel after the injection of local anesthetic.

b. Using sterile techniques the tract is followed, under direct vision, until its end is positively identified or penetration of the posterior abdominal wall fascia or peritoneum is visualized.

c. If the end of the tract cannot be identified, or posterior fascial penetration is noted, then the wound is closed; a DPL is then performed if the stab wound is anterior to the posterior axillary line, or a CT scan if the wound is posterior to the posterior axillary line.

J. GENITOURINARY TRAUMA SERIES. This includes an intravenous pyelogram (IVP), cystogram, and urethrogram.

1. A retrograde cystourethrogram is indicated in any patient with blunt trauma if there is difficulty in passing a urinary catheter or if the patient has a perineal hematoma, a scrotal hematoma, a high-riding prostate on rectal exam, or blood at the urethral meatus.

2. On examination of the urine, if there is gross or microscopic hematuria associated with hypotension, pelvic fracture, lower posterior rib or lumbar transverse process fractures, or any other suspected urinary tract injury, then an IVP (with a retrograde cystourethrogram as indicated) is performed.

3. If a retroperitoneal injury is suspected, a CT scan may be performed in place of the IVP.

4. Preoperative IVPs may be performed in the case of missile wounds to the chest or abdomen to evaluate kidney function.

K. DOPPLER STUDIES.

1. Useful for noninvasive, bedside evaluation of potential vascular injuries.

DIAGNOSTIC MODALITIES IN THE EMERGENCY DEPARTMENT

9

2. **Ankle brachial index (ABI)** of <0.9, or significant difference between right and left extremities, have a sensitivity of approximately 87% and specificity of 97% for arterial injury. The absence of a pulse, an expanding hematoma, or pulsatile bleeding warrants exploration.

L. ECHOCARDIOGRAPHY.

1. **Twenty per cent of patients with penetrating cardiac injuries** reaching the hospital alive will be in stable condition.
2. **This technique is useful in patients with penetrating cardiac injuries** (96% sensitive, 100% specific, 99.2% accurate) for detecting pericardial fluid.
3. **This test demonstrates reduced sensitivity** for the detection of cardiac injuries in patients with a hemothorax.
4. **Transesophageal echocardiography** may be useful for great vessel injury to the neck and chest (sensitivity 86%, specificity 90%). This method is best performed on patients who are intubated and sedated.

M. PERICARDIOCENTESIS AND PERICARDIAL WINDOW.

1. **Pericardiocentesis** is used in hemodynamically unstable patients with suspected cardiac tamponade both as a temporizing measure and a diagnostic study.
2. **The angiocath is left in place**, until the patient is taken to the operating room, if the study is positive. The syringe is connected to a stopcock which will allow repeated aspiration if necessary.
3. **A subxiphoid pericardial window** (accuracy 98%, sensitivity 100%, specificity 97.5%) is performed on patients suspected of having a cardiac injury.

III. DEPARTMENTAL DIAGNOSTIC STUDIES

Hemodynamic stability must be assured before patients are transferred to the radiology department.

A. CT SCAN OF THE HEAD.

1. **Indications** include history of loss of consciousness, altered mental status, GCS <13, abnormal neurological exam, and inability to obtain serial neurologic examinations (i.e. immediate operation or sedation required) (see Chapter 11, Head Injury).
2. **Does not rule out head injury** (i.e. CT scan may not show diffuse axonal injury), but does evaluate for presence of edema, midline shift, hematoma, contusion, foreign body, or fracture.

B. CT SCAN OF THE ABDOMEN.

1. **Indicated for suspected retroperitoneal injuries** – including stab wounds to the back with positive local exploration (see Chapter 25, Colon Injuries).
2. **Use following ultrasound** in stable patients as outlined in Figure 9.1.

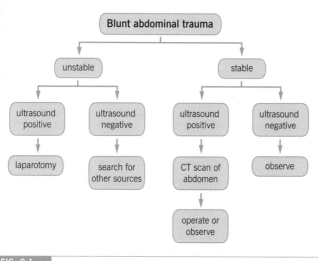

FIG. 9.1

Ultrasound plan for blunt abdominal trauma.

C. ANGIOGRAPHY.
1. **Used for suspected great vessel injury** following significant blunt trauma due to decelerating mechanism.
2. **Indicated for extremity trauma** following an abnormal examination or Doppler study. Exploration is preferable to arteriography if the patient is unstable, or has an expanding hematoma or a pulseless ischemic extremity.
3. **Useful in patients with penetrating neck trauma** in zones I or III. Arteriography is also used in patients with planned nonoperative management of zone II injuries.
4. **Other indications** include suspected renovascular or pelvic trauma. It is frequently used in patients with pelvic trauma or bleeding solid organ injuries who may benefit from embolization.
D. MAGNETIC RESONANCE IMAGING.
1. Rarely indicated in trauma patients.
2. **May be used to identify ligamentous injuries to the neck** within 72 hours of injury.

IV. FURTHER READING

Berquist TH. *Diagnostic imaging of the acutely injured patient*. Baltimore: Urban and Schwarzenberg; 1985:1–88, 195–241.

Brasel KJ, Weigelt JA. Blunt thoracic aortic trauma, a cost–utility approach for injury detection. *Arch Surg* 1996; 131:619–626.

Martin LC, McKenney MG, Sosa JL et al. Management of lower extremity arterial trauma. *J Trauma* 1994; 37(4):591–598.

McKenney MG, Martin L, Lentz K et al. 1000 consecutive ultrasounds for blunt abdominal trauma. *J Trauma* 1996; 40(4):607–610.

Meyer DM, Jessen ME, Grayburn PA et al. Use of echocardiography to detect occult cardiac injury after penetrating thoracic trauma: a prospective study. *J Trauma* 1995; 39(5):902–907.

Mirvis S. Trauma. *Radiol Clin North Am* 1996; 6:1225–1257.

Rizzo AG, Steinberg SM, Flint LM. Prospective assessment of the value of computed tomography for trauma. *J Trauma* 1995; 38(3):338–343.

Rozycki G. Abdominal ultrasonography in trauma. *Surg Clin North Am* 1995:75(2):175–191.

Shires GT, Thal ER, Jones RC et al. Trauma. In: Schwartz SI, Shires GT, Spencer FC, eds. *Principles of surgery*. New York: McGraw-Hill; 1994:175–224.

CATHETERS AND TUBES

I. ARTERIAL CATHETERS

A. INDICATIONS.

1. **Hemodynamic monitoring** in unstable patients (mean arterial blood pressure <80mmHg).
2. **Arterial blood sampling** in patients requiring frequent evaluation of blood gases (mechanical ventilation).

B. INSERTION SITES.

1. **The radial artery** is the most common site because of relative safety and ease of insertion.
2. **The dorsalis pedis** is relatively safe but congenitally absent in 12% of patients.
3. **Femoral arterial lines** are useful in patients who are in shock but may be difficult to cannulate in patients without a palpable pulse.
4. **Brachial arterial access** is rarely used because of the incidence of upper extremity ischemic complications.
5. **The axillary artery** is often difficult to access and proximity of neural structures may lead to complications.

C. CONTRAINDICATIONS.

1. **Positive Allen's test.** Occlude the radial and ulnar arteries simultaneously. Ask the patient to clench and unclench the fist until the palm becomes pale. Release the ulnar artery. If palmar blushing does not occur within 7 seconds, the Allen's test is positive. This indicates inadequate ulnar collateral circulation. Radial or brachial artery catheterization is contraindicated in this instance because of increased risk of distal ischemia. Similarly, a dorsalis pedis catheter insertion may be contraindicated because of inadequate posterior tibial artery flow.
2. **Lower extremity occlusive arterial disease**. The high rate of ischemic complications is a relative contraindication for dorsalis pedis catheterization in patients with known lower extremity arterial disease.
3. **Anticoagulation.** Increased bleeding and hematoma formation may complicate catheterization, especially in the brachial and femoral arteries.

D. INSERTION TECHNIQUE (RADIAL ARTERY).

a. Dorsiflex the wrist at 60°.
b. Palpate the radial artery pulse just proximal to the radial head.
c. Cleanse and drape the site using sterile technique.
d. Anesthetize the overlying skin with 1% lidocaine.
e. Insert a 20-gauge angiocatheter or Arrow catheter at a 30° angle to the skin.

f. Advance the needle until blood flows into the hub, then advance the catheter into the artery over the needle.
g. Withdraw the needle and attach the catheter to arterial tubing. If pulsatile blood flow is not seen upon needle removal, withdraw the catheter and make another attempt.
h. Secure the catheter with 3-0 silk suture and apply a sterile dressing.
i. Tape the wrist in neutral position on a rigid board.

E. COMPLICATIONS.

1. **Thrombosis** is the most common complication, with an incidence of 5–8%, though only 4% of these result in distal limb ischemia. Thrombosis is more common with large (20-gauge) catheters, catheters left in place for more than 4 days, catheters placed by surgical cutdown, and intermittent (rather than continuous) flushing. Catheter removal is usually all that is necessary for treatment.

2. **Infection** is the second most common complication and is associated with systemic infection, most common in catheters left in place for at least 4 days and catheters placed via a surgical cutdown. Gram-negative rods, *Enterococcus* sp., and Candida are the usual pathogens. Catheter removal and antimicrobial therapy is adequate for these patients.

3. **Embolism.** Emboli may migrate distally, causing limb ischemia, or proximally (as a result of forceful flushing) causing central nervous system deficits. Ischemic symptoms will resolve with short-term anticoagulation; if this fails then embolectomy may be indicated for large vessel occlusion.

4. **Ischemic necrosis of overlying skin** occurs in 3% of catheterizations and necessitates catheter removal.

II. SAPHENOUS VEIN CUTDOWN

A. INDICATIONS.

1. **The major indication** is failure to obtain upper extremity venous access.

2. **The saphenous vein is utilized liberally for resuscitation** at Parkland Memorial Hospital. When performed efficiently, saphenous cutdown will avoid delay in resuscitation which occurs while searching for a suitable vein. Also, rapid access can be gained with relative ease by the experienced physician.

B. ANATOMY. As a result of its constant location and subcutaneous course, the saphenous vein is ideally suited for rapid vascular access via the cutdown technique. It is most accessible in the ankle 1.5cm anterior and cephalad to the medial malleolus. At the level of the ankle the saphenous vein is exposed with minimal dissection and, owing to its predictable location, it is the classic pediatric cutdown site (Figure 10.1).

C. EQUIPMENT.
a. Curved hemostat..
b. Curved iris scissors.
c. Self-retaining tissue retractor .
d. Scalpel with no. 11 and 15 blades .
e. Small smooth forceps.
f. Needle holder.
g. Silk suture ties (4-0).
h. Nylon suture on a cutting needle (4-0).
i. Short large-bore catheter.
j. Plastic venous introducer.

D. TECHNIQUE.
1. **The area of skin to be incised**, around the medial malleolus, should be widely prepared with an antiseptic solution and draped with sterile towels.
2. **In the conscious patient** the site 1.5cm anterior and cephalad to the medial malleolus should be infiltrated with 1% lidocaine solution.
3. **A transverse incision is made** perpendicular to the course of the vessel at this level extending through the dermis into the subcutaneous tissue (Figure 10.1A).
4. **Bluntly dissect the subcutaneous tissue** by spreading with a curved hemostat in a direction parallel to the course of the vein. A length of vein 1–3cm is adequate for canalization. A self-retaining tissue retractor may be used at this time to facilitate exposure.
5. **Mobilize the vein** from the surrounding tissue by passing a hemostat under it and pass two silk ligatures around the vein – one proximally and the other distally (Figure 10.1B).
6. **With gentle traction on the proximal ligature**, incise the vessel at a 45° angle through one-third to one-half its diameter using either the no. 11 blade or the iris scissors (Figure 10.1C).

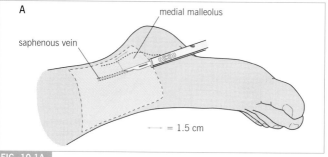

FIG. 10.1A
Saphenous vein cutdown procedure. See text for details.

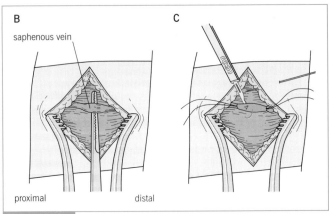

FIG. 10.1B&C

Saphenous vein cutdown procedure. See text for details.

7. **The large-bore catheter** may now be threaded into the lumen of the vessel using either the forceps or the plastic venous introducer (Figure 10.1D).

8. **Alternatively, an intravenous catheter and introducer needle complex** may be used simply to enter the vessel lumen through either the skin incision or a separate puncture site (Figure 10.1E).

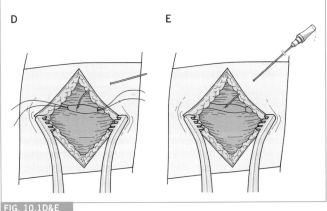

FIG. 10.1D&E

Saphenous vein cutdown procedure. See text for details.

9. **Once the catheter is advanced**, blood is allowed to backbleed from the cannula, which is then connected to the intravenous tubing.
10. **The proximal ligature is then tied** around the vessel and cannula, and the distal ligature is tied down as well.
11. **The skin is then closed** using nylon suture and the catheter is secured to the skin.
12. **Topical antibacterial ointment is applied** and a sterile dressing is placed over the catheter site (Figure 10.1F).

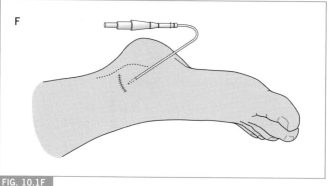

FIG. 10.1F
Saphenous vein cutdown procedure. See text for details.

D. **COMPLICATIONS AND TREATMENT.**
1. **Wound infection** – remove catheter; antimicrobial agents.
2. **Thrombophlebitis** – remove catheter; warm compresses; antimicrobial agents. Vein excision is indicated for suppuration.
3. **Hematoma** – incision and drainage of hematoma.
4. **Failure of wound healing** – common in diabetic patients with vascular insufficiency and is treated nonoperatively with topical dressings. Angiography and revascularization procedures are occasionally indicated.

III. URINARY CATHETERS
A. **INDICATIONS.**
1. **Monitoring of urine output.**
2. **Decompression of the bladder** prior to peritoneal lavage.
3. **Neurologic injury** resulting in inability to void spontaneously.
4. **Diagnosis of urinary tract trauma (hematuria).**

B. **TYPES OF CATHETERS.**

1. **Foley catheter** (most common): sizes 16F or 18F are those most commonly used (1F is equal to 0.33mm). The higher the number, the larger the size.

2. **Coude-tip catheter** is used primarily to negotiate the difficult male prostatic urethra when a round-tip Foley catheter will not pass and prostatic hypertrophy is suspected.

C. **CONTRAINDICATIONS TO URETHRAL CATHETERIZATION IN TRAUMA PATIENTS.**

1. **Signs of suspected urethral injury,** such as scrotal hematoma, blood at the male urethral meatus, or a high-riding or free-floating prostate on rectal examination.

2. **Known or suspected fracture** of the interior pelvic ring.

3. **Perineal hematomas.** A rectal examination must always be performed, prior to insertion of a urinary catheter, in patients with any possibility of urethral injury.

D. **EQUIPMENT.**

a. Sterile gloves.

b. Povidone–iodine solution (or other topical antimicrobial).

c. Cotton balls or gauze.

d. Sterile drapes.

e. Sterile lubricating jelly.

f. Urinary catheter (Foley or Coude).

g. A 10mL syringe, with sterile water for balloon inflation.

h. Urinary drainage bag (sterile system).

E. **TECHNIQUE.** Adherence to aseptic technique is mandatory for catheter placement.

1. **Male patient.**

a. Place the patient in the supine position.

b. Open the tray and put on sterile gloves.

c. Prepare tray prior to insertion.

d. Soak cotton balls with povidone–iodine solution.

e. Place lubricating jelly in tray.

f. Inflate Foley catheter balloon with sterile water to assure its integrity.

g. Apply sterile drapes over patient.

h. Penis is grasped with the nondominant hand. This hand should not touch the catheter and should not release the penis until the catheter is in position. If the patient is uncircumcised, the foreskin should be retracted prior to placement.

i. Glans and distal shaft of the penis are prepared with several cotton balls soaked in povidone–iodine solution.

j. The dominant hand holds catheter and generously lubricates (water-soluble lubricant jelly) the catheter to minimize insertion trauma.

k. Insert catheter in the urethral meatus.

l. Carefully stretch penis perpendicular to the body to eliminate urethral redundancy (Figure 10.2).

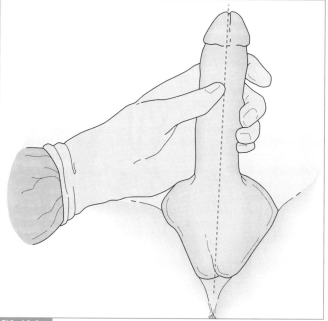

FIG. 10.2

Foley catheter insertion. Penis is held straight upward to provide the straightest course of the urethra that will allow the Foley access to the urinary bladder.

m. Advance catheter gently, but with firm pressure, inserting the entire catheter to the level where the sidearm is located. Do not force the catheter at any time during its insertion.

n. Inflate balloon with 10mL of sterile water and gently withdraw catheter until resistance of the bladder neck is encountered.

o. Attach to closed drainage bag.

p. Tape the tubing to the medial aspect of the thigh.

2. Female patient.

a. Place patient in the frog-leg position, with flexion of knees and hips and abduction of thighs.

b. Place sterile gloves and prepare tray as stated above.

c. Labia is separated with thumb and index finger of the nondominant hand. This hand is now considered contaminated (Figure 10.3).

d. Prepare urethral meatus with cotton balls soaked in povidone–iodine, in the pubis–anus direction using 3–4 passes with sterile cotton ball each pass.

e. Lubricate the distal third of the catheter generously.

f. Grasp catheter with the dominant hand and gently pass through the meatus into the bladder.

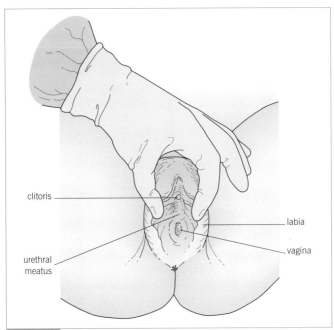

FIG. 10.3
Anatomical relationship of the female urethra. With the hips abducted, a gloved hand spreads the labia to expose the urethra. The other hand prepares the area and inserts the lubricated catheter. (From Lawrence PF. *Essentials of general surgery*. Baltimore: Williams and Wilkins; 1988.)

- g. Remember the female urethra is much shorter.
- h. Advance until the return of urine is seen, and then advance additional 3–4 cm further.
- i. Inflate balloon with 10mL of sterile water and gently withdraw catheter until resistance of the bladder neck is encountered.
- j. Attach to closed drainage bag.
- k. Tape the tubing to the medial aspect of the thigh.
- F. COMPLICATIONS AND TROUBLESHOOTING.
1. **Creation of false passages** usually occurs secondary to excessive force or inadequate amount of lubricant on the catheter.
2. **If resistance is encountered**, 5–10mL of sterile lubricant can be injected gently into the meatus. Also, if resistance is met close to the bladder, as judged by the length of catheter, possible prostatic obstruction may be present and the use of an 18F Coude-tip catheter may facilitate entry into the bladder.

3. **If no urine returns**, irrigation with 5–10mL of sterile saline may be tried. If this does not allow easy irrigation, the catheter is probably not in the correct position.
4. **Forceful inflation of balloon is contraindicated**. If the balloon does not inflate easily, try reinsertion or seek help.
5. **Infections and complications** may occur if one does not adhere to aseptic technique. This is mandatory as many trauma patients require long-term bladder catheterization.

G. PEARLS AND PITFALLS.
1. **Urine must be visualized** in tubing prior to balloon inflation.
2. **Insertion of the full length of the catheter** is recommended to assure placement into the bladder and avoid inflation of the balloon in the prostatomembranous urethra.
3. **If the patient is uncircumcised**, replace foreskin to prevent paraphimosis.
4. **Tape catheter loosely** to medial aspect of thigh to avoid dislodgment.

IV. NASOGASTRIC TUBES

A. INDICATIONS.
1. Gastrointestinal decompression to prevent aspiration.
2. Identification of injury to the upper gastrointestinal tract.
3. Decompression of the stomach prior to peritoneal lavage.

B. CONTRAINDICATIONS.
1. **Midface fractures**. The nasogastric tube may be inserted through a disrupted cribiform plate into the cranium.
2. **Suspected vascular neck injuries**. The coughing and retching caused by the nasogastric tube insertion may cause hemorrhage from a previously nonbleeding arterial injury.

C. TYPES OF NASOGASTRIC TUBES.
1. **Levin** – single-lumen tube with perforated tip and side-holes. Enables aspiration of gastric contents.
2. **Salem sump** – double-lumen tube with irrigation and air-intake ports, allowing continuous tube decompression. This tube is superior for gastric lavage.
3. **Dobhoff** – single-lumen duodenal feeding tube. Placing the tube distal to the pylorus prevents aspiration of feeds in obtunded patients.

D. INSERTION TECHNIQUE.
1. **Choose a 16F or 18F tube size**. Smaller tubes are useful for feedings; larger tubes are best for gastric lavage and decompression.
2. **Lubricate distal end of tube** with lidocaine or K-Y jelly.
3. **Insert the tube in the more patent nares** and guide posteriorly, not superiorly. (Temporary oral insertion may be necessary.)
4. **Have patient swallow repeatedly** to facilitate passage into esophagus.
5. **Confirm gastric placement** by injecting 50mL of air through the nasogastric tube while auscultating for gurgling over the stomach. If the tube is not in the stomach, it is either in the tracheobronchial tree or

curled in the mouth and reinsertion is necessary. A radiopaque marker indicates distal tube location on a radiograph.

6. **Tape the tube securely** to the nasal dorsum.

V. CLOSED-TUBE THORACOSTOMY DRAINAGE

A. INDICATIONS.

1. **Pneumothorax**. If a chest radiograph is not immediately available, trauma to one side of the chest associated with decreased or absent breath sounds or hypotension should be treated urgently with either needle thoracentesis or a chest tube.

2. **Hemothorax**.

3. **Empyema**.

4. **Chylothorax**.

B. TECHNIQUE FOR INSERTION OF A 36F CHEST TUBE.

1. **Site of insertion**. Identify the fifth or sixth intercostal space at the point in the midaxillary line. (Feel for space between the pectoralis and latissimus muscles.) This can be done quickly and will consistently place the chest tube above the diaphragm.

2. **Prepare the skin** with iodine solution and drape in a sterile fashion.

3. **Anesthetize** with 1–2% lidocaine with epinephrine. Create a skin weal to mark the site, then fan out over subcutaneous tissue and to the top of target rib.

4. **Use a scalpel to create an incision** large enough for fingers and chest tube (Figure 10.4A).

5. **Tunnel up one to two ribs from the margin** (especially important in thin patients) to create a soft tissue cover that will occlude the hole when the chest tube is removed (Figure 10.4B).

6. **Dissect over the top of the selected rib** with a large Kelly clamp (Figure 10.4C). Open it widely after it has penetrated the intercostal muscles and pleural space. The index finger should be inserted to confirm entry into the pleural space, break up loculations or adhesions, and demonstrate proper path of the tract.

7. **The chest tube can then be placed** in the Kelly clamp and guided into the pleural space.

8. **Movement of fluid and air** in the tube with respiration should be noted.

9. **Clamp the distal end of the tube** to prevent loss of fluid.

10. **Position the tube posteriorly** and attach tubing to suction and drainage device.

11. **Unclamp the tube**.

12. **Close the incision and secure the tube** to the chest wall with a 2-0 silk or nylon suture. Apply a sterile dressing.

13. **Each day the system should be checked** for amount of drainage, air leaks, presence of respiratory fluctuations (fluid column variation with respiration), and maintenance of the desired amount of suction.

C. **REMOVAL OF CHEST TUBE.**
1. **Materials**. Suture removal kit, wide gauze tape, Vaseline or petroleum gauze, 4-inch square gauze packs.
2. **Technique**. Instruct patient to take a deep breath and hold it as the tube is quickly removed. It is important to practice this with the patient a few times before removal. Place Vaseline gauze and 4-inch square gauze over the entrance site. Obtain a chest radiograph following removal.
D. **COMPLICATIONS AND TREATMENT.**
1. **Lung injury** is treated by tube removal and replacement.
2. **Diaphragm injury** is an indication for operative therapy and repair.
3. **Intra-abdominal solid organ injury** (e.g. liver, spleen) is treated by tube removal. Continuing hemorrhage from the injured organ is treated by operation and repair.
4. **Retained hemothorax or empyema** is a common complication of inadequate chest tube drainage. If the retained fluid is accessible, a second chest tube might provide complete drainage. However, most of these fluid collections are loculated or clotted, in which case thoracoscopy or thoracotomy and decortication will be necessary. The presence of fever and leukocytosis associated with an undrained thoracic collection is an indication for thoracoscopy or thoracotomy.
5. **Persistent pneumothorax or air leak.** In the absence of any leaks in the tubing and connection system, this is most likely due to an inadequately evacuated pneumothorax, parenchymal leaks from pulmonary lacerations, or large airway injuries. Air leaks can be managed with additional chest tubes; however, failure of these leaks to seal will require thoracoscopy and repair of parenchymal injuries.
6. **Rib fractures** will heal with adequate pain control.

VI. CENTRAL VENOUS CATHETERIZATION
A. **INDICATIONS.**
1. Volume resuscitation.
2. Monitoring of resuscitation.
B. **ANATOMY.**
1. Subclavian vein.
a. The subclavian vein begins as a continuation of the axillary vein at the outer edge of the first rib and, subsequently, joins the internal jugular vein to become the innominate vein.
b. The subclavian vein lies in close approximation to the posterior border of the medial third of the clavicle.
c. It is at this point that access to the subclavian vein is simplest and safest via the supraclavicular or infraclavicular approaches (Figure 10.5).

10

CATHETERS AND TUBES

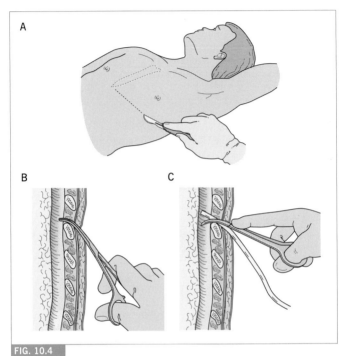

FIG. 10.4

Technique for closed-tube thoracostomy. See text for details.

2. **Internal jugular vein.**
a. The internal jugular vein emerges from beneath the apex of the two heads of the sternocleidomastoid muscle high in the lateral aspect of the neck.
b. It proceeds inferiorly to join the subclavian vein behind the medial third of the clavicle.
c. In the lower cervical region, where access is to be gained, the common carotid artery lies medial and deep to the internal jugular vein in a paratracheal location (Figure 10.5).

C. **CENTRAL VENOUS ACCESS CATHETERS.** There are three main types of intravenous access system.

1. **Catheter-over-the-needle technique.** There are two disadvantages to this technique.
a. First, once blood return is achieved, the catheter itself may still be outside the vessel. This will result in the catheter pushing the vein in front of it and never entering the lumen.

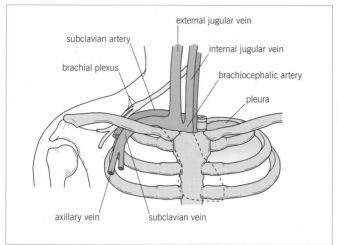

FIG. 10.5
Subclavian vein and local anatomy.

b. The second disadvantage is that a 14-gauge catheter requires a 14-gauge needle introducer, which is obviously unattractive when accessing vessels in the chest or neck region.

2. **Catheter-through-the-needle technique**. The main disadvantage of this technique is the risk of catheter shearing and embolism if attempts are made to withdraw it through the needle.

3. **Seldinger guide-wire technique**. The Seldinger technique, which is described here, offers rapid access without the aforementioned risks.

D. **TECHNIQUE.**

1. **Subclavian access – infraclavicular approach**

a. Prepare the area widely with antiseptic solution and drape the neck and shoulder region with sterile towels. Place patient in the Trendelenburg position – 10–15°.

b. The point of entry is generally the junction of the middle and medial third of the clavicle. In the conscious patient, the point of entry is anesthetized with 1% lidocaine along with subcutaneous infiltration of the tissue to the periosteum of the clavicle.

c. Align the bevel of the needle inferiorly to direct the guide-wire toward the innominate vein.

d. Place the left index finger on the suprasternal notch to facilitate as a reference point for the direction of needle (Figure 10.6).

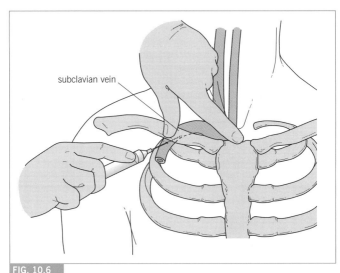

FIG. 10.6
Hand position during subclavian venipuncture.

e. Insert the introducer needle at the entry site approximately 2cm inferior
    to the clavicle and aim for the superior aspect of the left index finger. A
    flashback of blood usually occurs at a depth of 3–4cm. At this point
    detach the syringe and cover the needle hub with the thumb to prevent
    an air embolus.
f. The J-wire is then advanced into the needle, using the introducer
    sleeve. The wire should thread smoothly until at least one-quarter of
    the wire is within the subclavian vein.
g. The sleeve and introducer needle are subsequently removed, leaving
    only the guide-wire in the vessel.
h. A small incision is made at the entry site of the wire, approximately the
    size of the catheter to be introduced. When a standard central venous
    catheter is used, a dilator may be used first to introduce the catheter
    into the vessel over the guide-wire.
2. **Subclavian access – supraclavicular approach.** The main advantage of
    the supraclavicular approach is evident during cardiac arrest situations.
    Because the operator is located away from the area of sternal
    compression, this technique is superior to the infraclavicular method
    (Figure 10.7).
a. Prepare, drape, and infiltrate the site of entry over the lower
    neck region.
b. The point of entry is identified 1cm lateral to the clavicular head of the
    sternocleidomastoid and 1cm posterior to the clavicle.

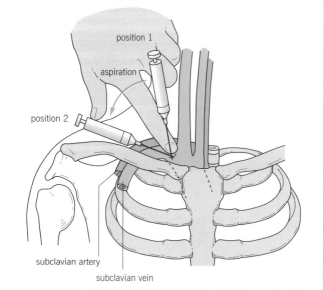

position 1

aspiration

position 2

subclavian artery

subclavian vein

FIG. 10.7
The junction of subclavian and internal jugular veins can be punctured supraclavicularly by advancing the needle medial to the inner edge of the first rib. This junction is larger than either vein and it can be distended further by asking the patient to do a Valsalva maneuver in a forced-expiration phase. The needle is advanced gradually with a constant negative pressure in the syringe. Once a blood flow is obtained, the needle is stabilized to prevent further advancement and entry into the pleural space. The catheter is then inserted. This technique should be avoided in the left side in cirrhotic patients.

c. The introducer needle is held 10–15° above the horizontal, pointing toward the contralateral nipple.
d. Successful access into the vessel occurs at a depth of 2–3cm.
e. The remainder of the supraclavicular access using the Seldinger technique is the same as described for the infraclavicular approach.

3. Internal jugular access – central approach.
a. In this approach, as in all three methods of internal jugular cannulation, the patient is placed in the Trendelenburg position with the head turned away from the side of access.
b. The patient's neck is prepared with an antiseptic solution and draped with sterile towels, as with all vascular access techniques.
c. The point of entry is identified by locating the apex of the triangle formed by the two heads of the sternocleidomastoid muscle and the clavicle (Figure 10.8). In the conscious patient, this area is infiltrated with 1% lidocaine solution.

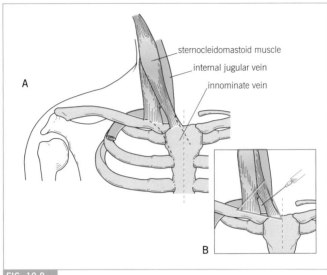

FIG. 10.8

Central approach to internal jugular vein. (A) Relationship of sternocleidomastoid muscle to chest. (B) Course of internal jugular vein; note its sagittal course.

d. The carotid pulse is then palpated with the left hand, when attempting a right-sided approach, and it is retracted medially away from the point of entry.

e. In nonemergency situations, a 22-gauge needle may be used as a guide to identify the location of the internal jugular vein. In emergency situations, this step should be deleted and the standard 16-gauge access needle should be used.

f. The needle is directed 30–40° off the supine plane aiming for the ipsilateral nipple. The internal jugular vein is usually found at a depth of 1–1.5cm. A depth of 4cm should not be exceeded, as this increases the risk for pneumothorax.

g. Once access to the vein is achieved, the Seldinger wire technique is carried out as noted in the section on infraclavicular access (see above).

4. Internal jugular access – anterior approach.

a. The anterior approach to internal jugular cannulation is very similar to the central approach with the exception of the location of entry and direction of needle travel.

b. The carotid artery is palpated with the left hand with a right-sided attempt, and it is retracted medially.

c. The needle entry point is along the medial border of the sternocleidomastoid at its midpoint.

d. The needle is held 30–45° off the supine plane, aiming toward the ipsilateral nipple.

e. After blood return is established, the remainder of the procedure is the same as described previously.

5. Internal jugular access – posterior approach.

a. The posterior approach differs primarily in the location of entry and the direction at which the needle travels.

b. The skin is entered along the lateral aspect of the sternocleidomastoid approximately one-third of the distance from the clavicle to the mastoid process, or at the level of the two heads of the sternocleidomastoid, aiming toward the sternal notch until blood return is obtained.

c. After this is performed, simply follow the steps in the Seldinger wire technique described previously (Figure 10.9).

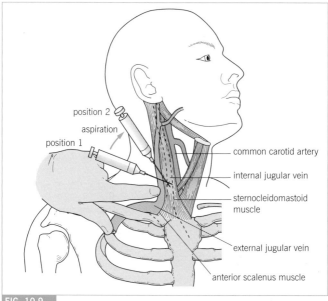

position 2
aspiration
position 1

common carotid artery
internal jugular vein
sternocleidomastoid muscle
external jugular vein
anterior scalenus muscle

FIG. 10.9

Illustration of the internal jugular puncture from the posterior border of the sternocleidomastoid muscle. The neck is turned 45° to the opposite side. The needle is inserted at the posterior border of the sternocleidomastoid muscle and advanced at a 45° angle to this border and 45° to the surface of the body. A gentle and constant negative pressure created by a syringe attached to the needle reveals the vein entry (position 1).

10

CATHETERS AND TUBES

6. **Femoral vein access – Seldinger technique.**

a. Prepare the entire groin area with povidone–iodine (Betadine) antiseptic solution and drape with either sterile towels or a prepackaged sterile paper drape.

b. Palpate the femoral artery 1cm below the inguinal ligament. The femoral vein is located 1cm medial to the arterial pulsations. If no palpable pulse is present then locate the femoral vein at a point midway between the anterior spine of the ileum and the pubic tubercle.

c. Anesthetize the skin and subcutaneous tissue over the femoral vein using 1% lidocaine.

d. With the 16-gauge introducer needle, held at a 45° angle, advance the needle cephalad until a flash of blood is obtained at a depth of 1.5–2cm.

e. The syringe is removed from the needle hub and the guide-wire is threaded into the vein for at least one-third to half its length.

f. A no. 11 blade is then used to incise the skin; subsequently, a dilator is used to dilate the subcutaneous tissue. The guide-wire should be visualized and controlled at all times to prevent embolization.

g. The 16-gauge catheter is then threaded into the femoral vein over the guide-wire, which is then removed. Blood is allowed to backbleed through the catheter prior to connecting it to the intravenous tubing.

h. The catheter is secured in place using either 2-0 silk or nylon suture to prevent dislodgment. Antibacterial ointment is placed over the entrance site and the wound dressed.

E. **COMPLICATIONS AND TREATMENT.**

1. **Overview.**

a. The complication rate of subclavian vein catheterization has generally ranged from 0.4% to 11.1% in most series, with the average rate being quoted as 4.8%.

2. The main complications are related to the structures that surround the subclavian vein (Figure 10.9).

c. Pneumothorax is reported as the most frequent complication of both subclavian and internal jugular cannulation.

d. This highlights the importance of obtaining a chest radiograph following all attempts at vascular access because up to 20% of pneumothoraces may not be clinically detectable.

e. The remainder of the complications associated with internal jugular catheterizations are similar to those with subclavian access.

2. **Pulmonary.**

a. Pneumothorax, hemothorax, hydrothorax, or chylothorax – insert chest tube for drainage or evacuation.

b. Hemomediastinum or hydromediastinum – observation, angiography, or exploration may be indicated for progressive hemomediastinum. Most cases will resolve spontaneously without intervention.

c. Tracheal perforation – observation in the absence of airway compromise.

d. Endotracheal cuff perforation – exchange endotracheal tube if air leak compromises adequate ventilation.

e. Intrathoracic catheter fragmentation – requires retrieval of fragment by fluoroscopy.

3. Infectious.

a. Generalized sepsis and local cellulitis – requires catheter removal and treatment with appropriate antimicrobial agents.

b. Osteomyelitis and septic arthritis – requires débridement, drainage, and adequate antimicrobial therapy.

c. Catheter sepsis is the most common complication of long-term catheter use. The incidence varies depending on the definition of catheter infection. Routine catheter changes every 72 hours can reduce the incidence of catheter infection when combined with a protocol for catheter care. However, this must be balanced against the risks of mechanical complications during multiple catheter insertions. At Parkland Memorial Hospital, catheters are not routinely changed every 72 hours in the intensive care unit.

4. Neurologic. These complications usually resolve with observation but occasionally will require nerve repair.

   a. Phrenic nerve injury.

   b. Brachial plexus injury.

5. Vascular.

a. Air embolus usually occurs during insertion of central lines. These patients undergo acute hemodynamic compromise and signs of acute heart failure. A continuous murmur is sometimes audible over the heart. Treatment is commenced by administering 100% oxygen, placing the patient in the left lateral decubitus position (right-side up) and attempting to aspirate the air out of their right atrium using the same central line.

b. Subclavian artery puncture responds to manual compression in the supraclavicular region. If this is unsuccessful, or the hematoma is expanding, exploration and repair of the arteriotomy is indicated. Pulse or pressure deficits in the arms is also an indication for vascular exploration.

c. Pericardial tamponade is treated expediently by pericardiocentesis and emergency sternotomy with repair of the vascular injury.

d. Septic thrombophlebitis is frequently fatal and associated with generalized sepsis. These patients are initially treated with antimicrobial agents. In severe cases, excision of the vein may be necessary.

e. Catheter embolus is a potentially fatal complication. Fortunately, most catheter fragments can be retrieved using fluoroscopy.

f. Arteriovenous fistula is treated by coil embolization or surgical ligation of the fistula. Distal emboli, high-output cardiac failure, or distal ischemic symptoms are all indications for intervention.

g. Superior vena cava thrombosis is managed by heparinization and ambulatory anticoagulation for 3–6 months. Serial duplex examination will confirm recanalization of these vessels, which is the norm.

6. Miscellaneous.

a. Dysrhythmias (atrial and ventricular) are treated by removal of the offending catheter. Hemodynamic instability will require anti-arrhythmic agents or electric cardioversion.

b. Ascites is managed nonoperatively with diuretics and sodium restriction.

c. Catheter knotting may be managed by untying the knot under fluoroscopy. Rarely is operation required to remove the knot.

d. Catheter malposition is treated by removing and replacing the catheter.

F. PEARLS AND PITFALLS.

1. Central access does not guarantee adequate flow. Flow rates through a peripheral 2-inch, 14-gauge catheter are approximately twice that of a centrally located 8-inch, 16-gauge catheter under identical pressure situations.

2. The 8F Swan–Ganz introducer is a useful tool for rapid infusion.

3. The guide-wire must be visualized at all times while introducing either the dilator, intravenous catheter, or dilator–introducer sheath combination. This is performed by always controlling the distal end of the wire before introducing these into the vessel. Once the vessel is dilated, either the catheter or the introducer sheath may be advanced over the wire into the vessel.

4. Connect to the infusion port once blood is allowed to backbleed from the catheter or introducer sheath.

5. Always obtain a chest radiograph even after unsuccessful attempts to cannulate a central vein.

VII. FURTHER READING

Bund J, Maki D. Infections caused by arterial catheters used for hemodynamic monitoring. *Am J Med* 1979, 67:735.

Collicott PE. Initial assessment of the trauma patient. In: Moore EE, Mattox

KL, Feliciano DV, eds. *Trauma,* 2nd edn. East Norwalk: Appleton and Lange; 1991: 119.

Etheredge E. *Management and techniques in surgery*. New York: Wiley; 1986: 399–402.

Gomella LG, Braen GR, Olding M. *Clinician's pocket reference*. Garden Grove: Prentice-Hall; 1981.

Orland MJ, Saltman RJ. *Manual of medical therapeutics*. Boston: Little, Brown; 1981.

NEUROLOGIC TRAUMA

I. INTRODUCTION

1. **There are approximately 150,000 deaths** every year from trauma and, of these, half are due to fatal head injury.
2. **In 5% of severe head injuries** there is an association with spinal cord injury.
3. **In addition, 10,000 people annually sustain spinal cord injury** without associated head injury.
4. **After injury, the central nervous system** requires weeks to months to achieve functional recovery.
5. **The goal in the acute management of severe head injury** is to provide immediate life-saving therapies and to arrange for appropriate transitional care to enhance functional recovery.
6. **Recently the American Association of Neurologic Surgeons (AANS) and the Joint Section on Neurotrauma and Critical Care** reviewed the available neurotrauma literature and established evidence-based practice guidelines.
a. Their recommendations were divided into three levels of certainty: standards, guidelines, and options; based on the type of literature supporting each recommendation.
b. Only three recommendations met the criteria required to be labeled a standard. They are:
   1) Chronic empirical hyperventilation should be avoided.
   2) Steroids do not improve outcome in patients with head injury and, as such, should be avoided in acute head trauma.
   3) Prophylactic antiseizure medication does not prevent late post-traumatic seizure disorder.

Despite the relatively few standards recommended by the AANS publication it provides well-documented guidelines and options for the treatment of head injury.

II. INITIAL EVALUATION

All patients, regardless of level of consciousness, should be evaluated using the ABC algorithm to avoid missed life-threatening injuries as the neurologic status is being addressed. After the primary survey, the physician should be able to determine if the patient is alert (A), responds only to verbal commands (V), or to pain (P), or is unresponsive (U). During the secondary survey, a neurologic examination should specifically evaluate the level of consciousness (Glasgow coma scale), cranial nerve function including pupillary size and reaction, and extremity motor and sensory function.

A. GLASGOW COMA SCALE.

1. The Glasgow coma scale (GCS) is an imperfect but objective method of rapidly assessing a patient's level of consciousness (Table 11.1).

2. The most important component in a head-injured patient is the motor component because these patients are generally intubated and eye-opening is least reliable.

3. Patients with a GCS <8 have a severe head injury and require intracranial pressure (ICP) monitoring and definitive control of their airway to prevent aspiration of oropharyngeal secretions.

4. GCS motor scores.

a. Follows commands.

b. Localizes to pain. To achieve this score the patient must acknowledge a painful stimulus and move toward its location. Generally, it is accepted that the patient must be able to cross the midline in so doing. Absent from the GCS motor score is a 'semipurposeful' response which is intermediate between localizing (5) and flexion withdrawal (4). In general, it is a meager response to central stimulation.

TABLE 11.1

GLASGOW COMA SCALE

Reaction	Score
Eyes open	
Spontaneously	4
To verbal command	3
To pain	2
No response	1
Best motor response	
To verbal command	
Obeys	6
To painful stimulus	
Localizes pain	5
Flexion withdrawal	4
Flexion abnormal	3
Extension	2
No response	1
Best verbal response	
Oriented and converses	5
Disoriented and converses	4
Inappropriate words	3
Incomprehensible	2
No response	1
Total score	1–15

c.   Flexion withdrawal (also called withdrawing to pain) is a clear
     response to a painful stimulus. However, it is not as clearly directed at
     removing the stimulus as is a localizing response. It often is only
     apparent when stimulating a distal extremity.
d.   Decorticate posturing (also called flexing) is the strong flexion of upper
     extremities with extension of the lower extremities. It is thought to be
     caused by removal of corticospinal inhibition of the midbrain. In
     classic downward herniation, it is a more rostral lesion than
     decerebrate posturing and may have a slightly better prognosis.
e.   Decerebrate posturing (also called extending) is the extension and
     internal rotation of both upper and lower extremities with flexion of
     wrists and fingers. This is felt to be a lower brain-stem injury based
     on animal studies.
f.   No motor response. Must insure no spinal cord injury is present.
B. CRANIAL NERVE EXAM
1.   **The cranial nerve I** is not frequently tested in the acute setting, but
     anosmia is sometimes associated with relatively minor injuries,
     particularly with falls on the occiput as a presumed consequence of
     contrecoup injury.
2.   **Assessment of the cranial nerve II is paramount.** The classic fixed,
     dilated pupil is typical of uncal herniation. Pupils that are only slightly
     asymmetric, but with the larger pupil being somewhat sluggish in its
     reaction to light, may be an early sign of herniation and demands
     immediate investigation.
     Traumatic mydriasis is a large, unreactive pupil associated with intact
     extraocular movement which may be observed in some individuals
     suffering direct blows to the orbit and globe who are fully awake, alert,
     and without neurologic deficit. The injury here is purely ocular. Testing
     gross visual acuity in the awake patient avoids discovering occult
     intraocular injuries later.
3.   **Cranial nerves III, IV, and VI.** Testing extraocular movements in the
     awake patient in the six cardinal fields of gaze may reveal a limitation
     of extraocular movement by entrapment of an extraocular muscle or
     other pathologic process.
4.   **Cranial nerve VII.** In the awake patient, testing sometimes reveals
     deficits in the individual with skull-base fractures or peripheral nerve
     injury.
5.   **Cranial nerve VIII.** Tinnitus and deafness may occur with skull-base
     fractures.
6.   **Cranial nerves IX, X, XI, and XII.** Patients incurring skull-base fractures
     severe enough to affect the lower four cranial nerves frequently
     succumb to their head injuries but, on occasion, isolated lower cranial
     nerve injuries can be detected.

11

NEUROLOGIC TRAUMA

III. IMAGING STUDIES

A. **COMPUTERIZED TOMOGRAPHY.** CT scans are invaluable: not only do they identify the specific pattern of the injury but also they are becoming more important in the decision-making process of operative versus observational therapy. They are also useful for planning surgical approaches and as such should be taken early in the care of patients suspected of having a head injury. Early surgical treatment and aggressive ICP management can definitely improve outcomes.

B. **ANGIOGRAPHY.** Indications for acute cerebral angiography include a large amount of subarachnoid blood, which suggests a cerebral aneurysm, and unilateral motor deficit with a normal CT scan, which is a common presentation for blunt carotid artery injury. Finally, basilar skull fractures involving the carotid canal constitute a relative indication for a cerebral arteriogram.

C. **PLAIN RADIOGRAPHY.** Skull radiographs are useful for assessing the presence of foreign bodies or tracking the path of missiles in penetrating injuries to the cranium. They are also sensitive for skull fractures (open or closed). Plain radiographs are not otherwise useful in the acute evaluation of head-injured patients.

IV. INITIAL MANAGEMENT

A. **MAINTAIN BLOOD PRESSURE.** Recent literature suggests that maintaining cerebral perfusion pressure (CPP = mean arterial pressure (MAP) – ICP) may be more important than controlling ICP alone. This is especially true in the initial management phase where no ICP monitor is present but many strategies are available to increase CPP by increasing MAP.

B. **HEAD-OF-BED ELEVATION.** The ICP difference between a flat and an elevated head is 10–15mmHg. Elevating the patient's head 30° is a simple, effective way to lower ICP. Obtaining plain films of the thoracolumbar spine in the emergency room excludes gross spinal injury and allows the bed head to be elevated early. Reverse Trendelenburg position is less effective.

C. **HYPERVENTILATION.** The use of prophylactic hyperventilation should be avoided during the initial management phase (i.e. keep P_{CO_2} 35–40mmHg). If acute deterioration is noted, hyperventilation can be used (i.e. P_{CO_2} 25–30mmHg) until an ICP monitor can be placed. In the presence of increased ICP detected by the monitor, hyperventilation may become part of the strategy to lower ICP. Excessive hyperventilation can impair cerebral perfusion by causing cerebrovascular vasoconstriction.

D. **MANNITOL.** Mannitol 250–1000mg/kg is effective in lowering ICP but it should be used only when an ICP monitor is in place. Two exceptions to this rule include acute neurologic deterioration and as a temporizing measure prior to a neurosurgical procedure. Recent evidence suggests that mannitol's mode of action alters blood viscosity, thus allowing blood to flow more easily through the vascular beds, rather then working as a diuretic to reduce brain edema. This difference in thinking about the mechanism of mannitol is more than academic and alters the way it is now used by most people. Currently, patients receiving mannitol are maintained in a euvolemic state: serum osmolarity is kept <310mOsm and serum sodium is kept <150mOsm. Mannitol seems most effective when given in boluses. The use of steroids does not appear to be beneficial for traumatic brain edema.

E. INDICATIONS FOR INTRACRANIAL PRESSURE MONITORING.

1. **An ICP monitor will usually need to be placed on patients with a GCS of 3–8** if they have abnormal CT scans. Patients with a GCS >8 generally have a motor exam which allows the patient to be serially examined clinically without an ICP monitor. This usually means they are localizing or better. Patients with a GCS of 7 or 8 and a normal CT scan can sometimes be managed without an ICP monitor.

2. **ICP monitor is recommended for patients with a normal CT scan** if two or more of the following are noted at admission:

a. Age over 40 years.

b. Unilateral or bilateral motor posturing.

c. Systolic blood pressure <90mmHg.

F. SEIZURE PROPHYLAXIS.

1. **There is a trend away from the use of prophylactic dilantin** in acute head trauma as there is a large amount of literature suggesting no benefit in the prevention of late post-traumatic seizures (>1 week). It is, however, quite effective in the prevention of seizures in the acute period. In this acute period, seizures can exacerbate pre-existing intracranial injury, transiently elevate ICP, and confuse the clinical picture when a previously lethargic patient becomes unresponsive in a postictal period. Thus, early empirical dilantin therapy may be indicated in many patients with head injury to prevent early seizure.

2. **Typically, two groups of patients receive empirical dilantin therapy**:

a. Patients with a high risk of seizure based on CT scan findings, such as temporal lobe contusions or large cortical contusions.

b. Patients in whom a seizure would be particularly deleterious.

3. **Empirical dilantin therapy is ceased** when the patient is transferred from the intensive care unit (ICU) or on discharge from the hospital.

G. COAGULOPATHY.

1. **Traumatic brain injuries are associated with coagulopathy**. This may be due to tissue factors released from the injured brain which interfere with normal coagulation. All patients should have coagulation profiles sent on admission and serially during the first 24 hours of admission.

NEUROLOGIC TRAUMA

11

Even a mildly prolonged prothrombin time or partial thromoboplastin time should be treated as a sign of early disseminated intravascular coagulation and not assumed to be a laboratory error.

2. **Correction of coagulopathy** will prevent exacerbation of intracranial bleeding.

V. ASSOCIATED SPINAL CORD INJURY

A. **ALL PATIENTS WHO ARE UNRESPONSIVE** should be treated as though they have a spine fracture.

B. **IN ADDITION TO THE USUAL CERVICAL SPINE FILMS**, the thoracic, lumbar, and a sacral spine should be viewed with both an anterior–posterior (AP) and lateral film. Obtaining these films early allows for early detection of potentially serious injuries. Furthermore, if the films are normal it decreases the nursing-care burden of these patients by easing spinal precautions.

C. **CLEARING THE CERVICAL SPINE** (i.e. removing the cervical collar) requires proof that no bony or ligamentous injury exists. Bony injuries can be identified with plain film and CT. Identifying ligamentous injury can be more difficult, as discussed below.

VI. SPECIFIC INJURIES

A. **SKULL FRACTURES.**

1. **The management of skull fractures** is related to their relationship to major dural sinuses and paranasal sinuses, the degree of displacement of the fracture, the presence of in-driven bone fragments, and the degree of underlying parenchymal injury. This range of consideration yields considerable variability in the management of skull fractures.

2. **As a general rule**, linear nondisplaced fractures require no operative treatment, while depressed fractures or fractures with in-driven bone frequently require operative repair (débridement and elevation).

B. **EPIDURAL HEMATOMA.**

1. **These are usually associated with a skull fracture and tearing of the underlying middle meningeal artery**; occasionally, however, they are associated with a tear of the venous sinus (the so-called venous epidural hematoma).

2. **The dura is tightly applied to the inner table of the skull**, and this accounts for the characteristic lenticular appearance of an epidural hematoma on CT.

3. **Diagnosis is suggested by focal neurologic signs** in the presence of an alteration in mental status.

4. **Occasionally, these patients present with a lucid interval** of several minutes to hours depending on the rate of expansion.

5. **Confirmation is by CT scan**.

6. **Treatment is by operative evacuation of the hematoma**.

C. SUBDURAL HEMATOMA.

1. **Impact from trauma may tear cortical bridging veins**, resulting in a subdural hematoma.

2. **The subdural hematoma usually has a crescent shape on CT scanning**, the clot spreading easily over the convexities.

3. **In addition to tearing of the bridging veins**, a subdural hematoma is usually associated with significant underlying parenchymal damage. This explains the overall 50% mortality rate with this lesion in spite of early clot evacuation.

4. **Operation is required for subdural hematomas**, with significant midline shift, large hematomas, or those collections associated with severe neurologic deficits.

D. CONTUSION.

1. **Bruising of the brain parenchyma** is usually prominent over the orbital portions of the frontal lobes and temporal poles.

2. **Although small contusions can be handled conservatively**, contusions characteristically evolve on serial CT scans, and consolidation and worsening of multiple small temporal lobe contusions can result in a life-threatening temporal lobe mass, with subsequent herniation and death. The dynamic nature of contusions, in any location, highlights the necessity for serial CT scans in the head-injured patient to assess their progression.

3. **These patients need to be observed in an ICU or step-down unit** until it can be reasonably concluded that the lesions are stable.

4. **Major non-neurosurgical operative procedures carry a high risk** of exacerbating these lesions and are best avoided in the acute period.

E. EDEMA.

1. **The edema that accompanies severe brain injury is poorly understood**, but probably represents both cytotoxic and vasogenic mechanisms.

2. **Brain swelling quickly results in increased ICP** because the cranium defines a fixed volume.

3. **Additionally, multiple dural reflections partition the brain into various compartments** – the falx cerebri lies between the cerebral hemispheres, while the tentorium separates the posterior fossa and cerebellum from supratentorial structures.

4. **These dural reflections complicate swelling**, as they create gradients between compartments and serve as rigid structures against which nerves, blood vessels, and critical structures can be compressed.

F. DIFFUSE AXONAL INJURY.

1. **It is not uncommon to see patients who have low GCS scores and minimal or no CT scan findings**. These patients are thought to have diffuse axonal injury.

2. **The proposed mechanism** is a shearing injury of the axons within the white matter. In reality, it is a histopathologic diagnosis made at autopsy.

3. **Numerous disruptions of axons** with characteristic spheroid formation on key stains are diagnostic.
4. **Nevertheless, the diagnosis is made clinically** when a patient's neurologic status is poor but the CT findings are minimal.
5. **Occasionally, magnetic resonance imaging (MRI)** in these patients will show a multitude of bright punctate lesions on T2-weighted images.

VII. OPERATIVE TREATMENT

The decision to operate on a head-injured patient depends not only on the CT scan appearance of the lesions but also on the presence of associated life-threatening injuries and overall clinical condition of the patient.

1. **Patients in good neurologic condition** can be managed nonoperatively even in the presence of small contusions or subdural hematoma.
2. **Some patients may have sustained such severe head trauma** that their clinical exam and CT scan may not be compatible with survival.
3. **The families of these patients must be counseled** in a caring and open but honest manner regarding the prognosis for meaningful, functional recovery. Allowing the family to see the patient early and the incorporation of nurse coordinators into the health care team greatly facilitate early decision-making in these complex situations.
A. **SURGERY.** Almost all epidural hematomas and most large subdural hematomas need to be evacuated early.
1. **An arterial line is necessary** for accurate blood pressure monitoring.
2. **A lateral cervical spine radiograph** is the minimal requirement to allow for safe positioning of the patient.
3. **A large question mark-shaped incision** is made in front of the ear, curving back and then forward again to midline.
4. **A large bone flap is fashioned.**
5. **Epidural hematomas are evacuated without opening the dura.**
6. **In the presence of a subdural hematoma,** the dura is opened and the clot and contused brain are removed.
7. **Fresh-frozen plasma is administered** early in the operation or preoperatively as coagulopathy is almost universal.
8. **Dural closure and replacement of the bone flap** are performed depending on the amount of brain removed and the potential for continued swelling.
9. **It is not uncommon to leave the bone flap out.**
10. **Tight skin closure is achieved and drains are frequently placed.** An ICP monitor, if not already present, is also placed.
11. **The patient is returned to the ICU for serial exam and CT scans.**

VIII. SPINAL CORD INJURIES AND EVALUATION OF THE VERTEBRAL COLUMN

A. GENERAL PRINCIPLES.

1. Spine fractures may be associated with as many as 10% of traumatic injuries.
2. The cervical spine should always be treated as if it were injured, even if suspicion is low, because the consequences of missing a cervical spine fracture can result in one of the most devastating iatrogenic injuries possible.
3. Spine fractures at one level raise suspicion for a second fracture elsewhere in the vertebral column.
4. Patients who are unresponsive should have plain radiographs of the entire axial spine as early as possible, preferably in the emergency room. This allows prompt diagnosis and treatment of injuries, allows for greater flexibility in positioning the patient for further workup and treatment, and, if negative, reduces the burden of nursing care by allowing spine precautions to be removed.
5. Spine precautions should be in place prior to complete evaluation of the patient and in the event of a spine fracture being detected.
6. Patients on spine precautions should still be removed from the backboard, however, the patient should be nursed flat in bed with the axial spine maintained in line. A hard cervical collar is left in place and flexion and extension are avoided. If the patient is moved, a minimum of three people are needed to assist: one to control the head, one to control the shoulders and hips, and one to control the lower extremities.
7. Examination of patients with suspected spine fracture should be performed as described below.

B. MOTOR EXAMINATION.

1. Awake patients can undergo testing of motor functions in the classic manner, including testing of drift (having the patient hold outstretched arms fully supinated with fingers extended and fully abducted so that subtle pronation or actual dropping of the extended arm occurs, indicating weakness).
2. The usual testing of the individual indicator muscle groups by spinal cord level can help detect the level of spinal cord dysfunction.
3. The spinal cord injury level is recorded as the lowest functioning level. Table 11.2 is a simple guide for determining cervical injury levels.

C. SENSORY EXAMINATION. These tests should be performed on all extremities.

1. Testing of pinprick sensation can help denote the level of spinal cord injury.
2. Testing of joint position sense can help detect posterior column lesions.

TABLE 11.2

DETERMINATION OF CERVICAL INJURY LEVELS

Vertebrae	Motor	Sensory	Reflex
C5	Deltoid	Region over the deltoid	Biceps
C6	Biceps	Thumb and index finger	Brachioradialis
C7	Triceps and wrist	Middle finger	Triceps and wrist extensors
C8	Finger flexion	Ring and fifth finger	None

D. REFLEXES

1. Generalities

a. The biceps jerk, brachioradialis, triceps jerk, ankle jerk, and knee jerk are listed and noted as absent, normal, or increased.

b. It is important to note the symmetry of the reflexes as well as the relationship of the upper to lower extremity reflexes.

c. Absent reflexes may indicate the presence of a lower motor neuron lesion (e.g. absent ankle jerks in cauda equina syndrome) or they can be associated with nerve root compression by a herniated intervertebral disk.

d. Absent reflexes may also be present in spinal shock – a state of areflexia and frequently impaired autonomic function in the acute phase of spinal cord injury which might normally be anticipated to be associated with increased reflexes.

e. Hyperreflexia suggests an upper motor neuron lesion (e.g. a high cervical cord injury leading to hyperreflexia in both arms and legs).

2. **The Babinski reflex** is elicited by a stroke of the reflex hammer from the lateral border of the sole across the ball of the foot. Extension or fanning of the toes indicates an upper motor neuron lesion (e.g. spinal cord or severe brain injury), while a flexor response is normal.

3. **Cremasteric reflex**: stroking the skin of the inner thigh results in elevation of the ipsilateral testicle, absent with lesions above L1 or L2.

4. **Superficial abdominal reflexes** are elicited by gently stroking the skin of the abdomen toward the umbilicus in a thin individual with good abdominal muscle tone and usually result in deviation of the umbilicus toward the stimulus. Its absence may indicate an upper motor neuron lesion.

5. **A decrease in rectal tone is a critical observation** to make when spinal cord injury is suspected. It is particularly important in the unresponsive patient where it may provide the first clue that a spinal cord injury is present.

6. **Bulbocavernous reflex**: a gentle pull on a Foley catheter results in a contraction of the anal sphincter. This is an easy reflex to test since most patients have a Foley catheter in place and it provides critical

information. If this reflex is present it suggests a spinal cord injury is incomplete. If absent it can confirm that decreased rectal tone is in fact due to a spinal cord injury.

E. **RADIOGRAPHIC STUDIES.**

1. **Plain films.** All patients with suspected spinal cord injury need AP, lateral, and odontoid films to identify bony injury. An adequate lateral C-spine film must visualize the C7–T1 interspace and the top of T1. A swimmer's view may be necessary to achieve this. Awake patients should have their axial spine palpated and plain films of any tender portion of the spine should be obtained (both AP and lateral). Unresponsive patients should have their entire axial spine imaged.

2. **A CT scan** should be obtained of any abnormality on plain film suspected of being a spine fracture. It may also be used to clear the odontoid or the C7–T1 junction in cases where multiple attempts at plain films have been inadequate.

3. **MRI is becoming increasingly used** in the acute trauma setting. It is thought to be useful in the detection of ligamentous injury, particularly in the unresponsive patient. Patients suspected of having prolonged periods of unresponsiveness will require an MRI. In this group of patients, physicians at Parkland Memorial Hospital obtain the MRI scan using a STIR sequence (similar to a T2-weighted image) within 48–72 hours to identify signal changes that signify ligamentous spinal injury. Bright signal in the posterior ligaments, particularly a signal extending to the posterior longitudinal ligament, is felt to be highly suggestive of ligamentous injury. Another use of MRI in trauma is for the evaluation of the spinal cord and spinal canal after a fracture is detected. While not as sensitive as CT scans for imaging bone, it can clearly demonstrate the presence of a spinal epidural hematoma or acute traumatic soft disk, which may serve as a contraindication for placement in traction or as an indication for urgent surgery.

F. **MANAGEMENT.**

1. **Remove the patient from backboard** (even those with fractures and neurologic deficits) and log roll every 2 hours to avoid skin breakdown even while in the emergency department.

2. **These patients are at risk of arriving in the ICU with early skin breakdown** already beginning to occur, depending on the time spent in the emergency department.

3. **Apply deep venous thrombosis prophylaxis early** as these patients are at high risk.

4. **Serial neurologic exams by the same person**. Initially, it is important to document the presence of a neurologic deficit early so that it is clear when the deficit occurred. Later, it is important to follow the deficit,

particularly a partial deficit, because progression of deficit is an indication for early surgery.

5. **Steroids are given to all patients** who arrive <6 hours post injury and have a neurologic deficit. The protocol used is 30mg/kg of methylprednisolone as an i.v. bolus, followed by 5.4 mg/kg per hour for 23 hours. If an accurate time is unknown it is probably best to err on the side of giving steroids. At Parkland Memorial Hospital we begin i.v. steroid protocol in the emergency department. There also may be some benefit, albeit less, when steroids are administered within 12 hours of injury. However, the increased risk of septic complications in the multiply injured patient receiving steroids must be balanced against the potential benefit of steroids in improving functional outcome in spinal cord injury.

G. SPINAL SHOCK.

1. **The sympathetic nervous system** regulates heart rate and blood pressure.
2. **The motor neurons** for the sympathetic nervous system are in the thoracic spinal cord.
3. **Cervical spinal cord injuries** can sever the communication between the brain and the sympathetics in the cord and result in hypotension and bradycardia.
4. **Spinal shock must be recognized** as the associated hypotension may not always respond to volume resuscitation.
5. **Continued fluid boluses** in these patients results in volume overload.
6. **Pressors should be used early** in these patients to maintain blood pressure.
7. **It is not clear what the goal blood pressure should be** in these patients. However, in general, systolic blood pressure >100mmHg or a mean arterial blood pressure of 75–90mmHg should be maintained, at least initially.

H. PULMONARY FUNCTION.

1. **Many factors place a spinal cord injury patient's pulmonary function at risk**.
2. **Patients with high lesions** have lost the use of their intercostal muscles and have only the diaphragm to generate inspiratory force.
3. **Pulmonary embolus is common** in this population.
4. **Volume overload** in spinal shock patients is common.
5. **Good ventilator management and excellent respiratory therapy** are critical for good outcomes.

I. SURGERY.

1. **In general, acute operations for spinal fractures are avoided** to allow time to evaluate other injuries.
2. **Progression of a partial neurologic deficit** is a common indication for acute surgery.

3. **Partial deficits caused by epidural hematomas or acute soft disk** are other indications for early operation.
4. **The goals of surgery** are to decompress the neural elements and restore spinal stability.
5. **Early (not acute) surgery** allows for early mobilization of the patient and helps avoid some of the pulmonary problems listed above.
6. **Surgery is often done** even in patients with complete neurologic deficit in whom little hope of recovery exists.
7. **The indication for surgery in these patients** is to decrease pain, prevent ascending neurologic deficit, and to provide mechanical stability to the spine to facilitate early mobilization and rehabilitation.
J. OUTCOMES.
1. **Patients with complete neurologic deficit** rarely regain function except in spinal shock.
2. **Patients with even a single modality preserved** have a better chance of regaining function.
3. **Sacral sparing of sensory loss and preserved dorsal column function** are common modalities present in patients who otherwise appear to have complete deficits.
4. **Patients with partial injuries,** who are weak but have some preserved strength, frequently improve dramatically.
5. **Completely paraplegic patients**, who have preserved upper extremity function, can live functional independent lives if they receive the appropriate rehabilitation.
6. **Patients with high cervical injury** (C5 and above) may lose innervation to the diaphragm and become ventilator dependent.

NEUROLOGIC TRAUMA

11

IX. FURTHER READING

Bullock R, Chesnut RM, Clifton G *et al*. Guidelines for the management of severe head injury. In: Trauma Foundation. *The Brain*. Park Ridge: American Association of Neurologic Surgeons; 1995.

Foulkes MA, Eisenberg HM, Jane JA, *et al*. The traumatic coma data bank: design, methods, and baseline characteristics. *J Neurosurg* 1991; 75:S8–S36.

Harvey SL, Gary HE, Eisenberg HM, *et al*. Neurobehavioral outcome 1 year after severe head injury. *J Neurosurg* 1990; 73:699–709.

Wilkins RH, Rengachary SS. *Neurosurgery*. New York: McGraw-Hill; 1985.

SOFT TISSUE INJURIES OF THE FACE

I. WOUND HEALING

A. **A CLEAR UNDERSTANDING OF WOUND HEALING** is important to approaching the repair of soft tissue injuries.

B. **WOUND REPAIR.** There are three phases:

1. **Inflammatory phase** (first 2–3 days): cellular infiltration.

2. **Proliferative phase** (established by day 3–5). Wound tensile strength increases secondary to the increasing levels of collagen within the wound and raised scar develops. The proliferative phase lasts approximately 2–4 weeks depending on the size and site of the wound.

3. **Maturation phase** (begins around 3 weeks after injury). The duration of this phase depends on several factors, including patient's age, type of wound, specific location on the body, and length and intensity of the inflammatory period.

C. **SURGICAL WOUND CLASSIFICATION.**

1. **Clean.**

a. <8 hours old and with minimal crush, contusion, or foreign body.

b. Bacterial contaminants are usually Gram positive with an infection frequency of 3%.

c. Can be meticulously debrided, copiously irrigated, and closed primarily without the need for antibiotic coverage.

d. Open wound treatment (healing by secondary intention) is rarely indicated.

2. **Clean-contaminated.**

a. Up to 3 days old.

b. Bacterial contaminants are polymicrobial with an infection frequency of 5–15%.

c. Treatment consists of thorough débridement with copious irrigation to remove all foreign bodies. May be left open (cover with antibiotic ointment and wet to dry dressings). Delayed primary closure can be performed in 3–7 days.

3. **Contaminated.**

a. Associated crush, contusion, or foreign body (e.g. dirt, gravel, saliva, teeth fragments, glass, wood, grass, etc.).

b. Bacterial contaminants are polymicrobial with an infection frequency of 15–40%.

c. Provide aggressive wound care for 7–10 days to try to get the wound into the clean-contaminated classification, then perform delayed primary closure.

4. **Dirty.**
a. Established infection usually associated with an abscess or the drainage of pus.
b. Infection is polymicrobial with a frequency of 40%.
c. Incision and drainage is the treatment of choice, with aggressive wound débridement and wet to dry dressing changes 2–3 times a day.
d. Intravenous antibiotics are advocated. The wound is allowed to heal by secondary intention with possible scar revision at a later time.

II. ANESTHESIA

The extent of injuries, general medical condition of the patient, psychological reaction to surgery, and ability to cooperate with a lengthy procedure are all factors when determining whether repair of soft tissue injuries may be carried out under local anesthesia in the emergency department or clinic, or in the operating room under general anesthesia.

A. **LOCAL ANESTHESIA.**
1. **Lidocaine 1–2%, with 1:100,000 epinephrine,** is the local anesthetic of choice at Parkland Memorial Hospital.
a. It decreases blood flow to the area of injection.
b. It provides 3–4 hours of soft tissue anesthesia. Limit epinephrine in sensitive patients.
c. It may be used in all areas of the head and neck.
2. **It is preferable to utilize regional nerve blocks whenever possible:**
a. To decrease the total dose of anesthetic.
b. To avoid distorting valuable landmarks necessary for aesthetic closure of wound edges.
c. To decrease edema at the wound edges, which will promote better healing.
3. **When local anesthesia is used in the face** it is usually injected around the nerve to the wounded area with a small gauge needle (25-gauge or 27-gauge) (Figures 12.1 and 12.2).

B. **SEDATION.**
1. **Sedation may be indicated depending on the extent of the injury and length of the repair.** All sedation must be monitored with pulse oximetry, blood pressure, EKG leads, supplemental oxygen, and with appropriate intubation equipment available.
2. **Midazolam (Versed).**
a. A patient's clinical response varies and may be unpredictable. Carefully titrate 1–2mg to achieve desired effect.
b. Antagonist. Flumazenil i.v. 0.2mg is titrated to a total dose of 1mg over a 5 minute interval.
3. **Fentanyl**
a. Administered intravenously.
b. Dosage for sedation is 2–8mcg/kg.

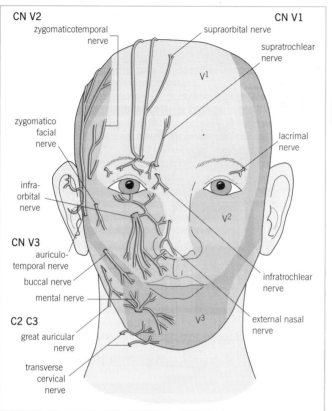

CN V2
zygomaticotemporal nerve

CN V1
supraorbital nerve

supratrochlear nerve

V¹

zygomatico facial nerve

lacrimal nerve

infra- orbital nerve

CN V3
auriculo- temporal nerve

buccal nerve

mental nerve

V²

infratrochlear nerve

C2 C3
great auricular nerve

V³

external nasal nerve

transverse cervical nerve

12

SOFT TISSUE INJURIES OF THE FACE

FIG. 12.1
Sensory nerves of the face. (From Agur A, Lee M. *Grant's atlas of anatomy,* 9th edn. Baltimore: Williams and Wilkins; 1990.)

c. May produce respiratory depression in a dose-dependent manner.
d. Antagonist. Naloxone i.v. bolus of 0.04mg every 2–3 minutes until desired effect.

III. BASIC MANAGEMENT

A   WOUND DEFINITIONS.

1. **A contusion** is usually produced by blunt trauma that ruptures subcutaneous vessels without disruption of the overlying skin.

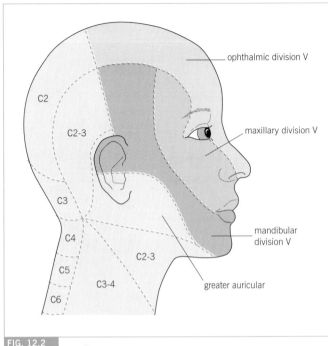

FIG. 12.2

Cutaneous sensory distribution of trigeminal nerve. (From Walker RV, Fonseca RJ. *Oral and maxillofacial trauma. Volume 1*. Philadelphia: WB Saunders; 1991:258.)

a. Results in extensive edema, ecchymosis, and hematoma.
b. Heals with conservative treatment.
c. May require débridement if associated with a laceration – unless vital areas (e.g. eyelid) are involved – or drainage of the hematoma.

2. **An abrasion** is an avulsion of the epithelial and papillary layers of the skin resulting from a shearing force to expose the reticular layer as a raw, bleeding surface.

a. Abrasions usually re-epithelialize within 7–10 days.
b. These injuries should be thoroughly scrubbed, irrigated, and coated with a thin layer of topical antibiotic ointment.
c. Inadequate débridement may result in an irregular scar or infection.
d. If the depth extends deep into the dermal layer, significant scarring may result.

e.   Sharp débridement, primary closure, or coverage with a thick, split-thickness, or full-thickness skin graft may improve cosmetic results.

3.   **Lacerations** may be simple, linear, jagged, or stellate; margins may be abraded, contused, or crushed.

a.   Following minimal débridement and copious irrigation, lacerations may be closed in layers using fine (5-0 to 6-0) chromic gut (less reactive) suture deep to approximate subcutaneous tissues and polypropylene (Prolene) suture, or nylon suture, for approximation of the skin edges.

b.   If meticulous subcuticular sutures are applied, the facial skin sutures may be removed in 3–5 days while supporting the wound with Steri-strips.

c.   Débridement or 'freshening' of the wound edges is often required in stellate, abraded, contused, or crushed lacerations.

d.   Flap-like lacerations require meticulous débridement and closure. Pressure dressings are important to avoid hematoma formation beneath the flap.

4.   **Large avulsions** of the soft tissue rarely occur in the maxillofacial region; they are most commonly associated with gunshot wounds or shotgun wounds.

a.   Apparent tissue loss is usually found in the form of rolled borders or retracted edges.

b.   Small avulsive defects of the face can usually be addressed by local undermining and advancement of adjacent tissue.

c.   Large avulsive defects should be approximated as closely as possible without creating tension. The exposed surfaces can then be addressed by skin grafts, local flaps, and other measures.

d.   Scar revisions may be necessary at a later date.

B.   RELAXED SKIN TENSION LINES.

1.   The relaxed skin tension lines **(RSTLs or Langer lines)** follow the furrows formed when the skin is relaxed. They are based on the orientation of the fibers in the reticular layer of the skin.

2.   **RSTLs run parallel to the principal fiber bundles** and thus place less tension on wound margins when incisions or lacerations lie parallel to the RSTLs.

3.   **Lacerations lying perpendicular to these lines** will tend to have greater tension on their margins and 'gape open'.

4.   **Lacerations and incisions that fall parallel to these lines** produce the most inconspicuous scars. If possible, the surgeon should attempt to place all incisions in the RSTLs, even if the tension-line incision is longer than the antitension-line incision.

C.   SKIN FLAPS. Local advancement skin flaps provide single stage repair of avulsion defects. The primary advantage is to cover defects that are difficult to approximate without distorting anatomy, or placing tension on the skin wound edges.

1. **Advantages of local skin flaps**
a. The flap carries its own blood supply.
b. It closely matches the skin color and texture of surrounding tissues.
c. Flap incisions can be hidden in RSTLs.
2. **Disadvantages of local skin flaps**
a. Additional incisions.
b. Increased scarring.
c. Excessive stretching, twisting, or kinking of the pedicle.
d. Creates a larger, more obvious defect than the defect to be covered.

IV. SPECIALIZED STRUCTURES

The facial region is blessed with an extensive primary and collateral blood supply that facilitates the rapid healing of even the most tenuous of flaps: yet accompanying this vascular network are a plethora of sensory and motor nerves, ducts, glands, and other structures. The repair of certain regions of the face requires special attention because of the functional and cosmetic problems that may occur from mismanagement.

A. SCALP.
1. **The anatomic layers of the scalp** can be remembered by the mnemonic SCALP (Figure 12.3).
2. **The high vascularity and inelasticity of the subcutaneous layer** reduces blood vessel retraction when lacerated, resulting in potential extensive blood loss.

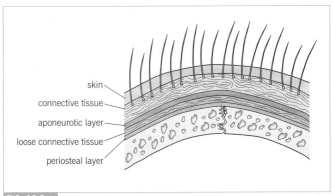

skin
connective tissue
aponeurotic layer
loose connective tissue
periosteal layer

FIG. 12.3
The scalp and forehead are portions of the same highly vascularized anatomic unit responsible for protection of the skull. They consist of five layers, best remembered by the mnemonic SCALP. In order, from skin to cranial bone, these layers are skin (S), subcutaneous tissue (C), aponeurosis layer (A), loose connective tissue (L), and pericranial layer (P). (From Walker RV, Fonseca RJ. *Oral and maxillofacial trauma. Volume 1.* Philadelphia:WB Saunders; 1991:643.)

3. **Management:** hemostasis, débridement, irrigation, and closure (two layers – galea aponeurosa and skin – or single layer which is a large suture through both the galea and skin).

4. **Significant subaponeurotic hematomas can develop** if hemorrhage is not adequately controlled at the time of closure.

5. **Large avulsions usually require extensive flap rotation or skin grafts** as a result of the inelasticity of the scalp.

B. **EYEBROW.**

1. **The eyebrow should never be shaved**; conservative clipping may be necessary, on rare occasions, to allow proper approximation of the skin edges.

2. **If débridement is necessary,** because of nonvital tissue, care should be taken to incise or cut parallel to the hair follicles so as not to damage the follicles of adjacent, viable tissue (this holds true for the scalp as well).

3. **Avulsive defects** may require hair transplantation as a secondary procedure.

C. **EYELIDS.**

1. **Injuries may result in cosmetic as well as functional defects** if not treated properly. Any injury of the eyelid should prompt a close examination of the globe for associated injuries.

2. **Simple lacerations to the upper lid** should be explored to rule out damage to the levator aponeurosis (especially if ptosis is present). If transection is present, meticulous approximation should follow to re-establish the upper lid fold and function.

3. **Simple lacerations to the lower lid** may be closed in layers. Care should be taken not to include the orbital septum in the suture, or cicatricial ectropion may result.

4. **Marginal lacerations** (those extending to the lid margin) require meticulous closure to prevent functional and cosmetic defects. Fine nylon sutures (6-0) are first used to approximate the lash line, meibomian glands, and gray line (junction of the skin and mucosa). Fine absorbable sutures (4-0, Vicryl) are used to approximate the fascia. The marginal sutures are left long and taped to the skin surface to prevent corneal abrasion. Through-and-through lacerations of the lid margin require closure in three layers: conjunctiva, orbicularis oculi muscle, and skin.

5. **Avulsive injuries to the eyelids** may be treated with full-thickness skin grafts (from postauricular area or contralateral eyelid). Marginal avulsions can be primarily closed if they constitute <25% of the lid length (lateral canthotomy may be required to achieve tension-free closure). Larger defects may require grafts or rotation flaps.

D. **LACRIMAL APPARATUS.**

1. **The lacrimal system** is composed of the medially located superior and inferior punctum, canaliculi, lacrimal sac, and duct. More than half of tear drainage is through the inferior canaliculus.

2. **Lacerations or fractures to the medial orbital area** may result in transection of the canaliculi or lacrimal sac. Damage to this system is usually apparent as epiphora (watering of the eye).

3. **Severed canaliculi can be primarily repaired** over fine Silastic tubing that extends to the inferior meatus of the nose.

4. **Nasolacrimal duct damage** may require dacryoadenectomy.

E. **NOSE.**

1. **Lacerations may involve the skin, vestibular lining, or nasal mucosa**.

2. **Inspection of the septum** is required to rule out septal hematoma (which requires prompt drainage) or laceration of the mucoperichondrium. Significant mucosal and vestibular lacerations should be closed with fine (4-0) chromic gut suture.

3. **Lacerations of the alar rim region** often violate the continuity of the supportive alar cartilage. Reapproximation of the cartilage with fine chromic gut suture is necessary to restore the structural support of the rim.

4. **The skin should be meticulously approximated** utilizing known landmarks (e.g. alar rim, tip) for proper orientation.

5. **Avulsive defects** may be treated with the avulsed segment being replaced if seen in a timely period (<1 hour). These rarely take and secondary reconstruction, with composite grafts or full-thickness skin grafts, is usually necessary.

F. **LIPS.**

1. **Anesthesia may be easily obtained** through bilateral mental nerve blocks for the lower lip and infraorbital nerve blocks for the upper lip.

2. **Superficial lacerations to the lip** may be closed in layers (muscle, subcutaneous tissue, and skin). The first suture should be placed at the vermilion border (junction of the skin and mucosa of the lip) to allow accurate closure without distortion of the tissue edges (Figure 12.4).

3. **Care should be taken to reapproximate muscle edges accurately** in order to avoid functional and cosmetic defects.

4. **Avulsive defects of the lip** may be closed primarily if <25% of the tissue is lost. More extensive tissue loss may require regional flap advancement for repair.

5. **Through-and-through lacerations** should be closed 'inside-out'. The oral mucosa should be closed 'water tight'. Thorough irrigation should follow this procedure, with closure of the remainder of the laceration as described earlier.

G. **PAROTID DUCT.** The parotid duct (Stensen's duct) exits the anterior aspect of the parotid gland at approximately the level of a line drawn from the tragus of the ear to the middle of the upper lip. The duct crosses superficially to the masseter muscle, then pierces the buccinator muscle to enter the oral cavity at approximately the level of the maxillary second molar tooth.

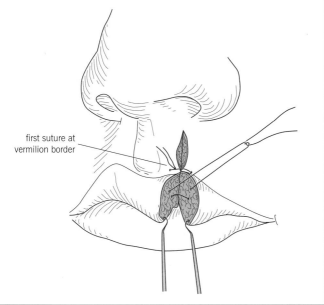

FIG. 12.4

Repair of a vertical laceration of the vermilion–cutaneous margin. First suture should be used for approximation of the vermilion–cutaneous border. Injection of a local anesthetic containing epinephrine might diminish ability to align this suture. Both edges of the vermilion, including that adjacent to the skin and white roll of the lip and that adjacent to the mucous membrane, should be carefully aligned. (From McCarthy JG. *Plastic surgery*. *Volume 2, part 1*. Philadelphia: WB Saunders; 1990:913.)

1. **Lacerations to the cheek area of the face** should arouse the suspicion of parotid duct injury (as well as facial nerve injury). Direct inspection of the wound may or may not reveal a lacerated duct. The intra-oral opening may be easily cannulated with a probe, followed by inspection for communication with the wound. Duct flow may be assessed by drying the oral opening with a gauze, then milking the gland clear. Smooth flow is usually indicative of a patent, intact duct. Sialography may be indicated.
2. **Lacerations of the duct** are primarily closed with absorbable suture (Vicryl, Monocryl or PDS) or over polyethylene tubing that remains in place for 5–7 days.

H. **EAR.**

1. **The external ear** (pinna helix, anthelix, lobule, and tragus) possesses an excellent blood supply that can maintain large areas on relatively small pedicles. Therefore, minimal débridement should be carried out. The wound should be copiously irrigated.

2. **The auricle of the ear** provides numerous landmarks that are helpful in the reapproximation of skin edges.

3. **Cartilage should not be left exposed**: it should be trimmed to the skin edges if needed.

4. **The sutures are placed through both sides of the skin**: no sutures are passed through cartilage.

5. **The cartilage may be approximated with fine chromic gut sutures** if needed for additional support and stability.

6. **A light pressure dressing** is helpful to prevent edema, seroma, and subperichondrial hematoma, which may lead to fibrosis and a 'cauliflower ear'.

7. **If a hematoma is present**, it should be aspirated using an 18-gauge needle under sterile conditions or drained promptly. A seroma may require daily drainage until the fluid collection stops.

8. **Avulsive defects** are managed by closure of the remaining skin and wound care of any exposed areas. Exposed cartilage is trimmed or covered with a skin flap.

9. **If the avulsed part of the ear is small** it may be replaced as a composite graft. Secondary reconstruction can be done with a local flap or composite graft from another donor site once the wound has healed and nonviable tissue has declared itself.

I. **ORAL MUCOSA AND TONGUE.**

1. **Mucosal lacerations** are meticulously debrided and inspected for foreign bodies, such as tooth restoration (amalgam) fragments. The lacerations are repaired with 3-0 chromic gut suture.

2. **The submandibular ducts (Wharton's ducts)** in the anterior floor of the mouth should be closely inspected for damage. Cannulation or sialography may be indicated if injury is suspected. Primary repair over a stent (5–7 days) or diversion of the proximal end is required if injury is present.

3. **Tongue lacerations** should be closed in layers utilizing 3-0 chromic catgut suture. Lingual nerve blocks are very helpful and prevent tissue distortion around wound edges.

4. **A documented neurosensory examination of the lingual nerve** (anterior two-thirds of the tongue) is imperative for any laceration of the floor of the mouth or tongue prior to the administration of local anesthetic and repair.

J. **PERIPHERAL NERVES.**

1. **Distal branches of either the trigeminal or the facial nerve** are generally not reapproximated primarily when injured. Accurate reapproximation of the tissue edges will allow regeneration.

2. **Identifiable lacerations of the trigeminal nerve** in the more proximal areas (near the mental foramen, infraorbital, foramen, or supraorbital notch) should be repaired at the time of injury utilizing microsurgical techniques.

3. **Named branches of the facial nerve** posterior to a vertical line drawn at the lateral canthus of the eye should be identified and primarily repaired within the first 2–3 days. It is generally not practical to repair injuries anterior to this line; these will most often regenerate with accurate tissue approximation (Figure 12.5).

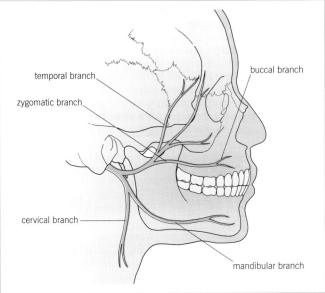

temporal branch

zygomatic branch

buccal branch

cervical branch

mandibular branch

FIG. 12.5

Distribution of facial nerve. Exact configuration can vary significantly and this illustration is only an example. (From Walker RV, Fonseca RJ. *Oral and maxillofacial trauma. Volume 1.* Philadelphia: WB Saunders; 1991:263.)

K. **ANIMAL BITES.**

1. **Primary closure** after copious irrigation and meticulous débridement is advocated in the facial region, unlike the rest of the body.

2. **An attempt is made to convert the wound from contaminated to clean.**

3. **Prophylactic antibiotics are generally indicated** to cover dog and cat flora (*Streptococcus* sp. and *Pasteurella* sp.). Penicillin or ampicillin–sulbactam usually provides good empirical coverage.

4. **Tetanus prophylaxis is indicated.**

V. FURTHER READING

Alling CC, Osborn DB. *Maxillofacial trauma.* Philadelphia: Lea and Febiger; 1988.

Borges AF. Relaxed skin tension lines. *Dermatol Clin* 1989; 7(1):169–177.

Kruger GW. *Textbook of oral and maxillofacial surgery,* 6th edn. St. Louis: Mosby; 1984.

McCarthy JG. *Volume 2, part 1: Plastic surgery.* Philadelphia: WB Saunders; 1990.

Rohrich RJ, Robinson JB. Wound healing and closure, abnormal scars, tattoos, envenomation, injuries. *Selected readings in plastic surgery.* Dallas: Univeristy of Texas Southwestern Center; 1992; 7(1).

Walker FV, Fonseca RJ. *Volume 1: Oral and maxillofacial trauma.* Philadelphia: WB Saunders; 1991.

INJURIES TO THE UPPER FACIAL SKELETON

I. FRONTAL SINUS FRACTURES

A. ANATOMY.

1. **The sinus is lined by respiratory epithelium** and communicates directly with the nose via the nasofrontal ducts.
2. **Variation in the anatomy of the nasofrontal duct is common**.
3. **Direct communication from the ductal lining to the subductal venous system** exists by way of the diploic veins of Breschet.
4. **Damage to the sinus** may predispose to pathologic sinus infection with intracranial extension.
5. Blood supply.
   a. Diploic branch of the supraorbital artery (major contribution).
   b. Anterior ethmoidal artery (minor contribution).
6. **Sensory innervation to the soft tissues of the frontal region** is supplied by the supraorbital and supratrochlear nerve (CN V).

B. CLINICAL PRESENTATION.

1. **Swelling and possible hematoma** of the glabellar region.
2. **Palpable depression** over the supraorbital region (swelling may mask this finding).
3. **Lacerations** over the glabellar region.
4. **Proptosis of the globe** downward and forward.
5. **Anesthesia and paresthesia** of the supraorbital and supratrochlear nerves.
6. **Cerebrospinal fluid (CSF) rhinorrhea.**
   a. CSF leak may occur secondary to a dural tear from fracturing the posterior table of the frontal sinus.
   b. A sample of nasal fluid that contains >30mg/dL glucose is CSF.
   c. Neurologic workup is essential.

C. RADIOGRAPHIC EVALUATION.

1. **Plain film radiographs** include facial series, anteroposterior (AP) skull, lateral skull, Waters' view, submentovertex, and Caldwell view.
2. CT scans
   a. Axial views and coronal views.
   b. Thin section (1.5–3.0mm) CT scanning is the imaging technique of choice.
3. **The presence of an intracranial pneumocele** is indicative of a dural tear, and neurosurgical consultation should be obtained.

D. MANAGEMENT.

1. Goals of treatment include
   a. Elimination of factors that predispose toward development of infection or mucocele formation.

    b. Restoration of normal sinus function, or complete obliteration if indicated.

    c. Repair of cosmetic defects.

  2. Definitive treatment may range from observation (as for nondisplaced anterior or posterior table fractures) to open reduction of displaced fractures and those involving the nasofrontal duct.

  3. Displaced fractures and those involving the nasofrontal ducts should be obliterated (Figure 13.1).

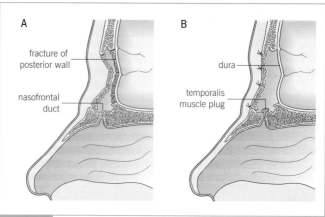

FIG. 13.1

(A) 'Cranialization' of a frontal sinus fracture with extensive comminution of the posterior wall. (B) Excision of the posterior wall plugging of the nasofrontal duct with temporalis muscle and interosseous fixation of the anterior wall. On occasion, primary bone grafting of the anterior wall may be necessary in addition. (From Luce D. Frontal Sinus Fractures: guidelines to management. *Plast Reconstr Surg* 1987; 80(4):506.)

    a. Obliteration of the sinus is achieved using any autogenous material (e.g., fat, bone, fascia, muscle).

    b. Prior to filling the sinus cavity, all of the lining mucosa is meticulously burred away in order to prevent future mucocele formation.

E. POSTOPERATIVE CARE.

  1. Postoperative antibiotics are administered as indicated.

  2. Systemic decongestants are indicated if the sinus remains patent (no surgical obliteration).

  3. Elevate head of bed 30–40° to:

    a. Decrease postoperative edema.

    b. Monitor CSF rhinorrhea if suspected.

    c. Create more dependent drainage of the sinus if nasofrontal stents are in place.

4. The patient is cautioned against nose blowing and sneezing.
5. **Irrigate nasofrontal stents** with sterile saline to decrease the incidence of infection and to maintain the patency of the stents.
G. **PEARLS AND PITFALLS.** When harvesting abdominal fat for sinus obliteration, the harvest site should not be located in the right lower quadrant. This may appear as an appendectomy scar to an unsuspecting emergency physician.

II. FRACTURES OF THE NASO-ORBITO-ETHMOID COMPLEX

A. **ANATOMY.**
1. **Bones.**
a. Nasal processes of the frontal bones.
b. Paired nasal bones.
c. Frontal processes of the maxilla.
d. Lacrimal bones.
e. Ethmoid bone.
f. Sphenoid bones.
g. Nasal septum and cartilages.
2. **Sinuses.**
a. Frontal.
b. Ethmoid.
c. Sphenoid.
3. **The medial canthal ligament**, a tendinous insertion of the orbicularis oculi, is composed of anterior and posterior attachments.
a. The anterior and posterior ligaments 'straddle' the lacrimal sac (Figure 13.2).

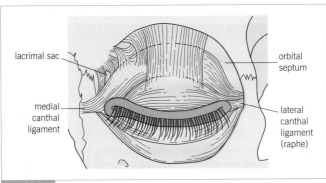

FIG. 13.2

Diagrammatic representation of attachment of the medial canthal ligament. Strong anterior head attached to the frontal process of the maxillary bone is emphasized. (From Walker RV, Fonseca RJ. *Oral and maxillofacial trauma. Volume 1*. Philadelphia: WB Saunders; 1991:399.)

13

INJURIES TO THE UPPER FACIAL SKELETON

b.   Instability of the bony insertions of these attachments results in lateral displacement of the medial corner of the eye(s) and telecanthus (Figure 13.3).

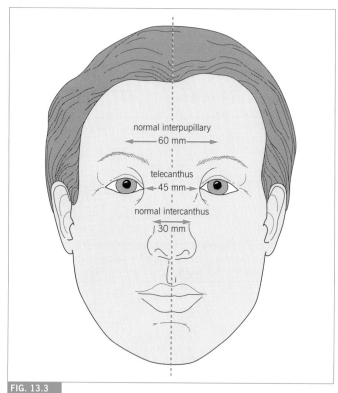

FIG. 13.3
Normal and pathologic distances of naso-orbital complex in traumatic telecanthus.
(From Holt GR. *Otolaryngol Clin North Am* 1985; 18:90.)

4.   **Blood is supplied** through the facial and maxillary branches of the external carotid artery.
5.   **Neurosensory.**
a.   Fifth and seventh cranial nerves.
b.   Close association with the first cranial nerve by way of the cribriform plate of the ethmoid places patients who suffer fractures of this region at risk for partial or complete loss of the sense of smell (anosmia).

B. CLINICAL PRESENTATION.

1. **Glabellar, periorbital, and nasal ecchymosis and edema,** and telecanthus (intercanthal distance greater than half of the interpupillary distance).

2. **Short and retruded nasal bridge.**
a. Traumatic telecanthus.
b. Enophthalmos.
c. Shortened palpebral fissure.

3. **Nasal exam.**
a. The external nasal dorsum may be flat or caved-in (saddle nose); crepitus can often be noted on palpation.
b. Epistaxis associated with septal displacement or hematoma is common. Septal hematomas require prompt drainage.
c. CSF fluid fistulae have been found in 10–30% of basilar skull fractures and CSF rhinorrhea is common after naso-orbito-ethmoid (NOE) fractures (secondary to fracture of the cribriform plate). This is often masked by initial epistaxis.
d. The 'double ring' test may be helpful (a drop of drainage is placed on a paper towel; the inner red ring is blood, the outer clear ring is CSF).

4. **Orbital exam.**
a. Telecanthus (intercanthal distance greater than half of the interpupillary distance).
   1) Average medial canthal distances are 33–34mm in men and 32–33mm in women.
   2) These distances are slightly greater in blacks.
   3) Soft tissue intercanthal distances >35mm are suggestive of a displaced NOE fracture.
   4) Soft tissue distances >40mm are typically diagnostic.
   5) The deformity can be unilateral; therefore, the distance from the nasal dorsum to each medial canthus should also be compared.
b. Lateral traction on the eyelids will often produce 'rounding' of the lax medial canthal tendon which has been detached; however, the 'eyelid traction test' misses all but the most comminuted of injuries (Figure 13.4).

5. **Ocular examination.**
a. Significant ocular injury in patients with complex facial fractures is 20–25%.
b. Ptosis of the upper eyelid may be present secondary to:
   1) Enopthalmos from medial wall collapse.
   2) Damage to the levator aponeurosis.
   3) Cranial nerve III injury.
   4) Intramuscular hematoma.
c. Epiphora (excessive tears) may be seen secondary to damage or obstruction of the nasolacrimal system. The patency of this system can be readily evaluated by placing fluorescein dye in the fornix of the eye

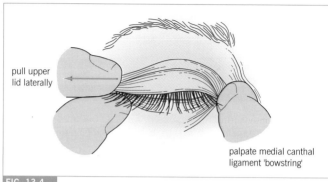

pull upper lid laterally

palpate medial canthal ligament 'bowstring'

FIG. 13.4

'Bowstring' test for medical canthal ligament integrity. Test is performed by pulling the lateral lid laterally and palpating the integrity of the medial canthal ligament. (From Foster CA, Sherman JE. *Surgery of facial bones fractures.* New York: Churchill Livingstone; 1987: 304.)

and observing for drainage on a cotton tip applicator placed below the inferior meatus.

6. **These patients should receive a complete neurologic examination** and consultation with neurosurgery as indicated.

C. RADIOGRAPHIC EVALUATION.

1. **Thin-section (1.5–3.0mm) axial and CT scan** is the imaging technique of choice for evaluation of fractures of this region.

2. Plain radiographs are rarely useful.

3. Fracture classification.

a. Type I – fractures are single-segment central fragment.

b. Type II – fractures are comminuted central-fragment fractures with fracture lines that do not extend into the area of medial canthal tendon insertion.

c. Type III – fractures exhibit bony comminution extending into the bony insertion of the medial canthal tendon. Canthal avulsion from bone may be present.

D. MANAGEMENT.

1. **Closed reduction.**

a. Intranasal and external manual manipulation.

b. Stabilization is achieved using external nasal plates (Figure 13.5).

c. Closed reduction frequently creates difficulty in establishing true anatomic relations and is generally not indicated.

2. **Open reduction** allows direct visualization of the fractured segments for alignment and stabilization. This can be achieved utilizing wire osteosynthesis or plate fixation.

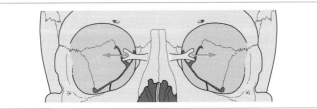

FIG. 13.5

Demonstration of technique used to repair telecanthus. (From Holt GR. Nasoethmoid complex injuries. *Otolaryngol Clin North Am* 1985; 18:90.)

3. **Primary reconstruction** of the dorsal nasal and medial orbital wall areas is indicated if severe comminution prevents stable anatomic reduction.
4. **External nasal splints and nasal packing** are often utilized after reduction to stabilize the segments further if severe comminution exists.
5. **Dacrocystorhinostomy** may be necessary if trauma to the lacrimal sac or duct exists.
6. **Treatment goals for NOE fractures include:**
   a. Anatomic reduction and stabilization of fractures.
   b. Re-establishment of normal intercanthal distance.
   c. Re-establishment of normal nasolacrimal drainage.
   d. Restoration of normal contours and cosmesis.
   e. Re-establishment of dorsal nasal height and projection.
   f. Elimination of CSF drainage.
E. **EARLY COMPLICATIONS.**
1. **CSF rhinorrhea** is usually self-limiting and ceases after 24–48 hours.
2. **Meningitis** (incidence 4–10%) – a neurologic consultation should be sought before beginning antibiotics for CSF fistulae.
3. **Postoperative proptosis of the globe** can be expected if primary grafting of the orbital wall was performed.
4. **Postoperative epiphora** should improve or cease as edema resolves.
5. **Post-traumatic telecanthus or canthal asymmetry:**
   a. Is difficult to repair secondarily.
   b. Should be treated early in the postoperative course if identified.
F. **LATE COMPLICATIONS.**
1. **Persistent CSF leakage** after fracture reduction requires additional surgical intervention.
2. **Persistent epiphora** requires re-evaluation of the nasolacrimal system for damage or obstruction.
3. **Late post-traumatic telecanthus or canthal asymmetry** may be difficult or impossible to repair adequately.
4. **Persistent nasal problems,** such as loss of dorsal support and airway obstruction, are addressed in secondary rhinoplasty procedures.

G. POSTOPERATIVE CARE.

1. **Elevate head of bed 30°** to decrease postoperative edema.
2. **Caution against nose blowing and sneezing** to prevent subcutaneous emphysema.
3. **Frequent ophthalmic examination** aids in early detection of ocular complications.
4. **CSF rhinorrhea** is common in the early postoperative phase and usually resolves with conservative management (head of bed elevated 60°, antibiotic coverage, no smoking, no nose blowing, and lumbar CSF drainage).

H. PEARLS AND PITFALLS. Facial CT scans should include the intracranial cavity.

III. NASAL TRAUMA

A. EPIDEMIOLOGY. The nose is the most frequently traumatized organ of the face and constitutes 39% of all facial fractures.

B. ANATOMY.

1. **Bones**
a. Nasal.
b. Perpendicular plate of the ethmoid.
c. Vomer.
2. **Cartilage**
a. Septum.
b. Paired upper lateral cartilage.
c. Paired lower alar cartilage.
3. **Blood supply**
a. Internal carotid artery – through the ophthalmic artery.
b. External carotid artery – through the facial and internal maxillary artery.
4. **Sensory innervation**
a. First and second division of the trigeminal nerve.
b. Primary innervation of the external nose:
   1) Infraorbital nerve.
   2) Anterior ethmoid nerve.
   3) Supratrochlear nerve.
c. Primary innervation of the internal nose:
i. Ethmoidal.
ii. Sphenoidal.
iii. Nasopalatine nerve.

C. CLINICAL PRESENTATION.

1. **Swelling and ecchymosis of external nose.**
2. **Epistaxis** – bleeding may be excessive.
3. **Pain on palpation.**
4. **Nasal deviation and deformity** with or without step deformity.

5. Septal hematoma.
6. Nasal obstruction.
7. Lacerations.
8. **Nasolacrimal damage or obstruction** presenting clinically as epiphora.

D. CLINICAL EXAMINATION.

1. **Palpation of the nasal bones** for mobility and crepitus.
2. **Direct visualization of the septum to note:**
a. Fracture.
b. Displacement.
c. Nasal obstruction.
d. Hematoma.
3. **Check for presence or absence of CSF leak.**
a. Ring test with gauze.
b. Check for glucose from nasal discharge.
4. **Measurement of intercanthal distance** – rule out possible NOE fractures.
5. **Assessment of lacerations.**

E. RADIOGRAPHIC EVALUATION.

1. **Radiologic documentation of nasal fractures** is not always necessary but it is useful to document the absence of injury to adjacent bones. Special nasal views may be obtained.
2. **CT scans** are rarely indicated for isolated nasal fractures.

F. MANAGEMENT.

1. **Epistaxis** may be controlled by:
a. Pressure.
b. Cauterization.
c. Topical vasoconstrictors.
d. Nasal packing.
e. Placement of a Foley catheter or Epistat balloons for significant nasal bleeding (described in maxillary-midface trauma section).
2. **Nasal and septal fractures.**
a. Treat promptly :
    1) Adults 7–10 days.
    2) Children 2–4 days
b. Most can be adequately managed by closed reduction:
    1) Blunt elevation of the nasal bones.
    2) Reduction of the nasal septum to the midline position.
c. Internal and external nasal support is achieved with nasal packs and splints, respectively.
d. Open reduction may be necessary if reduction of the bony fragments is not possible in a closed reduction or if significant septal displacement is present.
e. Anesthesia:
    1) Topical 4% cocaine is ideal because it provides excellent anesthesia as well as vasoconstriction.

2) Infiltration of 1–2% lidocaine with 1:100,000 epinephrine bilaterally at the infraorbital, supratrochlear, and intranasal nerves.
3) Sedation or general anesthesia may be indicated.

3. **Postoperative care.**
a. Nasal packing should be removed within 48–72 hours.
b. Nasal splints are usually maintained for 7–10 days.
c. The head of the bed should be elevated to reduce postoperative edema.
d. The nasal septum should be inspected after removal of the nasal packs to rule out postoperative septal hematoma formation.

G. PEARLS AND PITFALLS. Patients should be informed that post-traumatic nasal fractures may require revision rhinoplasty if unesthetic or poor functional healing occurs.

IV. FRACTURES OF THE ZYGOMATIC COMPLEX AND ARCH

A. ANATOMY.
1. **The zygomatic arch is a relatively thin structure** composed of the:
a. Articulating temporal process of the zygomatic bone.
b. Zygomatic process of the temporal bone.
2. **The arch commonly fractures at three sites**:
a. Zygomaticotemporal suture.
b. Temporal process of the zygoma.
c. Midportion of the arch anterior to the articular eminence.

B. CLINICAL PRESENTATION.
1. **Localized edema and ecchymosis** over the temporal and preauricular areas.
2. **Depression or 'dimple'** over the arch which may be masked by significant edema.
3. **Trismus secondary to masseter or temporalis muscle trauma** is present in up to 67% of patients with arch fractures.

C. RADIOGRAPHIC EVALUATION.
1. **Waters' and submental–vertex views** are obtained for suspected isolated zygomatic arch fractures.
2. **CT scans** rarely indicated.

D. MANAGEMENT. Isolated arch fractures can usually be treated by open reduction without internal fixation from either an extra-oral or intra-oral approach.

E. COMPLICATIONS. These may include:
a. Facial nerve injury.
b. Inadequate reduction.
c. Intraoperative oculocardiac reflex.
d. Hemorrhage.

F. POSTOPERATIVE CARE.
1. **A soft diet** is often required secondary to trismus or discomfort.
2. **A protective guard or splint over the arch** may be indicated to prevent postoperative traumatic displacement of the fracture.

V. ZYGOMATIC COMPLEX

A. ANATOMY.

1. The zygoma is the primary buttress between the midface and the cranium.
2. The zygomatic bone has four processes:
   a. Frontal.
   b. Maxillary.
   c. Temporal.
   d. Orbital.
3. These articulate with the frontal, maxillary, and zygomatic process of the temporal bone and sphenoid bones, respectively.
4. The zygomaticotemporal and zygomaticofacial branch of the second division of the trigeminal nerve pierce the zygoma to provide sensory innervation to the soft tissue of the malar region.
5. The zygomatic complex (ZMC) fracture (also referred to as tripod, zygomatic, zygomaticomaxillary, malar, or orbitozygomatic fracture) generally occurs at the:
   a. Zygomaticofrontal suture.
   b. Zygomaticosphenoid suture.
   c. Zygomatic arch.
   d. Infraorbital rim.
   e. Zygomaticomaxillary buttress.
6. Fracture displacement is usually downward and backward secondary to the vector of force and muscle pull.

B. CLINICAL PRESENTATION.

1. Periorbital edema and ecchymosis.
2. Subconjunctival and scleral hematoma.
3. Loss of cheek (malar) prominence.
4. Step defects of the bony lateral and infraorbital rim regions.
5. Intra-oral examination.
   a. Irregularity or defects at the zygomaticomaxillary buttress.
   b. Mucosal ecchymosis.
   c. Crepitus to palpation secondary to subcutaneous emphysema.
   d. Trismus secondary to masseter and temporalis trauma.
6. Ophthalmologic examination
   a. Diplopia due to disruption of normal intraocular muscle function.
   b. Dystopia (malposition of the globe) due to inferior and posterior displacement of the orbit.
   c. Inferior displacement of the lateral canthal tendon attachment resulting in downward deviation of the palpebral fissure, the so-called 'antimongoloid slant'.
   d. Restricted upward gaze – usually due to edema rather than entrapment.
   e. Periorbital fat or muscle entrapment (inferior rectus or inferior oblique muscles) as evidenced by a positive forced-duction test.

f.   Enophthalmos secondary to an increased orbital volume:
     1) Globe injuries.
     2) Traumatic mydriasis.
     3) Orbital apex syndrome.
     4) Superior orbital apex syndrome.
     5) Superior orbital fissure syndrome.
     6) Blindness.
7. **Neurologic examination**
a.   The infraorbital nerve may be damaged within the canal or at the foramen resulting in anesthesia or paresthesia of the anterior cheek, upper lip, and lateral aspect of the nose on the affected side.
b.   The anterior superior alveolar nerve may be traumatized resulting in anesthesia or paresthesias to the maxillary anterior teeth and gingiva of the anterior alveolus.
C. **RADIOGRAPHIC EVALUATION.**
1. **Axial and coronal CT** with thin sections (1.5–3mm) is the 'gold standard'.
2. **CT allows for rapid accurate assessment** of the bony orbit and adjacent structures as well as preoperative determination of the need for reconstruction of the orbital floor and walls.
3. **Other useful standard facial series studies are:**
a.   AP view.
b.   Lateral view.
c.   Waters' view.
d.   Submentovertex view.
4. **The Waters' view** is the single best plain film with which to evaluate the ZMC fracture.
D. **CLASSIFICATION.**
1. **High energy** – severely displaced, segmented, or comminuted.
2. **Middle energy** – mild to marked displacement with some comminution.
3. **Low energy** – minimal displacement.
E. **MANAGEMENT.**
1. **High-energy ZMC fractures:**
a.   Infrequently observed as an isolated injury.
b.   Usually associated with Le Fort or panfacial fractures.
c.   Frequently require extensive orbital reconstruction and rigid fixation.
2. **Middle-energy fractures** can be subdivided by CT scan into those which require orbital floor reconstruction and are treated similarly to high-energy fractures, and those that do not require orbital floor reconstruction and are treated similarly to low-energy fractures.
3. **Low-energy fracture** goals of treatment include:
a.   Restoration of normal contour and projection of the malar eminence.

b.   Restoration of the skeletal buttresses.
c.   Restoration of normal orbital contour and volume.
d.   Restoration of normal globe position and function.
e.   Decompression of the infraorbital nerve.

F.   **EARLY COMPLICATIONS.**
1.   Hemorrhage.
2.   Infection (rare).
3.   Diplopia – 42% and usually secondary to edema.
4.   Extraocular muscle entrapment.
5.   Superior orbital fissure syndrome.
6.   Orbital apex syndrome.
7.   Blindness
a.   0.5–2% usually secondary to hemorrhage and is preceded by pain, ophthalmoplegia, mydriasis, proptosis, and gradual loss of visual acuity.
b.   Irreversible damage can occur in 120 minutes.

G.   **LATE COMPLICATIONS.**
1.   Malunion and nonunion.
2.   Persistent diplopia.
3.   Persistent infraorbital nerve paresthesia – decompression may be indicated.
4.   Chronic maxillary sinusitis – may require nasal–antral window for adequate drainage.
5.   Enopthalmos – usually secondary to inadequate reduction.
6.   Ectropion and entropion.

H.   **POSTOPERATIVE CARE.**
1.   **Intra-oral topical antibiotic** (chlorohexidine) may be indicated if an intra-oral incision is used.
2.   **Systemic antibiotics** given perioperatively.
3.   **Topical ophthalmologic antibiotic ointment** on periorbital incisions.
4.   **Soft diet** may be necessary secondary to trismus and pain.
5.   **Daily ophthalmologic examination** is essential to assess changes in visual acuity.
6.   **Decongestants** may be indicated if maxillary congestion persists.
7.   **Instruct patient to avoid sleeping on the injured cheek**.

VI. FURTHER READING

Ellis E. Sequencing treatment for naso-orbito-ethmoid fractures. *J Oral Maxillofac Surg* 1993; 51:543–558.

Ellis E, Kittidumkerng W. Analysis of treatment for isolated zygomaticomaxillary complex fractures. *J Oral Maxillofac Surg* 1996; 54:386.

Fedok FG. Comprehensive management of naso-ethmoidorbital injuries. *J Oral Craniomaxillofac Surg* 1995, 1(4):36–48.

13

INJURIES TO THE UPPER FACIAL SKELETON

Ioannides CH, Freihofer HP, Friens J. Fractures of the frontal sinus: a rational for treatment. *Br J Plast Surg* 1993; 46(3):208–214.

Kruger GW. *Textbook of oral and maxillofacial surgery, 6th edn*. St. Louis: Mosby; 1984.

Manson PN, Morkowitz B, Mirvis S *et al*. Toward CT based facial fracture treatment. *Plast Reconstr Surg* 1990; 85:202–211.

Rohrich RJ, Mickel TJ. Frontal sinus obliteration: in search of the ideal autogenous material. *Plast Reconstr Surg* 1995, 95(3):580–585.

Walker RV, Fonseca RJ. *Oral and maxillofacial trauma. Volume 1.* Philadelphia: WB Saunders; 1991.

MAXILLARY, MIDFACIAL, AND MANDIBULAR INJURIES

I. MAXILLARY AND MIDFACE FRACTURES

A. **ANATOMY.** The midface begins at the supraorbital rims, extends to the mandible and is composed of nine bones (Figure 14.1):

a. Maxilla.
b. Zygomatic.
c. Lacrimal.
d. Nasal.
e. Ethmoid.
f. Sphenoid.
g. Palate.
h. Vomer.
i. Inferior turbinates.

14

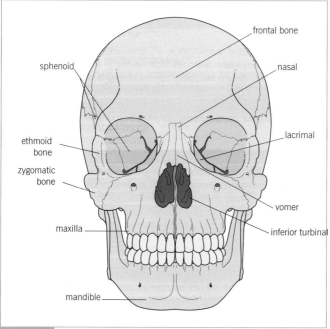

FIG. 14.1
Frontal view of skull.

2. **Three main buttresses provide support**:
a. Nasofrontal buttress.
b. Zygomatic buttress.
c. Pterygomaxillary buttress.
3. **Blood supply.**
a. Ethmoid artery – a branch of the internal carotid artery.
b. Facial artery.
c. Internal maxillary arteries – two branches from the external carotid artery.
4. **Innervation.**
a. Sensory – three branches of the second (maxillary) division of the trigeminal nerve (CN V):
   1) Pterygopalatine.
   2) Infraorbital.
   3) Zygomatic.
b. Motor – muscles of facial expression supplied by the facial nerve (CN VII).
B. EPIDEMIOLOGY.
1. **Motor vehicle collisions** are responsible for 50–70% of all maxillofacial fractures.
2. **Other causes** are sports-related accidents and gunshot injuries.
C. CLASSIFICATION OF MAXILLARY AND MIDFACE FRACTURES.
1. **Dento-alveolar fractures** (bony alveolus with teeth) account for 15% of all maxillary fractures.
2. **Le Fort I.**
a. The fracture line extends above the teeth, along the lateral maxilla from the anterior piriform rim posteriorly through the anterior and lateral wall of the maxillary sinus behind the maxillary tuberosity to the pterygomaxillary fissure or space (Figure 14.2).
b. Intranasally, the fracture extends through the vomer and usually disarticulates the cartilaginous septum from the maxilla.
3. **Le Fort II.**
a. The fracture extends from the nasofrontal suture line across the lacrimal bones and the anterior orbits through the infraorbital rim in the area of the zygomaticomaxillary suture (Figure 14.3).
b. The fracture line passes inferior to the zygoma and continues the path similar to a Le Fort I fracture in the posterior maxilla.
c. Intranasally, it passes through the superior cartilaginous septum and perpendicular plate of the ethmoid and across the middle of the vomer.
4. **Le Fort III.**
a. Occurs as a result of force delivered at the orbital level causing craniofacial disjunction.
b. Total disjunction of the midface from the cranial base occurs by a fracture at the nasofrontal and frontomaxillary sutures extending

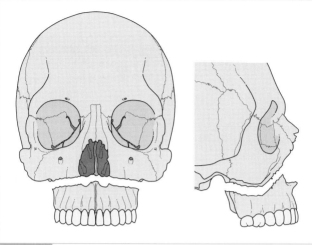

FIG. 14.2
Le Fort I fracture. (From Walker RV, Fonseca RJ. *Oral and maxillofacial trauma*, *Volume 1.* Philadelphia: WB Saunders; 1991.)

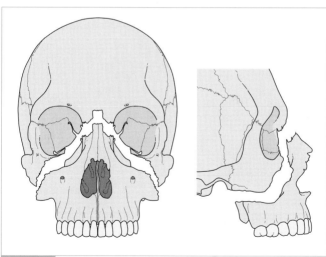

FIG. 14.3
Le fort II fracture. (From Walker RV, Fonseca RJ. *Oral and maxillofacial trauma*, *Volume 1.* Philadelphia: WB Saunders; 1991.)

posteriorly along the medial orbital wall through the lacrimals and ethmoids along the inferior orbital fissure laterally and through the lateral orbital rim (Figure 14.4).

c. The fracture passes through the pterygoids at a high level.

d. Intranasally, the fracture extends posteriorly along the ethmoid at the base of the cribriform plate, usually causing comminution, and through the sphenovomerine suture.

Isolated Le Fort I, II, and III level fractures are the exception rather than the rule. Multiple lines of fractures are the rule.

D. CLINICAL PRESENTATION.

1. Le Fort I fracture.

a. Facial edema and swelling.

b. Lacerations.

c. Epistaxis, common secondary to the fracture of the maxillary sinus walls, and tearing of the nasal mucosa (an understanding of the vascular supply to this region is essential for hemostasis).

d. Tenderness to palpation over the piriform rims and nasofrontal and zygomatic buttresses.

e. Subcutaneous emphysema and crepitance.

f. Fractured or avulsed teeth.

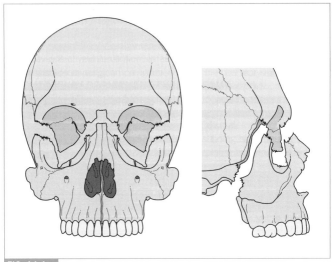

FIG. 14.4

Le fort III fracture. (From Walker RV, Fonseca RJ. *Oral and maxillofacial trauma*, *Volume 1.* Philadelphia: WB Saunders; 1991.)

g.   Malocclusion (anterior open bite secondary to posterior and inferior displacement of the maxilla related to the pull of the pterygoids) and palpable 'step-off' defects.

h.   Ecchymosis and palatal tear or laceration suggestive of a midline palatal fracture.

i.   Increased gross mobility of maxilla in the anteroposterior (AP), transverse, or vertical directions.

j.   Mucosal tears.

k.   Septal deviation or septal hematoma, which requires prompt incision and drainage.

2.   Le Fort II and III fractures.

a.   Similar to Le Fort I but with the addition of periorbital ecchymosis and edema.

b.   Palpable 'step-off' deformity or crepitus at nasofrontal region (II and III).

c.   Infraorbital defects and crepitus (II), and lateral orbital rim 'step-off' deformities.

d.   Crepitus (III).

e.   Subcutaneous emphysema.

f.   Intra-oral crepitus in zygomatic buttress area (II).

g.   Anterior open bite malocclusion (II and III).

h.   Traumatic telecanthus >45mm (normal intercanthal distance 30–35mm).

i.   Increased gross mobility of fractures in the AP, transverse, or vertical planes (attempt mobilization of the anterior maxilla with one hand, while palpating nasofrontal, infraorbital, then lateral orbital regions with the other hand).

j.   Nasal examination similar to that for Le Fort I level.

E.   **RADIOGRAPHIC EVALUATION.** CT scans with thin sections (1.5–3.0 mm) is the radiologic method of choice for all midface fractures and should include:

1.   Axial views to include the palate and extend superiorly to the level of the anterior cranial fossa.

2.   Coronal views to assess the orbital extent of injuries adequately.

3.   **Plain radiographs** – Waters' view if fractures are present.

F.   **ASSOCIATED INJURIES.** Up to 50% of adult and 70% of pediatric patients with maxillofacial injuries will show associated injuries of the cranium, cervical spine, orbit, chest, or abdomen.

1.   Craniofacial injuries include:

a.   Orbital (most commonly with Le Fort II and III).

b.   Superior orbital fissure syndrome – ophthalmoplegia, fixed and dilated pupil, increased consensual response in uninvolved eye, ptosis, and loss of corneal reflex.

  c. Orbital apex syndrome – superior orbital fissure syndrome with blindness.

2. Intracranial.

  a. Close observation for cerebrospinal fluid, otorrhea, and rhinorrhea.

  b. Close observation for skull defects and postauricular ecchymosis (Battle's sign).

G. MANAGEMENT.

1. Airway.

  a. Initial treatment is directed toward establishing a patent airway and removal of items that could potentially be aspirated, such as teeth, loose crowns and bridges, and dentures.

  b. Often simple débridement and placement of an oral or nasal airway is sufficient.

  c. Nasal trumpets are especially useful because they provide a patent nasal airway and can act as a tamponade for severe epistaxis.

2. Hemorrhage.

  a. Facial and scalp lacerations can usually be easily controlled with direct pressure bandages.

  b. Definitive control requires prompt débridement, ligation, and primary closure.

  c. Severe epistaxis can be controlled by:

    1) Bilateral nasal trumpet placement,.

    2) Balloon catheter tamponade.

    3) Nasal packing (Figure 14.5).

    4) Topical agents, such as Afrin (oxymetazoline) nasal spray.

    5) Fracture reduction.

    6) Selective embolization.

    7) Ligation of the external carotid system proximal to the site of hemorrhage.

3. Operative management.

  a. The primary goal is to restore form (normal facial height, width, and projection) and function (re-establish skeletal buttresses and preoperative occlusion).

  b. If the mandible is intact, returning the maxillary teeth to their pretraumatic occlusion is the key to reducing maxillary midfacial fractures.

  c. If significant delays in treatment are expected, simple maxillomandibular fixation (MMF) should be considered as an interim treatment in order to avoid scar contracture over a malformed facial skeleton.

  d. The indications for tooth extraction are the same as those used for mandibular fractures (Section II). Early open reduction with rigid internal fixation utilizing sophisticated plate and screw techniques is currently the treatment of choice for displaced maxillary midfacial

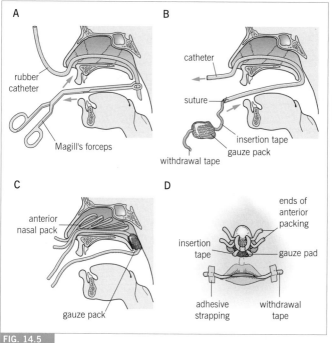

FIG. 14.5

Placement of posterior nasal pack. (From Rowe NL, Williams JL. *Maxillofacial injuries*. New York: Churchill Livingstone; 1986.)

fractures, although Le Fort I fractures can often be definitively treated with MMF.

e. Pediatric maxillary midfacial fractures are managed as conservatively as possible.

4. Postoperative care.

a. Airway patency is the primary postoperative concern.

b. Following extensive facial reconstructive surgery, the oropharyngeal and nasopharyngeal soft tissues are often sufficiently edematous to require prolonged postoperative intubation (3–5 days).

c. If intubation is to be anticipated to exceed 10–14 days, tracheostomy should be considered.

d. Nasogastric suction (placed under direct visualization in the operating room) should be maintained until the patient is awake and alert and clinical evidence of gastrointestinal function has returned. Routine nasal vasoconstriction and topical steroids will assist in maintaining a patent nasal airway.

e. Elevate the head of the bed at least 30° to decrease postoperative edema.

f. Perioperative systemic antibiotics should be given as indicated. A topical antibiotic rinse (chlorohexidine) is considered for all patients with MMF at Parkland Memorial Hospital.

II. MANDIBULAR TRAUMA

The mandible is involved in 10–25% of all facial fractures.

A. ANATOMY.

1. Bone structure.

a. The mandible is U-shaped with a horizontal bone component (body) and two vertical components (ramus) with an articulation to the skull base that will allow rotational and translational movements.

b. The mandible contains 16 teeth: six molars, four premolars, two canines, and four incisors (Figure 14.6).

c. The mandible is thinnest at the angle with a relatively high incidence of fracture in this region.

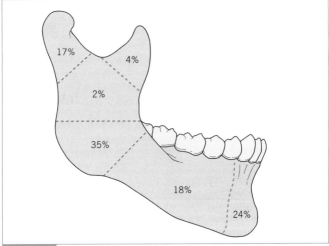

FIG. 14.6

Location of mandibular fractures seen at Parkland Memorial Hospital, Dallas, 1989. (From Sinn DP. Mandible fractures and midfacial trauma: diagnosis and management. In: Sinn DP, ed. *Selected readings in oral, maxillofacial surgery.* Dallas: Johnson Printing; 1990.)

2. **Blood supply.**
a. Inferior alveolar artery.
b. Muscular attachments.
3. **Innervation.**
a. The third division of the trigeminal nerve (CN V) provides sensory innervation to the mandibular complex.
b. The inferior alveolar nerve enters the mandibular ramus medially, where it courses within the mandibular canal to exit at the mental foramen.
B. **EPIDEMIOLOGY.** Statistics taken from Parkland Memorial Hospital, 1994.
1. **Mechanism.**
a. Aggravated assault 88%.
b. Motor vehicle accidents 8%.
c. Gunshot wounds 2%.
d. Sports or other injuries 2%.
2. **Location** (see Figure 14.6).
a. Angle 35%.
b. Symphysis 24%.
c. Body 18%.
d. Condyle 17%.
e. Coronoid 4%.
f. Ramus 2%.
3. **Classification.**
a. Mandibular symphysis: fractures occurring between the mental foramina.
b. Mandibular body: mental foramina to the area anterior to the third molar.
c. Mandibular angle: from third molar to the gonial angle.
d. Mandibular ramus: above the gonial angle, extending to the sigmoid notch.
e. Mandibular condyle: area superior to the ramus including the condylar process.
f. Mandibular coronoid: area superior to the ramus including the coronoid process.
g. Dento-alveolar: bony mandibular ridge (alveolar process) with teeth.
C. **CLINICAL PRESENTATION.**
1. **Localized mandibular pain and facial swelling.**
2. **Malocclusion.**
3. **Trismus.**
4. **Ecchymosis** of the vestibule or floor of mouth tissues.
5. **Mucosal or gingival lacerations.**
6. **Gross malalignment of segments.**
7. **Loose or fractured teeth.**

14

MAXILLARY, MIDFACIAL, AND MANDIBULAR INJURIES

8. Gross mobility of fractured segments
9. **Deviation of the chin** associated with displaced condylar fractures (Figure 14.7).

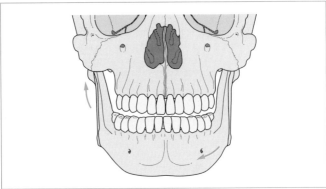

FIG. 14.7

Unilateral fracture of neck and condyle. (From Massler M, Schour I. *Atlas of the mouth,* 2nd edn. American Dental Association.)

10. **Anterior open bite** may occur with bilateral condyle fractures.
11. **Neurosensory deficits** secondary to fracture through the region of the mandible where communication of the inferior alveolar neurovascular bundle courses through the mandible.
D. RADIOGRAPHIC EVALUATION. The mandibular series includes:
1. Posterior–anterior skull.
2. Lateral skull.
3. Right and left lateral obliques.
4. Towne projections.
5. Submental vertex (SMV).
a. A panoramic radiograph is invaluable for diagnosis, evaluation, and treatment planning of mandibular fractures. This view allows visualization of virtually all fractures of the mandible and their relationship to the teeth.
b. CT scans are infrequently indicated for the evaluation of mandibular fractures.
E. MANAGEMENT.
1. Initial goals.
a. Secure airway and prevent aspiration.
b. Assess hemodynamic stability.
c. Evaluation of the cervical spine and possible closed head injuries.

d. Definitive treatment is often delayed secondary to associated life-threatening injuries.
e. Definitive treatment can be deferred by temporary immobilization.
   1) This can be accomplished through head wraps (Barton's bandage) or intra-oral stabilization wires placed on teeth adjacent to the fracture (bridle wire).
   2) Temporary immobilization will provide patient comfort, decrease risk of infection, and minimize additional damage to associated structures such as the inferior alveolar neurovascular bundle.

2. Definitive treatment goals.
a. Reduction and immobilization of the fracture (either open or closed).
b. Adequate duration of immobilization to allow osseous healing.
c. Prevention of infection.
d. Re-establishment of proper occlusion.
e. Restoration of contour and function.
f. Generally, teeth in the line of fractures are extracted if grossly mobile.
g. Minimally mobile and nonrestorable teeth may be retained if they play a key role in reduction of the fracture.

3. Indications for nonoperative management.
a. Nondisplaced and nonmobile fracture.
b. Normal occlusion.
c. Minimal patient discomfort.

4. Indications for closed reduction of mandibular fractures with arch bars, wires, and elastic bands – MMF:
a. Nondisplaced or minimally displaced fractures.
b. Reproducible occlusion.

5. Postoperative care.
a. Primary concern is the maintenance of a patent airway. If significant postoperative edema is present in the floor of the mouth or pharynx, prolonged endotracheal intubation may be necessary if the patient is in MMF.
b. Analgesics.
c. Wired-jaw diet with nutritional support for 4–6 weeks (arch bars and MMF).
d. Aggressive postoperative physiotherapy (jaw exercises) is essential to successful rehabilitation, whether open or closed reduction is utilized or whether the patient is an adult or child.
e. Oral hygiene is essential to reduce the risk of postoperative infection.
f. Nutritional assessment should be made to address diet concerns for adequate caloric intake.
   1) If MMF is used, patients will need to be maintained on full liquid diets.
   2) For the patient treated by open reduction and internal fixation (ORIF), soft mechanical diets are recommended.

MAXILLARY, MIDFACIAL, AND MANDIBULAR INJURIES   14

F. PEDIATRIC MANDIBLE FRACTURES.
1. **Mandible fractures in children** are best treated by closed reduction.
2. **In children aged 2–6 years**, sufficient primary dentition is usually present to facilitate arch bars and MMF with wires or elastics.
3. **Children aged 9–12 years** enter the stage of mixed dentition. There may be insufficient numbers of stable teeth present to facilitate placement of arch bars. Therefore, skeletal fixation or fixation with the aid of plastic splints, may be required.
4. **Rapid healing in children** means that immobilization of pediatric mandibular fractures is usually limited to 1–2 weeks (Figure 14.8).
5. **Open reduction** of pediatric mandibular fractures is infrequently indicated.

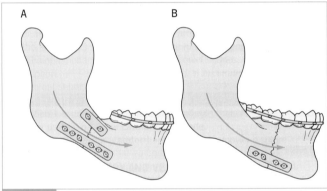

FIG. 14.8
(A) Stabilization plate in conjunction with tension band plate at superior border.
(B) Stabilization plate at inferior border with arch bar acting as a tension band. (From Sinn DP. Mandible fractures and midfacial trauma: diagnosis and management. In: Sinn DP, ed. *Selected readings in oral, maxillofacial surgery*. Dallas: Johnson Printing; 1990.)

III. PEARLS AND PITFALLS
1. **Sagittal or 'hemi-Le Fort' fractures** are not uncommon.
2. **The patient with nasal trumpets or a nasoendotracheal tube** who develops a fever should receive a prompt sinus evaluation if no other source of fever can be found. Maxillary sinus aspiration may be indicated as a diagnostic aid.
3. **Airway obstruction** can occur with bilateral mandibular body fractures secondary to posterior and inferior displacement of the tongue and floor of mouth structures.

4. **Preoperative documentation of neurosensory deficits** is imperative in patients with facial fractures to determine if postoperative deficits are truly a result of operative manipulation.
5. **Definitive treatment of mandible fractures may be postponed** for as long as 2 weeks with systemic or topical antibiotic coverage in the presence of life-threatening injuries.

IV. FURTHER READING

Alling CC, Osborn DB. *Maxillofacial trauma*. Philadelphia: Lea and Febiger; 1988.

Calloway DM, Anton MA, Jacobs JS. Changing concepts and controversies in the management of mandibular fractures. In: *Clinics in plastic surgery, Volume 19*. Philadelphia: WB Saunders; 1992.

Ellis E. Treatment of mandibular angle fractures using the AO reconstruction plate. *J Oral Maxillofac Surg* 1993; 51:250.

Ellis E, Dean JS. Rigid fixation of mandibular condyle fractures. *Oral Surg Oral Med Oral Pathol* 1993; 76:6–15.

Kruger GW. *Textbook of oral and maxillofacial surgery,* 6th edn. St. Louis: Mosby; 1984.

Sinn DP. Mandible fractures and midfacial trauma: diagnosis and management. In: Sinn DP, ed. *Selected readings in oral, maxillofacial surgery*. Dallas: Johnson Printing; 1990.

Walker RV, Fonseca RJ. *Oral and maxillofacial trauma, Volume 1.* 2nd edn. Philadelphia: Harcourt Brace & Co.

14

MAXILLARY, MIDFACIAL, AND MANDIBULAR INJURIES

OPHTHALMIC INJURIES

I. OVERVIEW
1. **Ocular trauma** is often associated with intracranial injuries.
2. **The examiner** should be familiar with the anatomy of the eye (Figure 15.1) and use of a slit lamp.
3. **An ophthalmologic consultation** must be obtained when the diagnosis or management is in question.

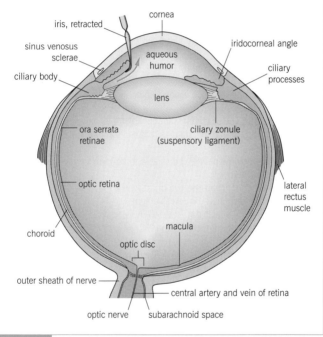

FIG. 15.1
Horizontal section of eyeball. Observe its three coats: external or fibrous coat (sclera and cornea), middle or vascular coat (choroid, ciliary body, and iris), and internal or retinal layer. The four refractive media are the cornea, aqueous humor, lens, and vitreous body. Arrow indicates flow of aqueous humor from the posterior chamber to the anterior chamber. Aqueous humor is a thin, watery medium formed in the posterior chamber by the ciliary process. (From Moore K. *Clinically oriented anatomy*, 3rd edn. Baltimore: William and Wilkins; 1992)

II. EXAMINATION

1. **Examination of the patient with multiple injuries** performed at the bedside is quite different from that of the medically stable patient who should be examined with the slit lamp.
2. **The functional state of the eye** must be determined prior to a detailed anatomical exam.
3. **The use of mydriatic agents** should be postponed until the patient is neurologically stable.
4. **Topical anesthetics** may be utilized to facilitate the exam. However, under no circumstance should the patient be allowed to use the medication for pain control, since repeated usage will lead to corneal decompensation.

A. VISUAL ACUITY.

1. **Always check visual acuity first** (with the exception of a chemical burn).
2. **Assess each eye individually**.
3. **Assess with a Snellen chart**.
4. **When evaluating distance vision**, a pinhole occluder is able to eliminate refractive error from patients who do not have their glasses.
5. **A near card is useful** when examining at the bedside.
6. **Document appropriately**, such as 'patient can read small print at 14 inches (35cm)'.
7. **The elderly presbyope** may be unable to perform a near-vision test without corrective lenses.
8. **If patients cannot read the eye chart**, see if they can count fingers, recognize hand motion, or perceive light.

B. VISUAL FIELDS. Each eye is tested individually as the patient is instructed to fixate on the examiner's nose as follows:

1. **To test the patient's right eye**, the left eye should be occluded.
2. **The examiner opens his or her left eye** while closing the right eye.
3. **Fingers are flashed in each quadrant** at a point halfway between the patient and the examiner.
4. **Visual field defects commonly seen in trauma patients include**:
a. Retinal detachment.
b. Vitreous hemorrhage.
c. Cerebral injuries.

C. EXTRAOCULAR MOVEMENTS.

1. **The six positions of cardinal gaze** need to be carefully evaluated.
2. **The oculomotor nerve** (CN III) innervates the superior rectus (SR), medial rectus (MR), inferior rectus (IR), inferior oblique (IO), and the levator muscle.
3. **The trochlear nerve** (CN IV) innervates the superior oblique (SO).
4. **The lateral rectus** (LR) is innervated by the abducens nerve (CN VII).

5. **Findings suggestive of injury:**
a. Double vision.
b. Pain when gaze is directed away from the trapped muscle.
c. Entrapment limiting mobility.

D. **PUPILS.**

1. **Pupillary reaction:** brisk, sluggish, or absent?
2. **Shape.** Is the pupil round or irregular?
3. **Determine if an afferent pupillary defect** (APD or Marcus Gunn pupil) is present.
a. This is accomplished by shining the light in one eye then quickly shining the light in the opposite eye. Repeat this as many times as it takes to obtain a consistent response.
b. In the normal patient, the direct response should cause the initial pupil to constrict; the response in the opposite eye will be to constrict.
c. When the light is quickly moved to the opposite eye, the pupil should remain constricted if light is being perceived equally in both eyes.
d. In the trauma patient with an APD, one would expect to see a sluggish reaction in the affected eye, a brisk reaction in a normal eye.
e. When light is moved from the sluggish pupil to the normal eye, constriction will occur, indicating presence of an APD.
4. **Causes of APD include:**
a. Traumatic optic neuropathy.
b. Retinal detachment.
c. Vitreous hemorrhage.
d. Retrobulbar hemorrhage.
e. Traumatic iritis.
f. Incarceration of iris in wound.

E. **ORBITAL RIM.**

1. **Examination.**
a. Feel for step-off deformity.
b. Evaluate for dystopia.
c. Determine if hypesthesia is present in VI, V2, and V3.
2. **Management.**
a. CT scan (see Section III, Imaging).
b. Blowout fractures can be associated with numerous injuries including extraocular muscle (EOM), entrapment, hyphema, ruptured globe, and traumatic optic neuropathy.
c. When superior roof fracture exists, combined operative repair with a neurosurgeon is necessary.
d. Surgical repair is often performed 2 weeks after injury when soft tissue swelling is minimized.
e. A medial wall blowout fracture may not require surgery unless entrapment or other complications exist.

15

OPHTHALMIC INJURIES

F. **EYELID.**

1. **Examination.**

a. Inability to open lid may indicate a CN III palsy or more commonly levator dehiscence (Figure 15.2).

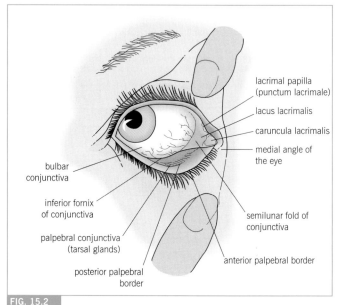

Right lower eyelid and medial angle. (From Clemente CD. *Anatomy: a regional atlas of the human body,* 3rd edn. Philadelphia: Lea & Febiger/Munich: Urban and Schwarzenberg; 1967.)

b. Inability to close the lid may indicate facial nerve involvement.
c. Identify foreign bodies and lacerations.
d. Examine under eyelids until cul-de-sacs are visualized, using a bent paper clip to evert the lid.
e. Avoid pressure on the globe.

2. **Management.**

a. Remove all foreign bodies and irrigate the cul-de-sacs with saline.
b. Lacerations involving the lacrimal sac should be repaired in the operating room.
c. Uncomplicated lacerations may be repaired with 6-0 nylon.
d. Care should be taken to prevent sutures from having contact with the cornea.

e. The tarsal plate must be appropriately realigned to prevent lid notching.

f. Excess tension can create an entropion, or an ectropion, or may induce lagophthalmos.

g. If fat is visualized at a laceration site, the orbital septum has been violated and closure of these wounds in the emergency room is ill-advised. Consultation with an ophthalmologist is essential since a large percentage of these patients will develop ptosis.

G. CONJUNCTIVA AND SCLERA.

1. Examination.

a. Evaluate for subconjunctival hemorrhage, injection, laceration, abrasion, foreign body.

b. Fluorescein. Wet a fluorescein strip, apply liberally, and place on conjunctival surface. A Wood's lamp or slit lamp will clearly show areas devoid of corneal epithelium. The entire surface of the globe should be evaluated. If aqueous humor is seen percolating through the fluorescein a ruptured globe exists (see Section IV Ruptured Globe).

2. Management.

a. Subconjunctival hemorrhage, which can exist without additional pathology, will resolve in approximately 2 weeks. If it is present and extends posteriorly, or is present in 360°, a retrobulbar hemorrhage must be ruled out (see Section IV, Retrobulbar Hemorrhage).

b. An injected eye may indicate venous congestion secondary to an obstructive phenomenon.

c. Conjunctival lacerations need to be evaluated with the slit lamp, if possible, to rule out scleral involvement. Small lacerations are frequently left unrepaired although antibiotic coverage is necessary.

H. CORNEA.

1. Examination.

a. Evaluate for clarity, foreign body, laceration, or abrasion.

b. Clarity. A cloudy cornea is usually the result of acute stromal edema often seen with elevated intraocular pressure.

c. Fluorescein (see Section II, Conjunctiva and Sclera).

2. Management.

a. A superficial foreign body imbedded in the cornea can be removed with a cotton tip applicator, a foreign body spud (a blunt needle), or a 25-gauge needle after instillation of topical anesthetic.

b. Bacitracin ointment (or other nonsteroidal ointments) can be applied 4 times a day.

c. Pressure patching is best avoided when abrasion is at high risk of infection.

d. Cycloplegic drops (cyclopentolate 2%) can be applied. The patient should be seen the next day by an ophthalmologist.

e. Laceration (see Section IV, Ruptured Globe).

I. **ANTERIOR CHAMBER.**
1. **Examination.**
a. Evaluate for hyphema, cell and flare, and depth. A flat anterior chamber is often seen with a ruptured globe.
b. The anterior chamber is difficult to evaluate without the use of the slit lamp.
2. **Management.**
a. If layered blood (hyphema) is present in the anterior chamber (AC) an ophthalmologist should be contacted regarding management. This would often include:
    1) Bed rest.
    2) Atropine.
    3) Topical steroids.
    4) Medications to control intra-ocular pressure.
b. Surgery may be necessary if the hyphema is large, slow to resolve, or if it creates corneal endothelial staining.
c. All dark-skinned patients should have a sickle cell prep performed.

J. **IRIS.**
1. **Examination.**
a. Traumatic iritis will show evidence of cells in the AC.
b. The patient will usually be extremely photophobic.
c. Irregularity may be present with a penetrating injury (see Section II, Pupil).
2. **Management.**
a. If there is no evidence of additional pathology the patient may be started on cyclopentolate 2% 4 times a day.
b. Consult an ophthalmologist prior to initiating topical steroids.

K. **LENS.**
1. **Disruption of lens material** will often produce a traumatic cataract.
2. **Occasionally the lens can dislocate.**
3. **Patients with trauma involving the lens** are at higher risk of endophthalmitis.

L. **VITREOUS AND RETINA.**
1. **Examination.**
a. The dilated exam must be deferred until the patient is neurologically stable.
b. When a vitreous hemorrhage is present the red reflex may appear darkened.
c. In patients with suspected traumatic optic neuropathy, it is imperative to examine the fundus to exclude a vitreous hemorrhage which can produce an APD and a decrease in visual acuity.
d. Most retinal detachments will not be visible by direct (and undilated) ophthalmoscopy although they can certainly cause an APD.
e. The patient who complains of recent onset of floaters and flashes of light is at risk of a retinal detachment.

f. Some patients will report a black spot in the affected region.
g. 'Tobacco dust' (pigment seen floating in the posterior chamber) can be seen with a retinal detachment.

2. Management.

a. Patients with a vitreous hemorrhage will often need constant bed rest with the head of the bed elevated to 30°.
b. Activity must be limited (no bending over, no heavy lifting) and close follow-up with ophthalmology is necessary.
c. Ultrasonography may need to be performed to determine if a coexisting retinal detachment is present.
d. If a retinal detachment is present it may or may not require immediate surgery.
e. Factors include location of the detachment, vision, and duration of detachment. Immediate consultation with an ophthalmologist is mandatory.

III. IMAGING

A. CT SCAN. This is the study of choice for patients with ocular trauma.

1. Coronal and axial views (1.5mm sections) should be obtained on all patients with ocular trauma.
2. Thin 1.5mm sections will facilitate identification of foreign bodies which may be missed on a standard head CT with 5mm sections.

B. EVALUATION.

1. Foreign bodies.
2. Orbital wall fracture.
3. Tenting of the optic nerve.
4. Retrobulbar hemorrhage.
5. Penetration of cornea, lens, or sclera.

IV. RECOGNITION OF VISION-THREATENING EMERGENCIES

The following instances require immediate recognition and intervention, including an urgent consultation with an ophthalmologist.

A. CHEMICAL BURN.

1. Perform irrigation immediately.
2. Apply anesthetic drops.
3. Irrigation with saline should be instituted and performed for at least 30 minutes.
4. Application of a lid speculum will allow effective cul-de-sac irrigation.
5. The pH should be checked, preferably 3–5 minutes after irrigation is complete. Irrigation should be reinstituted if pH is not between 7.3 and 7.6.
6. Alkali burns are much more serious than acid burns since they can directly penetrate the sclera and may require take longer to neutralize.
7. Once the pH is neutral, fluorescein should be instilled in the eye to evaluate if there are epithelial defects present. Cycloplegic drops

(scopolamine 0.25%), antibiotic ointment, and an eye patch should be applied.

B. TRAUMATIC OPTIC NEUROPATHY.

1. Evaluation.

a. In patients with orbital blowout fractures, traumatic optic neuropathy must excluded.

b. The swinging flashlight test is essential in determining the presence of an APD.

c. A decrease in visual acuity and poor color vision are other associated findings.

2. Management.

a. Use of high-dose steroids for traumatic optic neuropathy is controversial.

b. In many trauma cases with dirty wounds and open fractures high-dose steroids are relatively contraindicated.

c. These cases should be handled on an individual basis with ophthalmologic consultation.

C. RUPTURED GLOBE.

1. Corneal and scleral lacerations are often visualized with the penlight exam.

2. If an obvious laceration exists, the examination is terminated; the wound is covered with sterile gauze pending repair in the operating room.

3. Additional findings on slit-lamp exam include:

a. Subconjunctival hemorrhage.

b. Flat anterior chamber.

c. Hyphema.

d. Iris protrusion through cornea.

e. Irregular pupil.

4. Blunt injuries may produce lacerations which can occur under or adjacent to the rectus muscles.

5. Liberal application of fluorescein will aid in the diagnosis.

6. Fluorescein should be applied over the suspicious area. If a subtle laceration exists aqueous humor can be seen percolating through the fluorescein dye.

7. If an impaled object is present, do not remove.

D. RETROBULBAR HEMORRHAGE.

1. Two signs should always alert the examiner to the possibility of a retrobulbar hemorrhage.

a. Proptosis.

b. Subconjunctival hemorrhage.

2. Proptosis which shows resistance to retropulsion (retropulsion should not be attempted until a ruptured globe has been conclusively ruled out) may be associated with retrobulbar hemorrhage.

3. Other signs include increased intraocular pressure and venous congestion.

a. In some cases the pressure can become so high it can occlude the central retinal artery.

b. If the fundoscopic exam shows a pulsating arterial flow, a central retinal artery occlusion (CRAO) may be imminent.

c. A lateral canthotomy with cantholysis may be required to alleviate the pressure.

E. OTHER EMERGENT OPHTHALMOLOGIC CONDITIONS.

1. **Uncal herniation and aneurysm** – may see pupil involved and CN III palsy.

2. **Carotid–cavernous fistula** – congested eye with an ocular bruit.

3. **Cavemous sinus pathology** – EOM abnormalities with associated CN V involvement.

V. PEARLS AND PITFALLS

1. **Isolated cranial nerve injuries** can occur with closed-head trauma.

2. **When an oculomotor nerve palsy is present** with a pupil abnormality, an aneurysm or uncal herniation must be considered.

3. **Pathology involving the cavernous sinus** should be considered, particularly if there is trigeminal nerve involvement.

4. **When EOM abnormalities exist,** in the presence of dilated conjunctival vessels, the eye should be auscultated to see if a bruit exists – which may be heard when an arteriovenous fistula is present.

5. **An APD in a trauma patient** can be difficult to identify in a patient with swollen lids. Unless an equal amount of light can be presented in each eye, an accurate determination of an APD cannot be made. Lids can be manually separated. It is imperative to avoid putting pressure on the globe and this is best done using a lid speculum.

VI. FURTHER READING

American Academy of Ophthalmology Vol. I-XII, San Francisco. 1994.

Spoor TC, Hartel WC, Lensink DB et al. Treatment of traumatic optic neuropathy with corticosteroids. Am J Ophthalmol 1990; 110(6):665–669.

Steinsapir KD, Goldberg RA. Traumatic optic neuropathy. Surv Ophthalmol 1994; 38:487–518.

OPHTHALMIC INJURIES

15

NECK INJURIES

I. INTRODUCTION

A. **THE MECHANISM OF INJURY AND ANATOMIC LOCATION** frequently dictates the priorities in the evaluation and treatment of neck injuries.

1. **Penetrating injuries** constitute the vast majority and are more likely to injure the soft tissue, vascular, and aerodigestive organs, whereas blunt trauma has a greater predilection for musculoskeletal and neurological injuries.

2. **Neurologic and vascular injuries** incur the greatest morbidity and mortality.

B. **THE CERVICAL FASCIA** is of clinical and diagnostic importance.

1. **The deep layer of the superficial fascia contains the platysma muscle**, which completely encircles the neck.

2. **This structure is quite superficial** and its penetration indicates a significant possibility of injury to deeper structures, thus requiring the physician to determine the need for further diagnostic studies or surgical exploration.

II. INITIAL ASSESSMENT

A. **LIFE-THREATENING AIRWAY OBSTRUCTION OR EXSANGUINATING HEMORRHAGE** is addressed emergently.

B. **UPON COMPLETION OF THE PRIMARY SURVEY**, the stable patient is assessed for evidence of neck injury in the secondary survey.

C. **SIGNS AND SYMPTOMS**

1. Expanding hematoma.
2. Pulsatile bleeding.
3. Airway obstruction.
4. Sucking or bubbling neck wounds.
5. Instability of the laryngeal cartilage.
6. Thrills suggesting arteriovenous fistula.
7. Crepitus in patients with aerodigestive tract injury.
8. Bruits.

D. **LOW-VELOCITY PENETRATING INJURIES.** In patients with low-velocity penetrating injuries, such as stab wounds or shotgun wounds, determination of platysma muscle penetration is a crucial part of the initial evaluation.

1. **Penetrating injuries** which violate the platysma have a high incidence of involvement of deeper structures.

2. **These patients require further evaluation or therapy** while superficial wounds may be managed in an ambulatory setting.

3. **Platysma muscle penetration** is determined by local exploration of the

wound in the emergency department.

a. After sterile preparati`on of the wound, the practice at Parkland Memorial Hospital involves infiltration of the wound edges with 1% lidocaine and extension of the injury by 2–3cm.

b. A small rake retractor or self-retaining retractor is placed in the wound which will allow good visualization of the extent and depth.

c. We do not recommend probing the wound as this might dislodge clots and aggravate further bleeding in the emergency department.

E. FOREIGN BODIES which are lodged in the area are left in place and removed in the operating room where hemorrhage and airway compromise can be safely managed.

F. INSERTION OF A NASOGASTRIC TUBE is deferred in patients with suspected vascular injury in order to avoid the possibility of dislodging a clot or stimulating bleeding.

III. ZONES OF THE NECK

The neck is divided into three zones (Figure 16.1) for the purpose of determining priorities, obtaining diagnostic studies, and preoperative planning of surgical procedures.

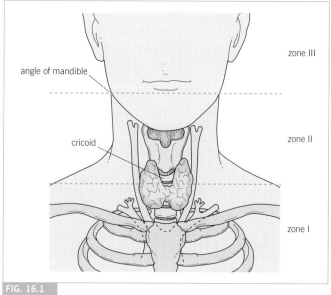

FIG. 16.1

Anatomic zones of the neck. (From Moore EE, Mattox KL, Feliciano DV, eds. *Trauma*. East Norwalk: Appleton and Lange; 1987:306.)

A. ZONE I. This is traversed by the great vessels, trachea, esophagus, and innominate vein at the thoracic outlet.

1. **The apices of both lungs** are also contained in zone I.

2. **Surface markings** for zone I extend from the clavicles to the cricoid cartilage superiorly.

3. **Penetrating injuries** in zone I usually require significant preoperative planning.

a. Surgical approaches have an increased morbidity and structures in zone I do not all lend themselves to easy access and repair.

b. At Parkland, multiple diagnostic studies are performed in these patients to identify injuries and appropriately plan surgical approaches.

4. **A hemodynamically stable patient** with a zone I injury will, at Parkland, undergo aortic arch and great vessel arteriography, bronchoscopy, and rigid esophagoscopy. In patients with a low suspicion for esophageal injury, cine-esophagography can be substituted for rigid esophagoscopy which requires general anesthesia.

5. **Injuries in zone I can be approached through a median sternotomy.** Proximal left subclavian artery injuries will require a left anterolateral thoracotomy for proximal control while a right thoracotomy may be required for high esophageal injuries.

B. ZONE II. This region contains the trachea, carotid artery, jugular vein, vertebral vessels, esophagus, and cervical spine.

1. **The surface markings** extend from the cricoid cartilage to the angle of the mandible.

2. **Anatomic structures** in zone II are easily accessible through an oblique neck incision with minimal morbidity.

3. **These reasons,** combined with the low cost of neck exploration, dictate the low threshold for operative exploration of zone II neck injuries.

4. **There are no significant differences in missed injuries** between surgical exploration and nonoperative evaluation by angiography, bronchoscopy, and esophagography. However, operative management has cost advantages and low morbidity; thus operative exploration of zone II injuries is favored at Parkland.

C. ZONE III. This area extends from the angle of the mandible to the base of the skull.

1. **The structures at risk** are mainly vascular, including the internal carotid and vertebral arteries.

2. **Operative exposure is frequently limited** and distal control of vascular injuries can be challenging, especially with high carotid lesions.

3. **Arteriography** is the preferred method of evaluation for stable patients at Parkland.

4. **Several maneuvers can improve exposure,** including mandibular subluxation; however, this needs to be achieved prior to making the

neck incision. At Parkland, mandibular osteotomy is rarely used to obtain distal exposure of the internal carotid artery, although this may be required if exposure is otherwise unattainable.

IV. SPECIFIC INJURIES
A. VASCULAR.
1. **Vascular and airway injuries** account for the majority of deaths due to neck trauma.
2. **The common carotid artery** is the most frequently injured structure in most series, injury occurring in about 10% of patients.
3. **The jugular vein** is the most frequently injured vein.
4. **A normal vascular examination** may be present in 10–30% of patients with vascular injuries, thus allowing for the possibility of missed injuries when relying solely on physical examination.
a.   Currently, arteriography remains the 'gold standard' for imaging the vascular system and allows reliable assessment of the presence of an injury.
b.   It also provides useful information regarding the collateral circulation and presence of vascular anomalies, which may affect the surgical management.
c.   Only 20% of all individuals have a complete circle of Willis, an important factor when contemplating ligation of the carotid artery.
d.   Approximately 3% of patients obtain blood supply to their spinal cord from the vertebral artery, thus rendering vertebral artery ligation a disastrous complication in this group of patients.
5. **Indications for neck exploration include:**
a.   Expanding hematoma.
b.   Pulsatile hemorrhage.
c.   Neurologic deficit.
d.   Presence of a thrill.
e.   Airway compromise.
6. **Although some centers advocate nonoperative management of injuries** thought to be minor on arteriography, we tend to operate on any patient with a radiographically proven injury to the common carotid or internal carotid artery.
7. **All carotid artery or internal jugular venous injuries** are repaired, when possible, with lateral arteriorrhaphy or venorrhaphy.
a.   Patients with severe venous injuries who have a patent contralateral jugular vein can undergo ligation of the injured jugular vein.
b.   Major carotid artery injuries may need a vein patch or interposition graft; thus the contralateral groin or ankle should be prepared and draped to allow simultaneous vein harvest.
c.   At Parkland, patients requiring prolonged reconstruction or additional repair of concomitant aerodigestive tract injuries should undergo routine vascular shunting.

8. **Ligation of the external carotid artery** may be considered in the unstable patient with multiple injuries. However, ligation of the internal carotid artery is fraught with severe neurologic complications and is generally avoided.

9. **Internal carotid artery ligation** may be considered in the patient with carotid injury, occlusion without distal flow, and a dense neurologic deficit.

a. A decision must be made regarding the safety of repair and restoration of flow in patients with a severe neurologic deficit.

b. This is made more difficult in the patient with a concomitant head injury as it is often not certain whether the deficit is due to the head injury or the vascular injury.

10. **In the past, concern was expressed** that if flow was restored an ischemic infarct may be converted to an hemorrhagic infarct, thereby increasing morbidity and mortality.

11. **Parkland recommends repair of most vascular injuries** in the presence of prograde flow. If the patient has evidence of a dense stroke and no prograde flow the risk of death may be increased; therefore, ligation without repair may be a satisfactory alternative.

12. **Distal internal carotid injuries** located near the base of the skull are often difficult to control. These may require ligation if collateral circulation is adequate and, if not, a subsequent extracranial–intracranial bypass procedure may be necessary in order to prevent neurological sequelae.

13. **An intraoperative completion angiography** is performed at Parkland to confirm a patent vascular repair without narrowing, as failure to do so may result in postoperative thrombosis.

14. **Vertebral artery injuries**, especially high distal arteriovenous fistulae, can be managed by embolization in the presence of adequate collateral circulation.

15. **Proximal vertebral artery injuries** can be managed by operative proximal and distal ligation.

B. PHARYNX.

1. **Pharyngeal injuries** generally occur as a result of penetrating trauma.

2. **These injuries may produce minimal signs and symptoms**; hence they are frequently missed, resulting in postinjury infections.

3. **These injuries are repaired** with at least two layers of monofilament absorbable suture and drained adequately.

4. **Proper mucosal apposition** will reduce the incidence of postoperative leaks.

5. **Cervical osteomyelitis** is a disastrous complication occasionally associated with pharyngo-esophageal injuries which occur in combination with penetrating cervical spine wounds. Contamination with pharyngeal flora is a contributing factor. However, this

16

NECK INJURIES

complication can be reduced by aggressive débridement, including diskal and ligamentous structures, stable spinal fixation, and appropriate antimicrobial therapy.

C. LARYNX.

1. **Laryngeal injuries** are usually mucosal tears, fractures of bony or cartilaginous structures, or avulsions and transections. They can be classified as supraglottic, transglottic, or cricoid in location. Indications for surgery include significant mucosal disruption or avulsion, arytenoid dislocation, and exposed cartilage.

2. **Timing of the operation is important**. Leopold[1] demonstrated improved results with early operation. In their study 87% of injuries repaired within 24 hours had a good airway, compared with 69% in patients treated within 2–7 days postinjury.

3. **The more common complications of laryngeal injury** are infection, airway stenosis or obstruction, and voice change.

a. Infection is treated by débridement, drainage, and antimicrobial therapy.

b. Airway stenosis is resolved by tracheal or laryngeal reconstruction.

D. TRACHEA.

1. **Isolated tracheal injuries** are rare with both blunt and penetrating trauma.

2. **The associated injuries** are often more dramatic and subtle trauma to the trachea may be overlooked.

3. **Indicators of possible tracheal injury** include sucking neck wounds, crepitus on examination, soft tissue air on plain radiographs, and hemoptysis.

4. **Bronchoscopy is accurate in identifying the injury**.

5. **One-layer repair** with absorbable monofilament suture is the preferred method of treatment at Parkland.

6. **In the presence of tissue loss**, mobilization of the trachea can obtain up to 5cm of length and achieve a tension-free repair.

E. ESOPHAGUS.

1. **Cervical esophageal injuries occur infrequently**.

a. During a 3-year prospective study at Parkland Memorial Hospital only 11 cervical esophageal injuries were identified.

b. Whereas penetrating trauma is the more common etiology, these injuries can be associated with blunt trauma, such as cervical spine fractures, blast effect, and crush injuries.

2. **Missed injuries are not uncommon** since they are often masked by trauma to surrounding organs that precludes their identification.

a. Although diagnostic studies, such as contrast radiography and endoscopy, are reliable, false-negative results occur.

b. Flexible endoscopy is much less reliable in identifying cervical esophageal injuries.

c. A study by Weigelt and co-authors[2] indicated that flexible endoscopy had a sensitivity of only 38% compared with 89% for rigid esophagoscopy.

3. **These injuries can also be elusive** at the operating table and a careful search must be made including the posterior aspect.

4. **Esophageal injuries should be repaired** in one or two layers.

a. Two-layer repairs may increase the incidence of postoperative dysphagia.

b. All repairs should have closed suction drainage and antibiotic prophylaxis.

c. Tenuous repairs are buttressed with a pleural or muscle flap.

5. **Massive injuries** may require esophagostomy, distal ligation, and gastrostomy tube placement.

6. **Missed injuries** can cause infectious complications, such as mediastinitis, cervical abscesses, and sepsis, but the more common problems seen following repair of these injuries are fistula formation and dysphagia.

7. **Esophageal leaks** are attributed to inadequate débridement, poor surgical technique when repairing the injury, and devascularization of the wall.

8. **Most patients with esophageal injury** have an uneventful postoperative convalescence.

9. **The incidence of esophagocutaneous fistula** is about 10–30%.

10. All patients should have a contrast study performed prior to starting an oral diet.

F. MUSCULOSKELETAL.

1. **Skeletal and ligamentous injuries** are more common following blunt trauma.

2. **Flexion and extension radiographs,** as well as other specialized imaging techniques, may need to be delayed while emergent problems are addressed.

3. **When evaluating potential skeletal injuries in the neck**, the physician must be compulsive in visualizing the C7–T1 interspace.

4. **Similarly, the odontoid must be seen in its entirety.**

5. **Occasionally, it will be necessary to obtain CT scans or magnetic resonance imaging (MRI) studies** to evaluate these areas completely. The importance of adequate visualization cannot be overemphasized as missed injuries in these areas may result in delayed and significant neurologic deficits.

6. **A stable burst fracture** (Jefferson fracture) of the atlas (C1) occurs from impaction of the ring of C1 against the occipital condyles. It is commonly seen with an axial load imparted to the top of the head.

7. **Odontoid fractures** are often associated with falls, blows on the head, vehicular collisions, and some sport, such as gymnastics. A type 1

fracture extends through the tip of the odontoid, type 2 extends through the body, and type 3 involves the base and the body of C2.

8. **Severe extension injuries** may cause a hangman's fracture (i.e. a fracture of the pedicle of the axis and a dislocation of C2 on C3). Owing to the large diameter of the spinal canal at this level, a neurologic injury may not occur.

9. **Treatment of skeletal and ligamentous injury** is by external stabilization or internal fixation, depending on stability of the fracture (see Chapter 11).

G. LYMPHATICS.

1. **The thoracic duct** is the most commonly injured lymphatic in the neck.

2. **These injuries may be identified during neck exploration**, but are usually discovered late in the hospital course.

3. **Unexplained fever, abscess formation, or abnormal fluid collections** should raise the suspicion of a thoracic duct injury. Drainage of milky white fluid from suction drains placed at the time of surgical exploration or aspiration of this material is often the first sign of a lymph fistula, lymphocele, or even a chylothorax.

4. **Conservative management** is usually adequate as these collections resolve spontaneously. However, if prolonged drainage continues, thoracic duct ligation is preferable to attempts at primary repair.

5. **Wide drainage** results in resolution of these complications.

6. **When these measures fail**, delayed ligation can be performed.

V. PEARLS AND PITFALLS

1. **Defer insertion of nasogastric tube** in patients with suspected vascular neck injuries.

2. **Do not remove impaled foreign bodies** in the emergency department. Removal may precipitate uncontrollable hemorrhage.

3. **Use liberal indications for four-vessel angiography** in patients with blunt neck injury to identify stretch injuries or intimal flaps.

4. **Intubate patients** with circumferential burns early to avoid a difficult airway.

VI. REFERENCES

1. Leopold DA. Laryngeal trauma. *Arch Otolaryngol* 1983; 109:106.
2. Weigelt JA, Thal ER, Snyder WH III et al. Diagnosis of penetrating cervical esophageal injuries. *Am J Surg* 1987; 154:619.

VII. FURTHER READING

Brown JM, Graham JM, Feliciano DV et al. Carotid artery injury. *Am J Surg* 1982; 144:748.

Liekweg WG Jr, Greenfield LJ. Management of penetrating carotid arterial injury. *Ann Surg* 1978, 188:587.

Rutherford RB, ed. *Vascular surgery,* 2nd edn. Philadelphia: WB Saunders; 1984:472.

Sheely CH II, Mattox KL, Reul GJ Jr et al. Current concepts in the management of penetrating neck trauma. *J Trauma* 1975, 15:895.

Thal ER, Snyder WH III, Hays RA et al. Management of carotid artery injuries. *Surgery* 1974, 76:955.

Unger SW, Tucker WS Jr, Mrdeza MA et al. Carotid arterial trauma. *Surgery* 1980, 87:477.

16

NECK INJURIES

I. INCIDENCE

Thoracic trauma accounts for 25% of the 150,000 annual trauma deaths in the United States.

II. ANATOMY

A. VITAL STRUCTURES.
1. **Thoracic outlet** (bounded by shoulder girdle).
2. **First rib.**
3. **Clavicles.**
4. **Manubrium.**

B. STRUCTURES AT RISK. These include:
1. **Vascular** – subclavian, carotid, jugular, and vertebral vessels.
2. **Nerves** – brachial plexus, vagus, recurrent laryngeal nerves, and phrenic nerves.
3. **Trachea.**
4. **Esophagus.**
5. **Thoracic duct.**

C. SURFACE MARKINGS.
1. **Angle of Louis** – 2nd intercostal space.
2. **Nipples** – 4th intercostal space.
3. **Scapular tip** – 7th intercostal space.
4. **'The Box'** – refers to the area bounded by the nipples laterally, the sternal notch, and the xiphoid process. A penetrating injury in this area mandates either subxiphoid exploration or transthoracic echocardiography (in the absence of a left hemothorax) to exclude an injury to the heart and great vessels.
5. **The plane created by the nipples anteriorly and the scapular tip posteriorly** represents the superior excursion of the diaphragm. Penetrating injuries below this level should raise suspicion for intra-abdominal injury.

D. STAB WOUNDS TO THE THORACO-ABDOMINAL AREA. If an abdominal injury has been excluded, evaluation of the diaphragm can be performed by video-assisted thoracoscopy (VAT) or abdominal exploration.

E. GUNSHOT WOUNDS TO THE THORACO-ABDOMINAL AREA. All these patients are operated upon provided that the following criteria are met: the wound or location of the missile is below the 4th intercostal space anteriorly, 6th intercostal space laterally, or 8th intercostal space (scapular tip) posteriorly.

III. MECHANISMS OF INJURY

A. BLUNT INJURY.
1. Most commonly associated with motor vehicle collisions and falls.
2. May result in chest wall contusions, fractures, cardiac or pulmonary contusions, hemothorax or pneumothorax, major vessel injury, or tracheal or esophageal injury.

B. PENETRATING INJURY.
1. May cause injury to any thoracic structure.
2. 80% will not require operative intervention.

C. IATROGENIC INJURY.
1. Pneumothorax from central venous access or barotrauma.
2. Esophageal or tracheobronchial perforation from endoscopy.
3. Cardiac or vascular perforation from venous access.

D. INGESTION. Esophageal burns from the ingestion of corrosives.

E. INHALATION. Smoke or other noxious gases inhalation.

IV. INITIAL MANAGEMENT

A. ABC. The establishment of an adequate airway with ventilation and appropriate resuscitation.

B. VENOUS ACCESS. Two large-bore upper extremity lines should be inserted.

C. CHEST-TUBE INSERTION. This is indicated prior to chest radiography when respiratory distress or diminished breath sounds are present.

D. PERICARDIOCENTESIS. Repeated aspirations will prevent hemodynamic deterioration prior to operation, but should not replace or delay operative intervention. In addition, results may be false-negative or false-positive.

E. EMERGENCY DEPARTMENT THORACOTOMY
1. This is usually reserved for patients with penetrating trauma, evidence of cardiac activity or signs of life, and unresponsive shock.
2. Salvage for patients with blunt trauma is dismal.
3. This procedure is not used in patients sustaining blunt trauma with no signs of life

V. DIAGNOSIS

A. HISTORY.
1. Obtain the history of the mechanism of injury – deceleration, ejection, seat-belt use, or broken steering wheel.
2. The symptoms may include:
a. Chest pain.
b. Shortness of breath.
c. Hoarseness.
d. Hemoptyis.
e. Stridor.
3. Past medical history – especially any cardiorespiratory diseases.

B. PHYSICAL SIGNS.
1. Abrasions.
2. Contusions.
3. Obvious fractures.
4. **Seat-belt marks** may suggest intrathoracic injury.
5. **Site of penetrating injury** (proximity).
6. **Beck's triad** – jugular vein distention, muffled heart sounds, and hypotension.
7. **Narrow pulse pressure.**
8. **Pulsus paradoxus.**
9. **Tracheal shift from midline.**
10. **Diminished or absent breath sounds.**
11. **Paradoxical chest motion.**
12. **Point tenderness** for sternum or rib fractures, crepitus, or deformity.

VI. SPECIFIC STUDIES

A. ARCH ARTERIOGRAM.
1. **Coupled with a suggestive mechanism of injury,** arteriograms are obtained when any of the following conditions are present on routine chest film:
a. Widened mediastinum.
b. First rib fracture.
c. Widening of the paraspinous stripe.
d. Shift of the trachea towards the right.
e. Deviation of the nasogastric tube.
f. Depression of the left mainstream bronchus.
g. Loss of aortic–pulmonary window.
h. Widening of the paratracheal stripe.
i. Abnormal aortic knob.
j. Apical capping.
k. Left hemothorax.
2. **Arch arteriograms are obtained** on patients with transmediastinal gunshot wounds in order to exclude great vessel injury.
B. ARTERIOGRAPHY. The indications for this technique include:
1. **Pulse deficit** or upper extremity pulse or blood pressure differential.
2. **Stable hematoma.**
3. **New peripheral nerve deficit.**
4. **Penetrating zone I neck injuries.**
C. BARIUM CINE-ESOPHAGOGRAM. The indications for this procedure include:
1. **Dysphagia.**
2. **Odynophagia.**
3. **Transmediastinal penetrating injuries.**
4. **Penetrating zone I neck injuries.**

17

THORACIC TRAUMA

D. ECHOCARDIOGRAM. This has limited utility except in patients with hemodynamic instability that is unresponsive to volume replacement. It can also exclude pericardial fluid, but is less sensitive when a left hemothorax is present.

VII. INDICATIONS FOR THORACOTOMY OR STERNOTOMY

1. Thoracic hemorrhage.
a. Initial chest-tube output of 1000–1500mL of blood.
b. 200mL per hour for ≥ 2 hours.
1. Cardiac tamponade or hemopericardium.
3. Acute hemodynamic decompensation following penetrating thoracic trauma with no other identifiable cause.
4. Transmediastinal wound with hemodynamic instability or positive findings on evaluation.
5. Large residual hemothorax after two well-placed 36F chest tubes (alternative is VAT for evacuation).
6. Massive air leak with respiratory distress.
7. Severe penetrating parenchyma lung injury.
8. Tracheal or bronchial disruption.
9. Esophageal perforation or disruption.
10. Aortic or other great vessel injury.
11. Central missile embolus.
12. Atrial–caval shunt placement for retrohepatic venous injuries.
13. Chronic chylous fistula.
14. Empyema secondary to remote trauma (the alternate is VAT surgery).

VIII. EXPOSURE CONSIDERATIONS

A. LEFT ANTEROLATERAL OR STANDARD POSTEROLATERAL THORACOTOMY.
1. Most versatile incision.
2. Easy to perform.
3. Expeditious.
4. Most cardiac injuries, as well as aortic and proximal left subclavian artery injuries, are approachable through this incision.
B. RIGHT THORACOTOMY. This procedure is useful for right-sided pulmonary parenchymal and tracheal injury.
C. MEDIAN STERNOTOMY.
1. Used for isolated cardiac trauma.
2. Good exposure for innominate and proximal left common carotid artery control.
3. Used for central pulmonary vascular injury.
4. Cannot expose posterior mediastinum, thus this technique is not indicated for aortic injury.

D. **LEFT SECOND INTERSPACE THORACOTOMY AND 'OPEN BOOK' THORACOTOMY.** These techniques can be used to control and expose the left subclavian artery.

IX. INTRAOPERATIVE MANAGEMENT

1. **Correction of physiologic derangement** including acidosis, coagulopathy, hypothermia, hypovolemia, and anemia.
2. **Autotransfusion of chest-tube drainage** can be helpful but should usually be stopped after 2L owing to the increased risk of coagulopathy.
3. **Cell-saver autotransfuser** use may be limited by the potential contamination in traumatic injuries. This is less of a problem with chest injuries than with abdominal injuries.

X. POSTOPERATIVE MANAGEMENT

1. **Patients who have undergone median sternotomy or thoracotomy** should be monitored in the intensive care unit.
2. **Pulmonary artery catheter** assists in volume management with severe cardiac or pulmonary injury.
3. **Cardiac arrhythmias** are common after thoracotomy.
   a. They may be a manifestation of an underlying cardiac disease.
   b. Supraventricular arrhythmias may occur in conjunction with thoracic trauma.
   c. Supraventricular or ventricular arrhythmias may occur after cardiac surgery.
   d. Verapamil β-blockers, or digoxin, may be used depending on the etiology of the arrhythmia.
   e. β-Blockers are contraindicated if cardiac dysfunction is present.
   f. Cardioversion for arrhythmias may be indicated for hemodynamic instability.
4. **When low cardiac output occurs** as a result of injury, inotropes can be used once hypovolemia, arrhythmias, and tamponade are excluded.
5. **Adequate analgesia** is essential for good pulmonary function.
6. **Control of secretions and avoidance of atelectasis** are crucial to avoid complications.

XI. INVASIVE PROCEDURES

A. **TUBE THORACOSTOMY.**
1. **Principles.**
   a. Indicated for pneumothorax or hemothorax.
   b. Location is usually the 5th or 6th intercostal space, midaxillary line.
   c. Elevate the patient on a rolled sheet.
   d. Prepare and drape the patient.
   e. Use 1% lidocaine liberally, infiltrating the skin, fascia, superior border of the rib, and the pleura.

THORACIC TRAUMA

17

f. In nonemergent situations, rib blocks may be placed prior to insertion.

g. A transverse incision (2–3cm) is made over the 6th or 7th rib.

h. Tunnel superiorly and posteriorly to enter the pleural space on the superior border of the 6th or 7th rib.

i. Digitally explore the chest to assure entrance into the thoracic and not abdominal cavity.

j. The goal is to place the tube in the posterior apex.

k. Insert a 36F tube in a superior posterior direction.

l. Make sure the most proximal hole is within the rib cage.

m. Place the tube on 20cm wall suction in a closed collection system.

n. Suture the tube to the skin with 2-0 silk.

o. Apply a sterile dressing.

2. Chest-tube management

a. The chest tube remains on 20cm wall suction until the lung has been fully expanded for 24 hours. Suction is then discontinued and the tube is placed on a water seal. If the lung remains inflated on subsequent radiography, the tube can be removed.

b. The practice at Parkland Memorial Hospital is to remove the tube after the lung is inflated on suction without placing the patient on a water seal.

c. Recurrent pneumothorax can be treated by placing the chest tube back on suction for 24–48 hours and repeating the cycle.

d. Inability to maintain lung reinflation suggests a nonhealing parenchymal injury or bronchial injury.

e. An air leak should be sealed and drainage should be <50mL per 8 hours prior to removing the tube.

f. Commercially available closed suction and collection systems are routinely used and can be connected to autotransfusion chambers (Figure 17.1).

g. Patients with chest tubes are placed on prophylactic first-generation cephalosporins for the duration of the chest tube.

h. Perioperative prophylaxis is adequate for thoracotomy.

3. Chest-tube removal

a. Cut the securing sutures.

b. Prepare a dressing of 4×4 gauze with petroleum jelly gauze to overlay the chest-tube site.

c. While holding the dressing over the chest-tube entry site, have the patient hold their breath and perform a Valsalva maneuver at maximal inspiration, helping to reduce the chance of recurrent pneumothorax.

d. Briskly pull out the tube in a single motion, while applying firm pressure on the dressing.

e. Apply tape to create a completely occlusive dressing, which should remain in place for at least 48 hours.

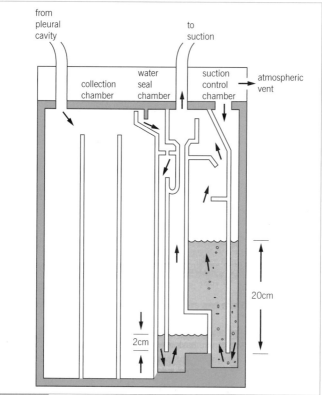

from
pleural
cavity

to
suction

water
seal
chamber

suction
control
chamber

atmospheric
vent

collection
chamber

20cm

2cm

FIG. 17.1

Commercially available apparatus for chest drainage. (From Symbas PN.
Cardiothoracic trauma. Philadelphia: WB Saunders; 1989.)

B. **PERICARDIOCENTESIS.**
1. **Prepare and drape** the xiphoid region.
2. **Use** a 30mL syringe and a 1.5–2 inch 18- or 20-gauge needle (not a
   spinal needle).
3. **Enter the left paraxiphoid region** with the needle at 45° to the plane of
   the anterior chest wall and at 45° to the sagittal plane (angle toward
   the left shoulder).
4. **Advance the catheter** while aspirating until blood is encountered.
5. **Aspirated blood should be nonclotting**, and the hemodynamics should
   immediately improve. Removal of as little as 20–30mL may relieve a
   tamponade.

6. **Repeat as necessary** or insert a Silastic pigtail catheter which can serve as a drain until surgery.

C. **EMERGENCY DEPARTMENT THORACOTOMY.**

1. **Prepare and drape** the left chest.
2. **Incise the sternum** to the posterior axillary line in the left inframammary fold toward the axilla (follow the course of the 5th rib).
3. **Enter the pleural cavity** along the superior margin of the 5th rib; watch for the internal mammary artery parasternally.
4. **Insert a self-retaining rib retractor**, and retract the lung to expose the pericardium.
5. **Assess the pericardium for tamponade**; if present, incise the pericardium longitudinally anterior to the phrenic nerve.
6. **Deliver the heart from the pericardium with care**, being careful not to impede venous return.
7. **Locate the cardiac wound** and repair with pledgetted sutures, or digitally control en route to the operating room.

D. **SUBXIPHOID EXPLORATION.**

1. **Prepare and drape** the entire chest and abdomen.
2. **Make a midline incision** over the xiphoid and upper epigastrium (3cm above and 5cm below the xiphoid). This should be made through the linea alba but not the peritoneum.
3. **Divide the xiphoid attachments of the diaphragm** with electrocautery. Hemostasis is very important so there is no question as to the nature of the pericardial fluid once the window is made.
4. **The xiphoid may be removed** if the costal margin is narrow.
5. **Bluntly dissect the pericardium** off the posterior sternum, being careful to stay directly under the sternum. Expose the pericardium by sweeping off the prepericardial fat.
6. **Grasp the pericardium** with Allis clamps.
7. **Once the operative field is dry**, open the pericardium between the clamps and note the nature of the fluid: if bloody, then proceed to a median sternotomy or left anterior thoracotomy; if clear, the wound may be closed.

E. **INTERCOSTAL NERVE BLOCK.**

1. **Used for analgesia** for rib fractures or chest-tube placement.
2. **With patient in the sitting position** and leaning slightly forward, the angles of the ribs to be blocked are identified, and this area is prepared (Figure 17.2).
3. **A 1:1 mixture** of 1% lidocaine and 0.5% bupivicaine is used and a skin weal made using a 25–27-gauge needle.
4. **The periosteum of the rib is then infiltrated** and the needle 'walked' down to the inferior border of the rib where it is advanced slightly while attempting aspiration.
5. **Care should be taken** to ensure that the pleural space and the intercostal vessels are not entered.

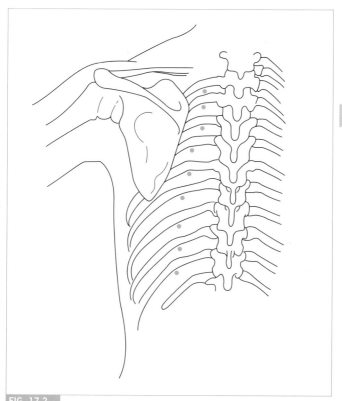

FIG. 17.2
Preferred site for intercostal block. Injection more medial poses risk of instilling the agent into the dural canal. (From Hood RM. Trauma to the chest. In: Sabiston DC, Spencer FC, eds. *Surgery of the chest,* 5th edn. Philadelphia: WB Saunders; 1990.)

6. **Once the needle is in the notch of the rib**, aspiration is again attempted and, if negative, 3–5mL of the lidocaine–bupivicaine mixture is injected.
7. **An intercostal block** is done for all fractured ribs at one space superior and inferior to the fractured ribs.
8. **When multiple fractured ribs are present** care should be taken not to exceed the maximum recommended doses for either lidocaine or bupivicaine (lidocaine 7mg/kg; bupivicaine 2mg/kg).

XII. SPECIFIC INJURIES

A. GREAT VESSEL INJURIES.

1. **Great vessel injury is seen** in <5% of patients arriving at trauma centers alive.
2. **Of the patients with thoracic aortic rupture**, 20% survive >1 hour.
3. **If not operated upon**, 40% of these patients die within 24 hours, 75% die by 3 weeks, and 90% die by 10 weeks.
4. **80–90% of aortic ruptures** occur at the aortic isthmus, with the second most common site being the proximal innominate artery.
5. **Maintain a high index of suspicion**, whether or not there is physical examination evidence of thoracic injury.
6. **Treatment is surgical repair** via a left anterior thoracotomy (3rd or 4th intercostal space).
7. **Adjuncts to repair** include:
a. Biomedicus centrifugal pump.
b. Maintenance of a distal blood pressure of 60–80mmHg under this type of assistance: left atrium to femoral artery or left atrium to distal thoracic aorta.
c. Cardiopulmonary bypass.
d. Heparin.
e. Internal shunts.

B. ASCENDING AORTA.

1. **Patients usually do not survive this injury.**
2. **They usually have pericardial tamponade.**
3. **Treatment is primary aortorrhaphy** with polypropylene suture (Prolene).

C. INNOMINATE ARTERY AND VEIN.

1. **Access** is via a median sternotomy.
2. **Repair**
a. Open pericardium first to ensure adequate proximal control.
b. Suture bypass graft to the ascending aorta.
c. Establish vascular control of distal innominate artery.
d. Use end-to-end anastomosis with the bypass graft.
e. Use lateral aortorrhaphy at take-off of innominate artery.
f. Use de-airing techniques to remove any clot or debris by back bleeding.
g. For penetrating injuries, lateral repair will control small injuries while complete transection requires anastomosis.
h. In cases of associated tracheal and esophageal injuries and vascular repair, interpose sternocleidomastoid muscle or strap muscles between repair of tracheal or esophageal injuries and vascular repair.
i. The innominate vein rarely requires repair and may be ligated without consequence.

D. **DESCENDING THORACIC AORTA.**

1. **Access** is through the left posterolateral thoracotomy (4th intercostal space) with a double-lumen endotracheal tube.
2. **Prepare femoral area into operative field**, with patient in the right lateral decubitus position with hips rolled back.
3. **Blunt injury.**
a. Achieve proximal and distal aortic control.
b. Proximal clamp may be between left carotid artery and left subclavian artery to provide additional exposure.
c. May encircle intercostals and temporarily occlude them.
d. Do not divide the intercostal vessels.
e. Partial tear of the aorta may sometimes be repaired primarily with 3-0 or 4-0 Prolene suture. Otherwise, a short segment of preclotted woven Dacron graft is necessary for repair.
f. Consider use of moderate hypothermia (32°C), but balance this decision with the inherent complications with hypothermia-related bleeding.
4. **Penetrating injuries** are primarily repaired with the use of pledgets.
5. **In patients who survive to the operating room**, mortality is 15% and paraplegia is 5–7%.

E. **PROXIMAL LEFT SUBCLAVIAN ARTERY.** A left anterior thoracotomy, at the 2nd or 3rd intercostal space, is indicated.

F. **DISTAL LEFT SUBCLAVIAN ARTERY.** Initial control is achieved with a left anterior lateral thoracotomy; then a subclavicular or supraclavicular incision is performed.

G. **PULMONARY ARTERY AND VEIN.**

1. **Access** is via a median sternotomy.
2. **A penetrating injury is more common.** Vascular clamps are used to control the hilus; this is a useful adjunct to help identify injury.
3. **Blunt trauma.**
a. Patients rarely survive.
b. Repair is the same as for penetrating injury.
4. **Repair is by lateral arteriorrhaphy** if anterior main pulmonary artery is injured.
a. The use of pledgets is important.
b. Use cardiopulmonary bypass if injury is extensive or if the posterior wall of main artery is involved.
5. **The intrapericardial pulmonary vein** is very difficult to explore and expose.
a. After controlling hemorrhage (consider Foley balloon catheter), the patient may require a cardiopulmonary bypass to decrease the size of heart (decompress) and expose the area of injury.
b. The use of vascular clamps to control the hilus is important.
c. The mortality rate is greater than 70–75%.

17

THORACIC TRAUMA

H. THORACIC VENA CAVA.

1. This is rarely an isolated injury.
2. Both the superior vena cava and inferior vena cava are intrapericardial in the thorax.
3. Access is via a median sternotomy.
4. Repair is with lateral venorrhaphy.
a. This may require isolation of injuries using intracaval shunt or snares, by way of the right atrial appendage.
b. A large defect may require pericardial patch reconstruction.
c. Posterior injuries of the vena cava may require cardiopulmonary bypass to access through the right atrium.
5. The mortality rate greater than 50% (high rate of associated injuries).

XIII. SPECIAL SITUATIONS

A. MULTIPLE INJURIES IN PATIENTS WITH WIDENED MEDIASTINUM.

1. Hemodynamically stable.
a. If the results of a diagnostic peritoneal lavage (DPL) or sonogram are negative, evaluate the aorta with aortography.
b. If abdominal evaluation is negative, evaluate aorta before celiotomy.
c. If abdominal evaluation reveals hemorrhage, celiotomy is followed by aortography.
2. Hemodynamically unstable.
a. For positive findings of abdominal hemorrhage, perform a rapid control celiotomy followed by aortography.
   1) Rapid-control celiotomy consists of rapid and simple control of blood loss and control of contamination followed by rapid closure of abdominal incision with towel clips and placement of adhesive dressing to cover operative area.
   2) Then address aortic injury with aortography (if not already performed) or thoracotomy.
   3) After aorta repair is complete, re-open celiotomy incision and complete the definitive repair of injuries.
b. The goal of a rapid-control celiotomy is to prevent exsanguination by controlling blood loss in the abdomen and then addressing the aortic rupture.

B. RIB FRACTURE.

1. Chest radiographs and a rib series document a fracture but have a false-negative rate up to 30–50%.
2. It is important to look for hemothorax or pneumothorax on presentation and during the initial 24–48 hours.
3. Treatment is supportive.
a. Control pain with oral, parenteral, or epidural analgesics or a rib block, depending on the individual patient's needs and associated injuries.

b.   Avoid binding the chest wall, as this contributes to ventilatory abnormality caused by splinting and may contribute to atelectasis and hypoxia.

c.   Focus on analgesia and pulmonary toilet (incentive spirometry and coughing).

C.   STERNAL FRACTURE.

1.   **Chest radiographs** may not show fracture.

a.   A lateral view or sternal view is more helpful but is often not possible to obtain in the multiply injured patient.

b.   Look for evidence of associated intrathoracic injuries.

2.   **Treatment focuses on associated injuries**, but urgent reduction of claviculosternal dislocation by placing a sandbag or rolled towel transversely under the upper thoracic spine may be necessary to relieve compression of airway, vessels, or nerves at the thoracic outlet.

a.   Analgesics or local injection may be used.

b.   Early wiring is beneficial if the patient's condition is stable and there is no need for mechanical ventilation.

c.   Sternal, 1st rib, or 2nd rib fractures should alert the physician to the possibility of associated intrathoracic injuries (bronchial or vascular rupture, myocardial or pulmonary contusion, or brachial plexus injury) and appropriate examination and workup should follow.

D.   FLAIL CHEST.

1.   **Occurs in 10–20% of trauma admissions.**

2.   **Paradoxical chest wall motion** that occurs with respirations.

3.   **Multiple contiguous rib fractures** may be present.

4.   **Morbidity and mortality** are related to underlying pulmonary parenchymal injury.

5.   **Treatment is supportive.**

a.   Intubation and positive pressure ventilation are undertaken for respiratory failure (progressive fatigue, Pco_2 50mmHg, Po_2 60mmHg on 100% oxygen by face mask, or negative inspiratory pressure 25mmHg).

b.   Avoid administration of excess fluid as this may exaggerate edema in underlying pulmonary contusion.

c.   Analgesia (oral, parenteral, epidural, or intercostal blocks) and pulmonary toilet (incentive spirometry, cough, humidification, and suctioning) are the most important factors in preventing further deterioration.

d.   Splinting or binding the chest wall may contribute to ventilatory abnormality.

e.   Internal fixation may help stabilize the chest wall earlier and should be considered in severe cases or when thoracotomy is performed for another reason.

E. **OPEN CHEST WOUND.**
1. **Beware of occlusive dressing** in the absence of a chest tube as this may precipitate a tension pneumothorax.
2. **A sucking chest wound** will lead to ineffectual ventilation of the ipsilateral lung when the cross-sectional area of the wound approaches that of the mainstem bronchus.
3. **On plain radiographs**, evaluate the extent of the chest wall injury and signs of associated injuries.
4. **Treat with occlusive dressing after chest-tube placement**, followed by débridement and closure of the wound if a large defect is present.
5. **Large wounds** may ultimately require a flap for coverage.
F. **HEMOPNEUMOTHORAX TREATMENT.**
1. **Closed-tube thoracostomy** is usually all that is required.
2. **If the patient has a stab wound to the chest** and is asymptomatic, and radiographs show no evidence of hemothorax or pneumothorax, a 6-hour chest study should be obtained and, if normal, the patient may be discharged (<1% will become symptomatic or develop delayed hemopneumothorax after a normal chest study 6 hours postinjury).
3. **The indications for thoracotomy** are listed above.
G. **THORACIC DUCT INJURIES.**
1. **A history** of recent retroperitoneal, posterior mediastinal, or cervical operation or trauma.
2. **Chylous effusion or chest-tube output** (a positive fat stain or a high level of triglycerides).
3. **Chest radiographs** may show pleural effusion.
4. **CT** may show mediastinal fluid collection.
5. **Lymphangiography** may assist with preoperative localization.
6. **Treatment.**
a. Most chyle leaks are self-limited and respond to nonoperative therapy (a low fat diet or total parenteral nutrition, if necessary, and drainage).
b. A severe fibrothorax may develop if chyle is allowed to collect in the pleural cavity.
c. Ligation of the thoracic duct should be performed during the initial operative procedure if the injury is recognized; collaterals are plentiful.
d. If delayed ligation, after failed conservative therapy, is to be performed, administration of a heavy fat (butter or cream) with dye may help with intraoperative identification.
e. If the injured duct cannot be found via a right posterolateral thoracotomy then multiple ligations of tissue anterior and to the right of T8–T9 at the level of the diaphragm should be performed.

XIV. PEARLS AND PITFALLS

1. **Inspiratory and expiratory upright chest radiographs** are necessary to help reveal occult pneumothorax.
2. **In patients with stab wounds and a normal first chest radiographs**, a 6-hour postinjury film can rule out delayed pneumothorax.

XV. FURTHER READING

Mattox KL. Thoracic great vessel injury. *Surg Clin North Am* 1988; 68:693–703.

Parmley LF. Nonpenetrating traumatic injury of the aorta. *Circulation* 1958; 17:1086.

Pate JW. Chest wall injuries. *Surg Clin North Am* 1989; 69:59.

Richardson JD, Wilson ME, Miller FB. The widened mediastinum. *Ann Surg* 1990; 211:731–737.

Shuck JM, Snow NJ. Injury to the chest wall. In: Moore EE, Mattox KL, Feliciano DV, eds. *Trauma,* 2nd edn. East Norwalk: Appleton and Lange; 1991:321.

Stubbs WK, Tabb HG. Thoracic duct injuries. *South Med J* 1977; 79:1962.

Townsend RN, Colella JJ, Diamond DL. Traumatic rupture of the aorta: critical decisions for trauma surgeons. *J Trauma* 1990; 30:1169–1174.

17

THORACIC TRAUMA

DIAPHRAGMATIC INJURY

18

I. INCIDENCE
1. **Diaphragmatic rupture** is present in 1% of all blunt trauma admissions and 7% of all blunt trauma fatalities.
2. **The incidence seems to be increasing,** probably owing to increased awareness and better diagnostic tests.
3. **Mortality rates** vary from 17% to 42%. Death is usually due to associated injuries, of which head injury is the most common.

II. MECHANISM
1. **Injury occurs** primarily as a result of lateral impact motor vehicle collisions or falls.
2. **Theories of mechanism** include the shearing of a stretched membrane, avulsion from attachments, and the sudden increase in intra-abdominal pressure.
3. **There is a predilection** (67–90%) for the left side to be injured.

III. ANATOMY
1. **The diaphragm is attached to the ribs** 11 through 12 posteriorly and laterally, and to the costal cartilages anteriorly.
2. **It is innervated by the phrenic nerve** (C3, C4, and C5).
3. **The anterior central portion** is the inferior wall of the pericardium.
4. **The arterial supply** is via the intercostal arteries.
5. **The venous return** is by way of the phrenic veins.
6. **During deep inspiration and forced exhalation** the dome moves from rib 12 to rib 7.
7. **Rupture is frequently associated with injuries** to the liver, aorta, and pelvic bones.

IV. CLINICAL MANIFESTATIONS
1. **One-half of patients with diaphragm injury** present in shock.
2. **Respiratory distress, abdominal pain, and shoulder pain** are common.
3. **Examination may reveal** a scaphoid abdomen or bowel sounds in the affected hemithorax.

V. DIAGNOSIS
1. **Diagnosis is made preoperatively** in only 30% of cases.
2. **30% of chest radiographs** suggest rupture.
3. **Placement of a nasogastric tube** with visualization of a thoracic location on a radiograph is diagnostic.
4. **Diaphragmatic rupture may also be diagnosed** incidentally at thoracotomy or celiotomy.

5. **Diagnosis can be made by return of lavage fluid** from a thoracostomy tube.
6. **Peritoneal lavage** is not a good diagnostic study for an injured diaphragm.
7. **CT** is also not a reliable study in the diagnosis of this injury.
8. **As a result of the poor yield for preoperative diagnosis**, at Parkland Memorial Hospital video-assisted thoracoscopy is performed in the operating room for the diagnosis of suspected diaphragmatic injuries. This technique is accurate for diagnosis and small injuries can also be repaired thoracoscopically.

VI. MANAGEMENT

1. **Respiratory distress**, secondary to a distended stomach, can be relieved with the insertion of a nasogastric tube.
2. **The abdominal approach to repair** is preferred because of the high incidence (70%) of associated abdominal injuries.
3. **Primary repair** is performed with permanent running or interrupted horizontal mattress sutures.
4. **The thoracic cavity** should be irrigated to avoid empyema.
5. **The necessity of a chest tube may be avoided** by aspirating the pleural space with a red Robinson catheter while the patient takes a deep breath.
6. **Sutures may have to be placed around the ribs** if the diaphragm is separated from its attachments.
7. **Chronic diaphragmatic ruptures** are better repaired through a transthoracic approach because of dense intrathoracic adhesions.
8. **Gore-Tex or Marlex can be used for the repair** of chronic ruptures.

VII. POSTOPERATIVE CARE AND PROGNOSIS

1. **The morbidity** associated with diaphragm injuries that are not repaired is significant.
2. **Patients require** an average of 4–5 days of mechanical ventilatory support.
3. **Temporary or permanent paresis** of the hemidiaphragm often occurs with large disruptions.

VIII. FURTHER READING

Spann J, Nwariaku F, Wait M. The role of video-assisted thoracoscopic surgery in the evaluation of diaphragmatic injuries. *Am J Surg* 1995; 170(6):628–631.

ESOPHAGEAL INJURY

I. ETIOLOGY

A. **CAUSE.** The most common causes of esophageal injury are:

1. **Iatrogenic perforation** (tracheal intubation, endoscopy, or dilatation).
2. **Penetrating trauma** (3.9–5.5%).

B. **LOCATION.** The most common location for injury after penetrating trauma is the cervical esophagus. Blunt esophageal trauma is extremely rare (<0.1%). This injury is usually located in the distal esophagus.

II. EVALUATION

A. **SIGNS AND SYMPTOMS.** Figure 19.1 outlines the method for diagnosis and the management of esophageal injuries.

1. Cervical dysphagia.
2. Chest pain.
3. Drooling.
4. Effusion.
5. Cough pneumomediastinum (crunch sound).
6. Hoarseness.
7. Pleural symptoms (pain on respiration).
8. Respiratory distress.
9. Stridor.
10. Shock.
11. Subcutaneous emphysema or crepitus.
12. Epigastric pain.
13. Pneumothorax.
14. Abdominal tenderness or rigidity.
15. Peritonitis.

B. **RADIOGRAPHS.**

1. **Cervical spine and chest film findings.**
   a. Para-esophageal air.
      1) Widening of the retrotracheal space.
      2) Cervical subcutaneous emphysema.
      3) Pneumomediastinum.
      4) Pneumothorax.
      5) Widened mediastinum.
      6) Pleural effusion.
   b. Air under the diaphragm.
2. **Esophagography**
   a. Two-plane cine-esophagography is more reliable than the conventional plain-film technique.

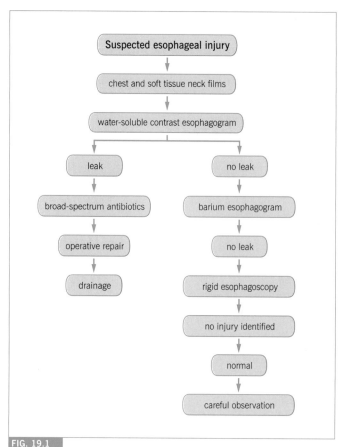

FIG. 19.1

Diagnosis and management of esophageal injury.

b. Use sterile water-soluble contrast, such as Gastrografin.
c. Accuracy approaches 90%.
d. If esophagography is equivocal, then esophagoscopy is warranted.

3. Esophagoscopy

a. Rigid esophagoscopy is more accurate than flexible esophagoscopy.
b. Flexible esophagoscopy is most likely to miss an injury at the level of the proximal cervical esophagus.

III. MANAGEMENT

A. **LIFE-THREATENING INJURIES.** These injuries should be addressed first.

1. **Proximal esophageal and gastric suction** help minimize leakage of oral and gastric secretions.
2. **Restore and maintain fluid and electrolyte balance**.
3. **Broad-spectrum antibiotics** are given.
4. **Nonoperative management** is reserved for minimal injuries with no extravasation or contamination.

B. **OPERATIVE MANAGEMENT PRINCIPLES.**

1. **Early surgical repair and drainage**.
2. **Careful and meticulous inspection** of esophagus at risk.
3. **Two-layer closure without tension**: mucosal layer with absorbable suture and muscular layer with monofilament suture.
4. **Viable interpositioning of tissue flap** (sternohyoid, sternothyroid, or sternocleidomastoid) between concomitant tracheal and esophageal, or carotid and esophageal, repairs to prevent fistula formation.
5. **Thoracic–esophageal repairs** should be reinforced with a pleural flap (Grillo patch) or intercostal muscle flap to decrease the incidence of anastomotic leaks.
6. **Abdominal–esophageal repairs** should be reinforced with a Thal patch or a Nissen fundoplication.
7. **Wide mediastinal and bilateral pleural drainage** is required for thoracic–esophageal injury.
8. **If primary repair is not possible** or if a major leak of the primary repair occurs, wide drainage should be achieved and control of the esophageal leak obtained by esophageal exclusion using the following:
   a. Lateral or end esophagostomy.
   b. Aspiration of secretions via a nasogastric tube with tip at level of repair.
   c. Temporary ligation of the esophagus distal to the repair to prevent gastroesophageal reflux with a temporary band (Urschel) or circumferential absorbable ligature (Popovsky) which allows restoration of esophageal continuity when the suture dissolves or is broken by dilatation if necessary.
   d. If extensive injury is present, end-cervical esophagostomy with delayed colon or small bowel interposition or gastric pull-up should be considered.
   e. A gastrostomy or jejunostomy tube should be considered for enteral feeding.
   f. Late repairs are more likely to fail.

C. **RESULTS.**

1. **Expeditious repair** (<12 hours) reduces the incidence of anastomotic leak, morbidity, and mortality.
2. **Overall mortality** is 2–30% and is often related to associated injuries.

19

ESOPHAGEAL INJURY

3. **Mortality of thoracic–esophageal injuries** (20–50%) is 3–5 times that of cervical or abdominal–esophageal injuries. This is a reflection of mediastinal and pleural sepsis, as well as associated injuries.
4. **Delay in diagnosis and treatment** (>12 hours) is associated with an unacceptably high mortality (nearly 100%).

IV. CAUSTIC INGESTION

A. INCIDENCE.

1. **Annually, 26,000 caustic injuries occur in the United States**.
2. **The majority of injuries are in infants and children** (80%), while the remainder are usually a result of suicide attempts.

B. AGENTS.

1. **Alkali (lye).**
a. 95% of cases.
b. Sodium and potassium hydroxide - drain and oven cleaners.
c. Rapid penetration with liquefaction necrosis.
d. Regurgitation into the esophagus is common.
2. **Acids.**
a. 5% of cases.
b. Sulfuric, hydrochloric, and phosphoric acids - lavatory bowl cleaners and battery fluids.
c. Rapidly produces coagulation necrosis; eschar limits penetration.
d. 80% of acid burns spare the esophagus.

C. CLASSIFICATION.

1. **First degree.**
a. Desquamation.
b. Mucosal edema and erythema.
2. **Second degree.**
a. Penetration into muscularis.
b. Ulceration.
c. Stricture in the esophagus at points where the caustic agents pool.
   1) Cricopharyngeus.
   2) Aortic arch.
   3) Tracheal bifurcation.
   4) Lower esophageal sphincter.
3. **Third degree.**
a. Transmural.
b. Leads to mediastinitis or peritonitis.

D. EVALUATION.

1. **Acute signs and symptoms.**
a. Dysphagia.
b. Odynophagia.
c. Epigastric pain.
d. Perioral pain.

e. Upper gastrointestinal bleed.
f. Stridor.
g. Fever.
h. Vomiting.
i. Drooling.
j. Burns on lips or oropharynx.
2. Late signs and symptoms.
a. Dysphagia.
b. Early satiety.
c. Weight loss.
d. Gastric outlet obstruction.
e. Stricture formation.
E. DIAGNOSTIC STUDIES.
1. Flexible endoscopy.
a. Limit advancement to site of injury.
b. Rigid esophagoscopy may lead to perforation.
c. May underestimate the severity of the injury.
d. Principal utility is to exclude patients without burns.
2. Radiologic studies.
a. Not sensitive in the acute setting.
b. Edema and irregularity persists for 2–3 weeks.
c. Chest radiographs and soft-tissue neck films may show evidence of perforation.
F. TREATMENT.
1. Emergency treatment.
a. Maintain control of airway.
b. Broad-spectrum antibiotics.
c. Intravenous steroids for 4–6 weeks.
d. Antacids or H_2-blockers while on steroids.
e. Neutralization with water or acid may release heat and further the injury with lye ingestion.
f. Water may dilute acid with minimal heat loss.
g. Emetics and gastric lavage increase risk of regurgitation.
h. Endoscopy.
2. Surgical exploration.
a. Utilized in the septic patient or patient demonstrating evidence of perforation.
b. Resection for perforation or transmural injury.
c. Esophagectomy and occasional partial gastrectomy may be necessary.
d. Formal reconstruction with stomach or colon is delayed until resolution of inflammation and sepsis.
3. Prevention of stricture.
a. Barium esophograms beginning at 2 weeks to evaluate for stricture if asymptomatic, earlier if indicated.

b. Dilatation.
   1) Recommend beginning 2–3 weeks after burn if stricture develops.
   2) Early dilatation may cause perforation or accelerated fibrosis.
   3) Pass string or nasogastric tube to maintain lumen for further dilatation.
c. Stents.
   1) Removed after 3 weeks if placed during surgery.
   2) May be of some benefit if placed endoscopically after dilatation to maintain patency.
G. COMPLICATIONS.
1. Mediastinitis.
2. Pneumonitis.
3. Laryngeal edema.
4. Perforation.
5. Tracheo-esophageal fistula.
6. Strictures – 18%.
7. **Antral stenosis** appears as early as 5–6 weeks. Treatment is vagotomy with gastroenterostomy or pyloroplasty.
8. Esophageal carcinoma.
a. One to three thousand-fold increase in squamous cell carcinoma.
b. No evidence of increased gastric carcinoma.
9. **Mortality** is 3–37%.

V. PEARLS AND PITFALLS

1. **Overzealous mobilization of the esophagus** may lead to devascularization and necrosis, or stricture formation.
2. **Prior to oral feeding** a barium swallow should document the absence of leaks.
3. **A high index of suspicion**, aggressive diagnostic evaluation, and expeditious repair and drainage are essential when managing a patient with a potential esophageal injury.

VI. FURTHER READING

Feliciano DV. *Trauma,* 3rd edn. Stamford: Appleton and Lange; 1995:375–385.
Hood RM. *Thoracic trauma*. Philadelphia: WB Saunders: 1989:290–322.
Zuidema GD. *The management of trauma,* 4th edn. Philadelphia: WB Saunders; 1985:368–372.

GASTRIC TRAUMA

20

1. EPIDEMIOLOGY

1. **Gastric injuries** occur in 7–20% of cases of penetrating abdominal trauma.
2. **Blunt gastric trauma** is rare, occurring in only 0.4–1.7% of blunt abdominal injuries, but the incidence is increasing.
3. **Gastric trauma is more common in children than adults**.

II. ANATOMY

A. THE STOMACH lies well protected in the intrathoracic portion of the abdominal cavity.

B. THE GASTRIC WALL consists of the following layers:

1. **Serosa.**
2. **Muscularis mucosa.**
3. **Strong, well-vascularized submucosa.**
4. **Thick mucosa.**

C. BLOOD SUPPLY.

Common hepatic [handwritten annotation]

1. **Right gastric artery** – from the ~~splenic~~ artery; provides branches to the first portion of the duodenum and the pylorus.
2. **Left gastric artery** – branch of the celiac axis; primarily supplies the lesser curve of the stomach.
3. **Right gastroepiploic artery** – from the gastroduodenal artery; supplies the greater curve of the stomach.
4. **Left gastroepiploic artery** – from the splenic artery; supplies the greater curve of the stomach.
5. **Extensive collaterals** exist among these four vessels such that three of the four vessels can be ligated without necrosis or significant dysfunction.

III. MECHANISM OF INJURY

A. PENETRATING INJURY. Most penetrating injuries are secondary to stab wounds or gunshot wounds with only mild-to-moderate tissue destruction.

B. BLUNT INJURY.

1. **Blunt injuries occur** most commonly following motor vehicle collisions, motor–pedestrian collisions, or falls.
2. **Gastric distention** with a sudden increase in intraluminal pressure (as caused by compression of the abdominal wall by a seat belt during a deceleration injury) is felt to predispose to blunt gastric rupture. 60% of patients with blunt gastric injuries give a history of recent ingestion of a meal. (The benefits of seat belts have clearly been documented and outweigh the risk demonstrated here.)

3. **The most common sites** for blunt gastric injury are along the anterior surface of the stomach or the greater curvature.

IV. DIAGNOSIS
A. PENETRATING GASTRIC TRAUMA.
1. **All patients with gunshot wounds to the abdomen** undergo exploratory celiotomy at Parkland Memorial Hospital.
2. **Patients with abdominal stab wounds** are managed as follows:
a. Exploratory celiotomy without further workup in patients with evisceration, peritonitis, or hemodynamic instability.
b. Local wound exploration in stable patients, with an abdominal wound located anterior to the anterior axillary line and in whom it cannot be determined if fascial penetration has occurred. If the local exploration is equivocal or positive (i.e. fascial penetration has been identified or the end of the tract is not seen), the patient undergoes a diagnostic peritoneal lavage (DPL). If the DPL is positive, the patient then undergoes an exploratory celiotomy.
c. If the local wound exploration is negative, the wound may be thoroughly irrigated and closed.
3. **The presence of gross blood** in the nasogastric aspirate is suggestive of, but not diagnostic of, a gastric injury.
4. **The diagnosis of a gastric injury** is usually made at celiotomy.
5. **Penetrating gastric injuries** are frequently associated with liver, diaphragm, and colon injuries.
B. BLUNT GASTRIC TRAUMA.
1. **A high index of suspicion is required**. Many patients have associated head trauma, are impaired, or have distracting injuries making their physical examination unreliable.
2. **50–80% of patients** present with signs of shock or peritonitis.
3. **The diagnostic procedures available** for identifying blunt abdominal trauma in an unstable patient are:
a. Abdominal ultrasound.
b. DPL – if ultrasound is equivocal or not immediately available.
c. Four-quadrant paracentesis – used rarely.
d. Exploratory celiotomy – if reliable examination demonstrates peritonitis.
4. **Stable patients at risk for abdominal injury** are evaluated in one of three ways:
a. Abdominal ultrasound.
b. Abdominal CT.
c. DPL.
5. **Both CT and ultrasound lack adequate sensitivity** for identifying hollow viscus injury unless there is a large amount of free

intraperitoneal air or fluid. If the patient has an equivocal examination, ultrasound is repeated at 2–4 hours after the original examination.

6. **Free intraperitoneal air is not a constant finding** and is found in only 16–66% of blunt trauma patients with an abdominal injury.
7. **Associated injuries occur frequently with blunt gastric injury**. They are generally severe because of the amount of force needed to produce a gastric blowout. The organs commonly injured include the spleen, the liver, bone, and thoracic cavity structures.

V. MANAGEMENT

1. **Operative management is the rule** – there is no role for observation in the treatment of suspected gastric trauma.
a. Control of hemorrhage is the first priority.
b. Control of contamination, especially colonic, is the second priority.
c. Definitive control of specific organ injuries then follows.
2. **Sites of commonly missed gastric injuries** include:
a. The gastroesophageal junction.
b. The lesser and greater curves at the sites of omental or ligamentous attachments.
c. The posterior gastric wall – therefore, all omental and ligamentous attachments should be mobilized, if necessary for adequate visualization.
3. **Most gastric injuries** (98%) can be treated by simple débridement and primary repair.
a. Repair is usually performed with a two-layer closure.
b. The inner layer is closed with a running absorbable suture.
c. The outer layer is closed with interrupted silk Lembert sutures.
4. **If a gastroesophageal junction injury is suspected**, injuries to the aorta or the celiac plexus should also be anticipated.
a. If these are identified, vascular isolation should be performed before the gastroesophageal junction is exposed.
b. Vagus nerve injury should also be considered and, if necessary, a pyloroplasty performed.
5. **Distal antral injuries** can be treated by:
a. Simple two-layer closure.
b. Vagotomy and antrectomy if the injury is severe. The gastroduodenal anastomosis is a Billroth I or II, depending on the viability of the proximal duodenum.
6. **Care should be taken not to narrow the lumen** at the pylorus or gastroesophageal junction when performing a closure.
7. **Antibiotics are given at the time of surgery** and continued for 24 hours.
8. **Primary closure of the celiotomy incision** is the rule for isolated gastric injuries.

VI. POSTOPERATIVE CARE

1. **Associated injuries** cause the majority of complications and deaths.
2. **Short-term nasogastric suction** is generally required in patients with gastric injuries.
3. **Neutralization of gastric pH** is not necessary for isolated gastric injuries.

VII. PEARLS AND PITFALLS

1. **In the nondiseased state, the stomach contains few bacteria** secondary to its acid environment. Most trauma patients have normal gastric physiology and are, therefore, at very low risk for bacterial contamination from a gastric perforation alone. Patients on antacids or H_2-blockers, however, may have increased intraluminal bacterial counts and increased risk of intra-abdominal contamination.
2. **The lesser sac should be entered for visualization of the posterior gastric wall.** This step is mandatory in cases of anterior gastric wall injuries.

VIII. FURTHER READING

Durham R. Management of gastric injuries. *Surg Clin North Am* 1990; 70:517–528.

Wisner DH. Injury to the stomach and small bowel. In: Feliciano DV, Moore EE, Mattox, KL, eds. *Trauma,* 3rd edn. Stamford: Appleton and Lange; 1996:551–571.

PANCREATIC AND DUODENAL TRAUMA

I. EPIDEMIOLOGY

1. **Pancreatic injuries** occur in 3–12% of all abdominal trauma.
2. **Duodenal injuries** occur in 3–5% of all abdominal trauma.
3. **Penetrating injuries** are more common than blunt injuries in both pancreatic and duodenal trauma.

II. ANATOMY OF THE PANCREAS

A. ENTIRELY RETROPERITONEAL.

B. FOUR DIVISIONS.

1. **Head** (including the uncinate process) – lies within the duodenal C-loop.
2. **Neck** – portion anterior to the superior mesenteric vessels.
3. **Body** – crosses the spine.
4. **Tail** – lies within the splenic hilum.
5. **There are no distinct anatomic definitions of the four divisions**, but the proximal–distal division is defined where the superior mesenteric vessels cross the gland posteriorly.

C. DUCTAL SYSTEM.

1. **Main pancreatic duct of Wirsung.**
   a. Usually traverses the length of the entire gland.
   b. Shares a common channel with the common bile duct in 85% of patients.
2. **Accessory duct of Santorini.**
   a. Absent in 10% of patients.
   b. May serve as the main duct in 8–10% of patients.
   c. Empties into the duodenum approximately 2.5cm superior to the ampulla of Vater.

D. ARTERIAL SUPPLY.

1. **Gastroduodenal branches.**
   a. Anterior superior pancreaticoduodenal artery.
   b. Posterior superior pancreaticoduodenal artery.
2. **Superior mesenteric artery branches.**
   a. Anterior inferior pancreaticoduodenal artery.
   b. Posterior inferior pancreaticoduodenal artery.
3. **Short branches from the splenic and left gastroepiploic arteries.**
4. **Superior pancreatic artery** – origin variable.
5. **Inferior pancreatic artery**.

E. VENOUS DRAINAGE.

1. **Corresponds to arterial supply.**
2. **Empties into the portal vein.**

III. ANATOMY OF THE DUODENUM

A. **EXTENDS FROM THE PYLORUS** to the ligament of Treitz.

B. **FOUR PORTIONS.**

1. **Superior or 1st portion** – the only intraperitoneal portion.
2. **Descending or 2nd portion** – contains the entrance of common bile duct.
3. **Transverse or 3rd portion.**
4. **Ascending or 4th portion.**

C. **ARTERIAL SUPPLY.** This is the same as for the head of the pancreas.

IV. PANCREATIC INJURIES

A. **MECHANISM OF INJURY.**

1. **Approximately two-thirds of all pancreatic injuries** are the result of penetrating trauma.
2. **Blunt abdominal trauma** accounts for one-third of pancreatic injuries.
3. **Blunt injuries are usually secondary** to direct compression of the pancreas against the spinal column.
4. **The following mechanisms of injury** are associated with pancreatic trauma:
a. Direct blows to the upper abdomen – impact with the steering wheel is responsible for 60% of pancreatic injuries following motor vehicle collisions.
b. Bicycle handlebar injury.
c. High-riding lap restraining belts.

B. **ASSOCIATED INJURIES.**

1. **The majority of early morbidity and mortality** is related to exsanguination from associated vascular, liver, or splenic injuries.
2. **Major vascular injuries** occur in approximately 40% of patients with penetrating pancreatic trauma and in approximately 12% of patients with blunt pancreatic trauma.
3. **The most frequently associated organ injuries** are:
a. Liver.
b. Stomach.
c. Major arteries and veins.

C. **DIAGNOSIS.**

1. **Penetrating trauma.**
a. If the patient's hemodynamic status is stable, an abdominal radiograph obtained preoperatively for localization of the bullet may provide useful information.
b. The diagnosis of penetrating pancreatic injury is made at the time of abdominal exploration.
c. Clues suggesting potential injury include:
   1) Central retroperitoneal hematoma.

2) Peripancreatic or lesser sac edema.
3) Bile staining of the lesser sac, retroperitoneum, or peritoneal cavity.

2. Blunt trauma.

a. Patients with clear indications (e.g. peritonitis, or positive ultrasound or diagnostic peritoneal lavage) for exploratory celiotomy require no further evaluation.

b. Preoperative evaluation of hemodynamically stable patients is more challenging.

c. Physical signs and symptoms related to pancreatic injury include:
1) Epigastric pain out of proportion to examination in a reliable patient.
2) Contusion or abrasion across the upper abdomen.
3) Lower rib or costal cartilage separation.

d. Serum amylase, with or without fractionation, has not proven beneficial in aiding diagnosis.

e. Abdominal radiographs are suggestive of pancreatic injury if the following findings are present:
1) Ground-glass appearance in midabdomen, indicative of fluid or edema in the lesser sac.
2) Retroperitoneal air.
3) Obliteration of the psoas shadow.

f. Diagnostic peritoneal lavage is generally poor for diagnosing retroperitoneal injuries.

3. Abdominal ultrasound may suggest pancreatic injury if the following findings are present:

a. Fluid in the Morrison's pouch.

b. Fluid in the retroperitoneum.

4. Abdominal CT scans have a specificity and sensitivity of approximately 80% for pancreatic injuries. The following findings may be seen with pancreatic injury:

a. Pancreatic parenchyma disruption.

b. Areas of diminished pancreatic enhancement.

c. Peripancreatic fluid.

d. Fluid between the pancreas and splenic vein.

e. Fluid in the lesser sac.

f. Thickening of the left anterior renal fascia (Gerota's fascia).

5. Endoscopic retrograde cholangiopancreatography (ERCP) is performed in stable patients and may be of benefit in the following situations:

a. When CT has identified a pancreatic injury with questionable ductal integrity and the patient has no other injuries requiring abdominal exploration.

b. If a patient is unstable intraoperatively (hypotensive, hypothermic, coagulopathic) before an evaluation of the ductal system can be

PANCREATIC AND DUODENAL TRAUMA 21

performed, ERCP can be performed postoperatively after the patient has been stabilized.

6. **Intra-abdominal findings** suggestive of pancreatic injury are:
a. Central retroperitoneal hematoma.
b. Peripancreatic or lesser sac edema.
c. Bile staining of the lesser sac, retroperitoneum, or peritoneal cavity.

D. OPERATIVE EVALUATION.

1. **This requires that the entire gland be exposed.**
2. **The following maneuvers will facilitate exposure.**
a. Opening of the lesser sac exposes the anterior pancreatic surface.
b. Extended Kocher maneuver (extend medially to the superior mesenteric vessels) exposes the head of the pancreas and the uncinate process.
c. Mobilization of the hepatic flexure allows better inspection of the pancreatic head.
d. Mobilization of the splenocolic and gastrolienic ligaments allows forward and medial rotation of the spleen and facilitates inspection of the pancreatic tail and the posterior surface.
3. **Findings indicative of ductal injury** include:
a. Direct visualization of ductal disruption.
b. Complete or near-complete transection of the gland.
c. Laceration involving >50% of the gland diameter.
d. Central pancreatic perforation.
e. Severe maceration of the pancreas.
f. Blunt trauma may result in ductal injury without transection of the gland.
g. An intact pancreatic capsule does not ensure ductal integrity.
4. **Intraoperative techniques for pancreatography** include:
a. Needle cholecystocholangiogram.
b. A 16-18 gauge angiocath is inserted into the gallbladder (or the cystic duct) and 20–30mL of water-soluble contrast is injected.
c. Prevention of contrast reflux and better visualization of the pancreatic duct may be provided by contracture of the sphincter of Oddi with i.v. morphine or by direct finger compression of the proximal common bile duct.
5. **Duodenotomy.**
a. The major and minor papilla are directly cannulated.
b. 2–5 mL of water-soluble contrast is injected.
6. **Distal pancreatectomy.**
a. Two to five mL of water-soluble contrast is injected into the duct.
b. This procedure is rarely done because of the small size of the duct at this location and occasional excessive bleeding.
7. **Intraoperative ERCP** is a very useful test, but it is often difficult to obtain on a emergency basis.

8. **Secretin stimulation.**
a. Secretin is given i.v. at $1\mu g/kg$.
b. Direct visualization of pancreatic secretions from the site of suspected injury indicates ductal disruption.

E. **INJURY CLASSIFICATION.**

1. **Grade I hematoma** – minor contusion without duct injury.
2. **Grade II laceration** – superficial laceration without duct injury.
3. **Grade II hematoma** – major contusion without duct injury or tissue loss.
4. **Grade II laceration** – major laceration without duct injury or tissue loss.
5. **Grade III laceration** – distal transection or parenchymal injury with duct injury.
6. **Grade IV laceration** – proximal (medial to the mesenteric vessels) transection or parenchymal injury involving ampulla.
7. **Grade V** – massive disruption of pancreatic head.
8. **Advance one grade for multiple injuries** to the same organ.

F. **TREATMENT.**

1. **Treatment follows five basic principles** once the diagnosis of pancreatic injury has been made.
a. Control pancreatic bleeding.
   1) Electrocautery.
   2) Topical hemostatic agents.
   3) Direct suture ligation, with care taken to avoid ductal injury or ductal ligation.
b. Debride devitalized pancreas. The débridement should be minimal to avoid excessive hemorrhage and to allow time for demarcation of necrotic vs viable pancreas.
c. Identify ductal injuries.
d. Preserve at least 20% of functional pancreatic tissue if possible.
e. Provide adequate internal and external drainage of pancreatic injuries or resections.
   1) Internal drainage is provided by restoration of gastrointestinal and ductal anatomy where applicable.
   2) External drainage is best provided by closed-suction drainage. Sump drainage may also be used if necessary.
   3) The majority of complications following pancreatic injury result from failure to identify and control ductal injuries.

2. **Grade I and II injuries.**
a. Account for 80% of all pancreatic injuries.
b. Require only hemostasis and adequate external drainage.
c. Drains are generally left in place for 7–10 days with the following criteria required for removal:
   1) Patient tolerating oral feedings.
   2) Drain effluent <200mL per day.
   3) Drain amylase <serum amylase.

PANCREATIC AND DUODENAL TRAUMA

21

d. Feeding jejunostomy should be considered for any multiply injured trauma patient with even minor pancreatic injuries.

3. Grade III injuries.

a. Best treated by distal pancreatectomy.

b. Splenic salvage can be attempted in the stable patient.

c. Distal pancreatic resection may be performed with:
   1) A stapling device (e.g. TA-55). The duct should be oversewn with nonabsorbable monofilament suture.
   2) Sharp transection and suture control.

d. The duct should be identified and individually ligated with nonabsorbable monofilament suture using a 'U' stitch or 'figure of 8'.

e. Mattress sutures are used to control the parenchymal hemorrhage.

f. Omentum may be used to buttress the stump closure.

g. A closed-suction drain should be left near the suture or staple line and drain management is as above.

h. Feeding jejunostomy.

4. Grade IV and V injuries.

a. Evaluation of the pancreatic and common bile ducts is essential.

b. Injuries to the proximal gland without ductal injury are best managed by external drainage.

c. Injuries to the proximal gland and duct that spare the ampulla and the duodenum can be treated by:
   1) Distal pancreatectomy if the residual proximal gland size approximates to 20%.
   2) Transection of the pancreas at the site of injury, proximal duct ligation, and distal pancreaticojejunostomy if there is concern about the proximal gland being able to meet the necessary exocrine and endocrine functions (i.e. proximal gland size <20%).
   3) Pancreaticoduodenectomy is reserved for devascularization injuries or severe crush injuries with involvement of the ampulla or the duodenum.

G. COMPLICATIONS.

1. Injury to the pancreatic duct is the single most important determinant of outcome in patients with pancreatic injury.

2. Multiple organ failure and sepsis result in 30% of deaths in pancreatic trauma.

3. Fistula.

a. This is the most common complication, occurring in 10–35% of significant pancreatic injuries.

b. The majority are minor (<200mL per day) and resolve spontaneously in 2–4 weeks.

c. High-output fistulae (>700mL per day) are rare and may require surgical intervention for resolution.

d. If a high-output fistula persists for more than a few days, ERCP is indicated to determine if ductal obstruction is the cause.

e.   Somatostatin 50µg subcutaneously every 12 hours has a variable
     response in decreasing the fistula output and aiding fistula closure, but
     only after duct obstruction and infection have been ruled out as causes
     of the persistent fistula.

4. Abscesses.

a.   Occur in 10–25% of pancreatic trauma patients.
b.   Early drainage, either surgical or percutaneous, is essential.
c.   Mortality rate for these patients is 25%.

5. Pancreatitis.

a.   Occurs in 8–18% of patients after pancreatic surgery.
b.   Treated with nasogastric decompression, bowel rest, and nutritional
     support.
c.   If there is any question that necrotic pancreas remains, repeat
     exploration and débridement may be necessary.
d.   Hemorrhagic pancreatitis may be indicated by bloody drain effluent or
     a decrease in serum hemoglobin; the mortality rate may be as high as
     80%.
e.   May have secondary hemorrhage requiring transfusion.
f.   Occurs in 5–10% of pancreatic trauma patients.
g.   Generally occurs when pancreatic drainage after débridement is
     inadequate or when infection develops.
h.   May require reoperation or angiographic embolization for control.

6. Pseudocysts.

a.   May result from blunt pancreatic injuries that are overlooked or treated
     nonoperatively.
b.   Status of the pancreatic duct dictates the treatment.
c.   ERCP to determine the integrity of the duct should precede any
     intervention.
d.   If the duct is intact, percutaneous drainage should be sufficient therapy.
e.   If the duct is injured or stenosed, the treatment options include:
     1) Re-exploration and partial gland resection (preferred).
     2) Internal roux-en-Y drainage of the distal gland.
     3) Endoscopic transpapillary stenting of the injured duct.

V.   DUODENAL INJURIES

A.   MECHANISM OF INJURY.

1.   Approximately 85% of duodenal injuries result from penetrating
     trauma and 15% from blunt abdominal trauma.

2.   Blunt injury to the duodenum occurs by one of the following
     mechanisms.

a.   Crushing injury – occurs when a direct blow to the upper abdomen
     crushes the duodenum against the vertebral column (e.g. impact of
     steering wheel or bicycle handlebars into the abdomen).
b.   Bursting injury – occurs when the intraluminal pressure is greater than
     the bowel wall strength (e.g. seat belt obstruction of a loop of bowel).

   c. Shearing injury – occurs when the force of the deceleration exceeds the stabilizing force of the duodenum at the ligament of Treitz.

3. Blunt duodenal injuries have a higher mortality than penetrating injuries.

B. ASSOCIATED INJURIES.

1. The most common cause of early death in patients with duodenal injuries is exsanguinating hemorrhage from associated vascular, liver, or splenic injuries.

2. The most frequently associated organ injuries are:

a. Liver.

b. Major arteries and veins.

c. Colon.

C. DIAGNOSIS.

1. Penetrating trauma.

a. The diagnosis of penetrating duodenal injury is generally made at the time of abdominal exploration.

b. With gunshot injuries, a preoperative abdominal radiograph (if the patient's hemodynamic status allows) may be helpful for localization of the bullet.

2. Blunt trauma.

a. Blunt injuries to the duodenum are more difficult to diagnose than penetrating injuries.

b. Presenting symptoms may be vague, poorly localized, and delayed for 6–72 hours secondary to retroperitoneal location.

c. Physical findings may also be nonspecific, but may include contusions or abrasions across the upper abdomen, steering wheel or seat-belt marks, and midepigastric tenderness.

3. Serum amylase.

a. Poor indicator.

b. Only 53% of duodenal injuries have abnormal serum amylase determinations.

4. Abdominal radiographs may show:

a. Location of bullet or foreign body.

b. Mild scoliosis of lumbar spine to left.

c. Obliteration of right psoas shadow.

d. Retroperitoneal air along the lateral aspect of duodenum, superomedially to right kidney.

5. Upper gastrointestinal series.

a. May localize site of injury.

b. Initial study is performed with water-soluble contrast (Gastrografin) and, if negative, may be repeated with barium.

c. Intramural hematoma is suggested by a 'coiled spring' or 'stacked coin' appearance of the involved segment.

6. Diagnostic peritoneal lavage.

a. Poor test for retroperitoneal organ injury.

b. Amylase, bile, or food particles in lavage is suggestive of injury.

7. CT.

a. Use i.v. and oral contrast.

b. May demonstrate retroperitoneal air or edema, or extravasation of contrast.

c. May also demonstrate an intramural hematoma.

D. INTRAOPERATIVE EVALUATION.

1. Findings suggestive of duodenal injury are:

a. Central or right upper quadrant retroperitoneal hematoma.

b. Bile staining of peritoneal cavity, retroperitoneum, or lesser sac.

c. Retroperitoneal or peripancreatic fluid or edema.

d. Air or crepitus anterior or lateral to duodenum, or in the transverse mesocolon.

2. Injury classification.

a. Grade I hematoma – involving single portion of duodenum.

b. Grade I laceration – partial thickness, no perforation.

c. Grade II hematoma – involving more than one portion.

d. Grade II laceration – disruption <50% of circumference.

e. Grade III laceration – disruption 50–75% circumference of D2; disruption 50–100% circumference of D1, D3, and D4.

f. Grade IV laceration – disruption >75% circumference of D2; involving ampulla or distal common bile duct.

g. Grade V laceration – massive disruption of duodenopancreatic complex.

h. Grade V vascular – devascularization of duodenum.

E. TREATMENT.

1. Duodenorrhaphy is successful treatment in 70–85% of all duodenal wounds.

2. Grade I laceration.

a. Primary closure with care taken to avoid narrowing of the lumen.

b. Absorbable monofilament suture is preferred.

c. Intramural hematoma.

1) If diagnosed preoperatively and is an isolated injury, management is nonoperative using the following measures: nasogastric decompression, total parenteral nutrition, and serial Gastrografin studies every 5–7 days if there are no signs of resolving the obstruction. A celiotomy, with evacuation of the hematoma, should be considered if the signs of obstruction persist after 14–21 days of conservative therapy. Coagulation disorders are associated with this injury and should be evaluated with appropriate tests.

2) If diagnosed intraoperatively, the duodenum must be adequately inspected to rule out perforation. A Kocher maneuver may evacuate the hematoma although controversy exists over the intentional incision of the serosa to facilitate the evacuation. Either a gastrojejunostomy or feeding-tube jejunostomy should be considered at the time of exploration.

3. **Grade II lacerations.**
a. Treated by primary closure after minimal débridement.
b. The inner layer is closed with a running absorbable suture and the outer layer with an interrupted nonabsorbable suture.
c. The laceration is closed in a transverse direction if possible, to prevent narrowing of the duodenal lumen.
d. If the injury dictates longitudinal closure, a one-layer closure incorporating serosa, muscularis, and submucosa may prevent narrowing.

4. **Grade III injuries.**
a. Primary end-to-end anastomosis is procedure of choice.
b. Two-layer closure is advocated.
c. If the duodenum cannot be adequately mobilized for primary repair, a roux-en-Y jejunal limb can be anastomosed to the proximal duodenal limb with oversewing of the distal injury.
d. The use of gastric diversion or duodenal decompression via tube duodenostomy is controversial in these injuries. At Parkland Memorial Hospital, these techniques are generally reserved for more severe injuries.

5. **Grade IV injuries.**
a. Primary closure is rarely possible.
b. If the ampulla and bile duct are intact, a roux-en-Y duodenojejunostomy is the procedure of choice.
c. When the ampulla is disrupted, the choices for repair are reimplantation of the ducts or pancreaticoduodenectomy.
d. Reimplantation is performed as follows:
   1) The bile and pancreatic ducts are approximated using interrupted absorbable suture.
   2) An opening is made in the posterior duodenal wall.
   3) The joined bile and pancreatic ducts are approximated to the duodenum with interrupted full-thickness absorbable suture.
   4) The ductal repair should be stented and the duodenal repair diverted or decompressed.
e. Most commonly a pancreaticoduodenectomy is required for these injuries.

6. **Grade V injuries.**
a. Requires pancreaticoduodenectomy.
b. Drainage of the anastomotic sites and feeding jejunostomy are essential.

7. **Duodenal diversion and decompression.**
a. These are adjunctive procedures designed to protect the duodenal repair.
   1) Pyloric exclusion.

    2) Duodenal diverticulization.

    3) Tube duodenostomy.

b. Pyloric exclusion is performed with absorbable 3-0 suture or alternatively a TA-55 stapling device.

    1) The staple line should be just distal to the pylorus to avoid retained gastric antrum within the duodenum.

    2) Side-to-side gastrojejunostomy is performed at the site of the gastrotomy.

    3) The pylorus re-opens in 90% of patients within 2–3 weeks.

c. Feeding jejunostomy tubes should be placed in all patients requiring duodenal diversion.

    1) Grade I and II injuries do not require diversion or decompression.

    2) Controversy exists over use of these techniques in Grade III injuries, but if deemed necessary, tube duodenostomy is recommended.

    3) Grade IV and V injuries should have diversion or drainage.

8. **Duodenal injuries** are categorized as mild or severe.

a. Mild injuries generally undergo primary repair.

    1) Stab wounds.

    2) <75% of duodenal wall involved.

    3) Third or fourth portion injury.

    4) Injury-to-repair interval is <24 hours.

    5) No common bile duct injury.

b. Severe injuries require more complex repairs and may benefit from diversion or decompression.

    1) Blunt or missile injuries.

    2) 75% or more of duodenal wall involved.

    3) First or second portion injury.

    4) Injury-to-repair interval is >24 hours.

    5) Common bile duct injury present.

F. **POSTOPERATIVE CARE.**

1. **Postoperative management** follows the same guidelines as pancreatic injuries.

2. **Prior to resuming oral feeding**, the duodenal repair should be studied with an upper gastrointestinal series.

G. **COMPLICATIONS.**

1. **Postoperative complications are common** in duodenal injuries with only about one-third having an uncomplicated recovery.

2. **Duodenal fistula** is one of the two major complications after injury.

a. Usually presents after 5th postoperative day.

b. Signs indicating fistula are:

    1) Bilious drainage at drain site.

    2) Deterioration in patient status with fever, hypotension, and increased abdominal tenderness.

    c. Diagnosis is made by an upper gastrointestinal series in patients with an intact pylorus or through the drain or duodenostomy tube.

    d. Treatment is nonoperative initially, with bowel rest and adequate nutrition.

    e. If surgical intervention is required, the following procedures may be used:

        1) Duodenal exclusion.

        2) Roux-en-Y drainage.

        3) Duodenal diverticulization.

3. Duodenal obstruction is the other major complication after duodenal injury.

    a. Partial obstruction requires nonoperative treatment for at least 3–4 weeks.

    b. Complete obstruction.

        1) Nonoperative treatment initially.

        2) If no improvement after 1 week, consider operation.

        3) Gastrojejunostomy is most commonly used.

    c. Mortality within the 1st 72 hours is usually related to associated injuries.

        1) The overall mortality rate for duodenal injuries is around 20%.

        2) The duodenal injury itself is responsible for only 2% of these deaths.

VI. FURTHER READING

Credi RG. Pancreatic and duodenal trauma. In: Lopez-Viego MA, ed. *The Parkland trauma handbook*. St Louis: Mosby; 1994:243–264.

Jurkovich GJ. Injury to the duodenum and pancreas. In: Mattox KL, Feliciano DV, eds. *Trauma*. East Norwalk: Appleton and Lange; 1996:573–594.

Jurkovich GJ, Carrico CJ. Pancreatic trauma. *Surg Clin North Am* **1990,** 70(3):575–593.

Weigelt JA. Duodenal injuries. *Surg Clin North Am* 1990, 70(3):529–539.

SMALL BOWEL TRAUMA

I. EPIDEMIOLOGY

1. **The incidence of small bowel injury from penetrating trauma** exceeds 80%. Gunshot wounds account for the majority (80%), while the remainder (20%) are caused by stab wounds, etc.
2. **Together, the stomach and small bowel** represent the most commonly injured organs in penetrating trauma.
3. **The incidence of small bowel injury from blunt trauma** is 5–15%.

II. ANATOMY

1. **The small bowel**, from the ligament of Treitz to the ileocecal valve, has an average length of 250–260cm (160% of body height).
2. **The jejunum** is 105cm long
3. **The ileum** is 155cm long.
4. **The mesentery** extends from the left side of the L2 vertebral body downward to the right sacro-iliac joint. It crosses the:
   a. Third portion of the duodenum.
   b. Aorta.
   c. Inferior vena cava.
   d. Right gonadal vessels.
   e. Right ureter.
5. **The superior mesenteric artery** (SMA) is the main blood supply giving off the following branches:
   a. Numerous small intestinal branches.
   b. Ileocolic artery.
   c. Right colic artery.
   d. Middle colic artery.
6. **There are no major (named) blood vessels** connecting the root of the mesentery and the retroperitoneum. This allows mobilization of the entire small bowel and right colon mesentery cephalad to the inferior surface of the pancreas (Cattel maneuver).
7. **The superior mesenteric vein** corresponds to the SMA and receives branches from the small bowel and colon. It passes under the pancreas to join the inferior mesenteric vein and the splenic vein forming the portal vein.

III. MECHANISM OF INJURY

A. **PENETRATING INJURY.** Most penetrating injuries are secondary to stab wounds or gunshot wounds.
1. **Firearms cause damage** by direct force and by a lateral blast effect. Therefore, organ injury cannot be predicted by mentally constructing a line connecting entrance and exit wounds.

2. **Stab injuries** are usually less severe than gunshot wounds because the mobility of the small bowel allows the intestine to slide away from the offending object.
B. BLUNT INJURY. The mechanisms of injury are more varied and sometimes less obvious in blunt trauma. They include:
1. **Crushing injury** – violent force directly applied to the abdomen can crush the intestine between a firm object and the lumbosacral spine.
2. **Shearing injury** – with sudden deceleration, avulsion of the small bowel from fixed points of attachment (ligament of Treitz, ileocecal valve) may occur.
3. **Bursting (blowout) injury** (very rare) – rupture of a segment of the small bowel due to a sudden increase in intra-abdominal pressure and the occlusion of that segment of bowel both proximally and distally.
4. **There is a strong association between blunt intestinal injury and chance fractures** – transverse fracture through a lower thoracic or lumbar vertebral body caused by a flexion–distraction mechanism.
a. Chance fractures are usually caused by seat belts.
b. 25% of patients with small bowel injury requiring operative intervention will have multiple small bowel injuries, emphasizing the need to examine the entire small bowel at exploration.

IV. DIAGNOSIS
The diagnosis of small bowel injuries is similar to that of other abdominal trauma.
A. PENETRATING TRAUMA.
1. **All patients with gunshot wounds to the abdomen** undergo exploratory celiotomy. Exploratory celiotomy is indicated without further evaluation in patients with evisceration, peritonitis, or hemodynamic instability.
2. **Local wound exploration for anterior stab wounds** is indicated in stable patients, as outlined in Chapter 9. Positive local exploration mandates further evaluation, such as diagnostic peritoneal lavage (DPL). If DPL identifies a possible injury, the patient undergoes exploratory celiotomy.
B. BLUNT TRAUMA. The diagnostic procedures available for identifying blunt abdominal trauma in an unstable patient are:
1. **Abdominal ultrasound.**
2. **DPL** – if ultrasound is equivocal or not immediately available.
3. **Four-quadrant paracentesis** – used rarely.
4. **Exploratory celiotomy** – if reliable examination demonstrates peritonitis.
C. STABLE PATIENTS. Those patients at risk for abdominal injury are managed in one of three ways:
1. **Abdominal ultrasound.**

2. Abdominal CT.
3. DPL.

1. **Both CT and ultrasound lack adequate sensitivity** for identifying hollow viscus injury unless there is a large amount of free intraperitoneal air or fluid.
2. **If the patient has an equivocal physical examination**, and the original study was negative for injury, ultrasound is repeated in 2–4 hours from the original examination.

V. MANAGEMENT PRINCIPLES

1. **Operative management is the rule** – there is no role for observation in the treatment of suspected intestinal trauma.
2. **Preoperative antibiotics** effective against enteric flora are administered.
3. **Exploration is rapid and systematic** through a midline incision. Priorities are (listed in descending order):
   a. Locate and control hemorrhage.
   b. Control enteric contamination.
   c. Identify and repair injuries to abdominal organs and structures.
4. **The bowel is eviscerated** and both sides are examined in a systematic fashion (direction is irrelevant, but is generally from proximal to distal).
5. **Repair of injuries should not occur** until the entire small and large bowel have been inspected as these repairs may have to be resected if other injuries are identified that require resection of the involved segment.
6. **Mesenteric bleeding should be controlled** with suture ligation of the bleeding vessel only, with care not to compromise the blood supply to the bowel by taking deep mesenteric stitches.
7. **All but 50cm of the small bowel may be resected** without compromising bowel function. It is more important to preserve the ileum than the jejunum.
8. **Simple perforations and small lacerations are closed** using silk suture to perform a single-layer closure with Lembert sutures.
9. **Multiple small perforations should be repaired** in a distal to proximal fashion to minimize contamination.
10. **All wounds should be closed transversely** so that the bowel lumen is not compromised. Large serosal injuries should be repaired with a single layer of interrupted silk Lembert sutures. Small serosal injuries do not necessitate repair.
11. **Bowel of questionable viability should be resected** when possible, otherwise re-exploration within 24 hours is mandatory.
12. **In patients with multiple injuries** (including head trauma), a feeding jejunostomy tube should be considered.

22

SMALL BOWEL TRAUMA

13. **Resection and primary anastomosis is indicated** in the following situations:
a. Through-and-through wounds.
b. Devascularized segments.
c. Wounds >50% of the bowel diameter.
d. Multiple wounds in close proximity such that primary repair of all wounds would compromise the diameter of the bowel lumen.

VI. POSTOPERATIVE CARE

1. **Antibiotics are continued** for 24 hours postoperatively.
2. **Nasogastric suction is continued** until bowel function returns.
3. **Enteral feedings are started** as soon as possible.
4. **Patients are monitored closely** for early signs and symptoms of postoperative complications.

VII. COMPLICATIONS

1. **Bleeding** requires re-exploration.
2. **Wound and intraperitoneal infection and abscess** – intra-abdominal abscess requires open or percutaneous drainage.
3. **Fistula** – may be managed nonoperatively in the absence of distal obstruction, generalized peritonitis, signs of systemic sepsis, or high output.
4. **Anastomotic dehiscence** – rare (0.5–1% of all cases), but catastrophic if missed.
5. **Ischemic bowel** – may lead to obstruction or progress to necrosis with perforation.
6. **Missed injuries.**
7. **Short-gut syndrome.**

VIII. PEARLS AND PITFALLS

1. **Bacterial counts in the proximal small bowel** are $<10^4$ organisms/mL. Therefore, distal small bowel perforation carries a greater risk of intra-abdominal or wound infection than proximal small bowel perforation.
2. **A high index of suspicion with early operation is the key to avoiding serious consequences.** The peritoneal cavity can overcome contamination if the source of contamination is controlled, but it does not tolerate continued contamination.

IX. FURTHER READING

Blaisdell FW, Trunkey DD. Abdominal trauma. In: *Trauma management*. *Volume 1*. Thieme-Stratton; 1982:149–163.

Fayiga Y. Small bowel trauma. In: Lopez-Viego MA, ed. *The Parkland trauma handbook,* 1st edn. St Louis: Mosby; 1994:265–270.

Wisner DH. Injury to the stomach and small bowel. In: Feliciano DV, Moore EE, Mattox, KL, eds. *Trauma,* 3rd edn. Stamford: Appleton and Lange; 1996:551–571.

22

SMALL BOWEL TRAUMA

LIVER AND BILIARY TRACT TRAUMA

I. OVERVIEW

1. Hepatic injury is more common in patients with penetrating injuries (30%) than in patients with blunt abdominal trauma (15–20%).
2. **The overall mortality of liver trauma is approximately 10%.** Blunt injuries are usually more complex and result in mortality rates approaching 25%.
3. **Most deaths occur in the early postoperative period** (<48 hours) from shock and transfusion-related coagulopathies.

II. ANATOMY

1. **The right and left lobes of the liver** are separated by a plane from the gallbladder fossa to the inferior vena cava (IVC).
2. **The right and left hepatic veins are intraparenchymal** except for 1–2cm prior to entering the IVC.
3. **The middle hepatic vein** usually joins the left hepatic vein in the parenchyma of the liver (85%).
4. **The retrohepatic IVC** is 8–10cm in length and, along with the major hepatic veins, receives blood directly from numerous small hepatic veins.
5. **To mobilize the liver adequately,** its numerous ligamentous attachments must be incised. These include:
a. The falciform ligament.
b. The right and left triangular ligaments.
c. The coronary ligament.
   Care must be taken when incising these ligaments not to damage the phrenic or hepatic veins.

III. CLASSIFICATION OF HEPATIC INJURIES

The most recent and comprehensive classification system has been compiled by the Organ Injury Scaling Committee of the American Association for the Surgery of Trauma and includes findings on both the preoperative CT and intraoperative assessment of hepatic injuries (Table 23.1).

IV. INITIAL MANAGEMENT

A. **BLUNT OR PENETRATING INJURY.** Patients with severe blunt or penetrating injury usually present with hypotension or a distended abdomen. They require rapid resuscitation and should be taken immediately to the operating room (OR).
B. **GUNSHOT OR SHOTGUN WOUND.** The hemodynamically stable patient with an isolated gunshot wound or shotgun wound to the

TABLE 23.1

LIVER INJURY SCALE[a]

Grade		Injury description
I	Hematoma	Subcapsular, nonexpanding, <10% surface area
	Laceration	Capsular tear, nonbleeding, <1cm parenchymal depth
II	Hematoma	Subcapsular, nonexpanding, 10–50% surface area; intraparenchymal, nonexpanding, <2cm in diameter
	Laceration	Capsular tear, active bleeding, 1–3cm parenchymal depth, <10cm in length
III	Hematoma	Subcapsular, >50% surface area or expanding; ruptured subcapsular hematoma with active bleeding; intraparenchymal hematoma >2cm or expanding
	Laceration	>3cm parenchymal depth
IV	Hematoma	Ruptured intraparenchymal hematoma with active bleeding
	Laceration	Parenchymal disruption involving 25–50% of hepatic lobe
V	Laceration	Parenchymal disruption involving >50% of hepatic lobe
	Vascular	Juxtahepatic venous injuries, i.e. retrohepatic vena cava and major hepatic veins
VI	Vascular	Hepatic avulsion

[a]From the American Association for the Surgery of Trauma Classification System.

abdomen or chest (below the nipple) requires minimal preoperative studies. Initial resuscitation should include intubation and chest tubes as necessary, two large-bore upper extremity intravenous lines (i.v.s), Foley catheter, and a nasogastric tube. After marking the entrance and exit wounds, a scout film may be helpful to locate the presence of missiles.

V. DIAGNOSIS AND ASSESSMENT

1. **After completion of the primary and secondary surveys** the decision is made to explore the abdomen or perform further diagnostic studies.
a. If the patient has sustained a gunshot wound to the abdomen, exhibits signs of peritonitis, hemodynamic instability, or a distended abdomen then emergent surgical exploration is required.
b. Further evaluation should address other life-threatening injuries, but should not delay operative intervention.
2. **In the stable patient with a stab wound to the abdomen** and an otherwise normal abdominal examination further evaluation is undertaken to plan treatment.
3. **If the stab wound is anterior or in the flanks** (and tracks anteriorly) initial workup should include local exploration to document penetration of the posterior muscle fascia (see Chapter 9).
4. **If the local exploration is equivocal or positive** a diagnostic peritoneal lavage (DPL) is performed in the absence of any other indication for operation.

5. **Under these circumstances,** at Parkland Memorial Hospital, all patients with a positive DPL are taken to the OR.
6. **Diagnostic peritoneal lavage.**
1. **The principal disadvantages** of DPL include its invasiveness and, in patients with minor injuries, the test is positive even in the presence of minimal bleeding (20mL of blood in peritoneal cavity). Bleeding may have ceased at the time of celiotomy.
2. **This has led to the use of the CT scan** to evaluate patients for hepatic and other abdominal organ injuries after blunt trauma.
3. **Another modality being evaluated** in many centers is abdominal sonography to detect free fluid (presumably blood) in the peritoneum.

VI. NONOPERATIVE MANAGEMENT
1. **As a result of the significant incidence of nontherapeutic celiotomies,** isolated blunt hepatic injury is now frequently managed nonoperatively.
2. **The criteria for nonoperative management include:**
   a. Hemodynamic stability.
   b. Absence of abdominal tenderness.
   c. Ability for the surgeon to follow serial physical examinations (i.e. the patient is neurologically intact).
   d. Minimal transfusion requirements (2–4 units packed red blood cells).
3. **This approach requires careful observation of the patient,** usually in the intensive care unit, with serial examinations and hematocrits. These injuries may bleed slowly and physical signs may be evident only when the patient becomes hemodynamically unstable.
4. **Nonoperative management should not be viewed as conservative management.** It is clearly more difficult to manage the patients without knowing the full extent of their injuries.
5. **Nonoperative management should not lead to excessive blood transfusions** or delay in operative intervention should the clinical situation change.

VII. OPERATIVE MANAGEMENT
A. INITIAL MANAGEMENT.
1. **Initial preparations** should include measures to prevent hypothermia. A warmed OR, warm i.v. fluids, and a heating pad on the OR table are important considerations.
2. **The patient should be prepared and draped from the neck to the midthigh** to allow access to the chest, if necessary, and to allow access to the upper leg for harvesting a saphenous vein for a vascular injury.
3. **Prophylactic antibiotics are given** and a midline incision made from the xiphoid to the pubis if maximum exposure is deemed necessary. The incision may be extended to include a sternotomy if a retrohepatic vena cava or hepatic vein injury is present.

4. **All intraperitoneal blood should be quickly evacuated** and bleeding sources controlled with packs. The source of bleeding is then located by rapid examination of the liver, spleen, mesentery, bowel, and retroperitoneum.
5. **In patients with blunt trauma**, solid organ injuries are usually the source of bleeding and the gastrointestinal tract or retroperitoneal vascular injuries are less common.
6. **In patients with penetrating trauma**, however, injuries to the small bowel (60%), colon (40%), liver (30%), vascular structures (25%), and stomach (20%) are all common.

B. SIMPLE INJURIES (GRADES I AND II).

1. **The majority of hepatic injuries** (blunt 60% and penetrating 90%) are minor (grades I and II) and will have stopped bleeding at the time of operation. If bleeding persists in these minor injuries it can usually be managed by simple techniques, such as suture hepatorrhaphy, application of topical agents, or electrocautery.
2. **For 1–3cm deep bleeding lacerations**, suture hepatorrhaphy generally suffices.
   a. Finger fracture and direct ligation of the bleeding vessels is the most direct method of obtaining hemostasis.
   b. Horizontal mattress sutures of 0 chromic on a large blunt needle can be used to loosely approximate the liver parenchyma.
   c. Care must be taken not to strangulate (and subsequently necrose) the hepatic tissue.
3. **Topical agents**, such as Surgicel or Avitene, as well as others are useful once major hemorrhage is controlled. They are applied to the raw hepatic surfaces and compressed with laparotomy pads for 5–15 minutes and repeated as necessary.
4. **Fibrin glue** is not used at Parkland. There have been reports of severe adverse reactions when it is injected into injured hepatic parenchyma.

C. COMPLEX HEPATIC INJURIES (GRADE III OR GREATER).

1. **In the presence of extensive hepatic injury** and massive hemorrhage, the initial management of complex hepatic injuries should be the control of the hemorrhage with manual compression of the injury using laparotomy pads. This allows the anesthesiologist time to correct the hypovolemia and acidosis. After completion of intraoperative resuscitation, the liver is released and the injury is further addressed.
2. **Prior to definitive hemostatic control** of the liver injury, the portal triad should be occluded with either manual compression, a Rumel tourniquet, or an atraumatic vascular clamp (the Pringle maneuver) (Figure 23.1). This should control most bleeding unless there is a major retrohepatic venous injury.
3. **The liver can tolerate** up to 90 minutes of warm ischemia during elective liver resections without subsequent complication. This

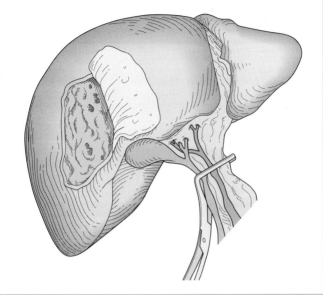

FIG. 23.1

Pringle maneuver using an atraumatic vascular clamp. (From Walt AJ, Levison MA. Hepatic trauma: juxtahepatic vena cava injury. In: Champion HR, Robbs JV, Trunkey DD, eds. *Rob and Smith's Operative Surgery*, 4th edn. London: Butterworths; 1983:378.)

experience cannot be extrapolated to the trauma setting, but it does suggest that the upper limit of warm ischemia is much longer than the 15–20 minutes previously reported.

D. **HEPATOTOMY.** Hepatotomy with selective vascular ligation is the most widely used method to control extensive bleeding in the depths of a laceration or in the tract of a penetrating wound.

1. **Glisson's capsule is incised.**

2. **The liver is finger fractured** through the parenchyma in the line of the laceration. The position of the left and right hepatic ducts must be visualized to avoid injuring them.

3. **Thin Deaver retractors are then inserted** into the open laceration and the bile ducts and vessels are selectively clipped or ligated.

4. **Large intrahepatic branches** of the portal or hepatic veins can be repaired using 5-0 or 6-0 monofilament suture.

5. **After hemorrhage is controlled** and necrotic parenchyma debrided, the resulting hepatotomy site can be filled with a pedicle of omentum based on the right gastroepiploic vessel (Figure 23.2).

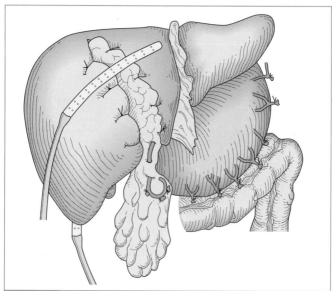

FIG. 23.2

Omental pedicle based on right gastro-epiploic artery packing a hapatotomy. (From Pachter HL, Liang HG, Hofstetter SR. Liver and biliary tract trauma. In: Moore EE, Mattox KL, Feliciano DV, eds. *Trauma,* 2nd edn. East Norwalk: Appleton and Lange; 1991:450.)

6. The liver edges are then loosely approximated with 0 chromic liver sutures.
7. The omentum will tamponade minor oozing, decrease dead space, and increase absorption of small amounts of blood and bile.
E. **DEEP LIVER SUTURING.** This technique, using mattress or simple sutures through uninjured liver to compress the area of injury, may control hemorrhage. However, deep liver suturing is not generally recommended because it fails to control bleeding which is deep to the sutures and may lead to liver necrosis and subsequent abscess.
F. **RESECTIONAL DÉBRIDEMENT.** This technique, which should not be confused with anatomic resection, is indicated when there is partially devascularized tissue on the liver edge or in a laceration.
1. Adequate débridement is essential to decrease the incidence of abscess formation.
2. If resectional débridement is used on the edge of a hepatic lobe it is not necessary to use an omental cover since it tends to trap fluid between it and the raw surface of the liver.

3. **Hepatic resection** refers to anatomic removal of a segment (or lobe) and is used in those patients with total destruction of a segment (or lobe) or when needed to control exsanguinating hemorrhage.

4. **Formal resection** is rarely used in trauma patients.

G. **SELECTIVE HEPATIC ARTERY LIGATION.** This specific type of ligation can be used to control arterial hemorrhage from the liver parenchyma.

1. **This maneuver is usually tolerated** because of the high oxygen saturation of the portal blood and it can be performed without subsequent hepatic necrosis.

2. **However, it is seldom used** since more selective intraparenchymal vessel ligation is preferable and it is ineffective in controlling bleeding from the portal and hepatic veins.

3. **Interventional radiology** has essentially replaced the need for hepatic artery ligation.

4. **This technique is indicated** in the rare instance when selective clamping of an extrahepatic artery causes cessation of arterial bleeding in a hepatotomy or laceration and the bleeding vessel cannot be seen inside the liver.

5. **A cholecystectomy** is recommended if the right hepatic artery is sacrificed.

H. **PERIHEPATIC PACKING.** This is indicated in patients with extensive uncontrolled lacerations, expanding subcapsular hematomas, transfusion-induced coagulopathy, severe hypothermia (<32°C), or acidemia (pH<7.2).

1. **The technique involves** placing either a small 30–45cm Steri-Drape which has been folded back onto itself or a vinyl or Dexon mesh directly on top of the liver surface.

2. **Multiple dry lap pads** are then placed on top of the drape or mesh until the ipsilateral hemidiaphragm is reached (Figure 23.3).

3. **Additional dry laps** may be inserted beneath the injured lobe as necessary.

4. **The abdomen is then closed** temporarily in a rapid fashion.

5. **The packing should be removed** after the patient has stabilized hemodynamically and the hypothermia, acidemia, or coagulopathy have been corrected. This usually occurs 24–72 hours after the initial operation.

6. **Re-operation after stabilization** also allows débridement of nonviable hepatic tissue, removal of clots, irrigation of the abdomen, and establishment of new drainage.

7. **The survival rate** with perihepatic packing approaches 75%, which is excellent in this group of high-risk patients. However, a 10–25% incidence of intra-abdominal sepsis (mainly subphrenic abscess) can be expected.

LIVER AND BILIARY TRACT TRAUMA

23

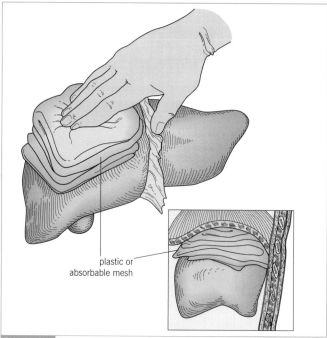

plastic or
absorbable mesh

FIG. 23.3

Perihepatic packing using a folded Steri-Drape and laparotomy pads. (From Feliciano DV et al. Packing for control of hepatic hemorrhage. *J Trauma* 1986; 26(8):738–743.)

I.   **INTERNAL TAMPONADE.** An internal tamponade of through-and-through liver injuries may be employed in patients who would otherwise require extensive hepatotomy and débridement.

1.   This is especially true in patients with extensive associated injuries and coagulopathy.

2.   The method involves passing a red rubber catheter through the missile tract.

a.   A pack made of several Penrose drains is tied to the end of the catheter and pulled back through the tract and left within the substance of the liver.

b.   The end of the Penrose pack is then brought through the skin.

c.   The pack tamponades the bleeding and serves as a drain.

3.   A similar situation can be achieved with a sterilized Sengstaken–Blakemore tube passed through the tract and inflated.

4. **Finally, a technique of balloon tamponade** can be performed utilizing a red rubber catheter and a Penrose drain tied at each end (Figure 23.4).
5. **Radiopaque contrast** can be instilled through the red rubber catheter to distend the Penrose drain and tamponade the bleeding.
J. **DRAINAGE.** For many years, drainage following liver injury was standard practice.
1. **It is now clear** that, if there are no apparent bile leaks, grade I or II injuries (see Table 23.1) usually do not require drainage.
2. **A simple method to evaluate the injury** is to place a lap pad over the area for several minutes and then examine it for bile staining.
3. **Complex hepatic injuries**, however, should be drained.
4. **Closed suction drainage** (Jackson–Pratt drain) is preferable for egress of blood and bile.
5. **Prospective trials** have shown conflicting results with both open and closed drains; therefore, it is important to individualize drainage in each patient.

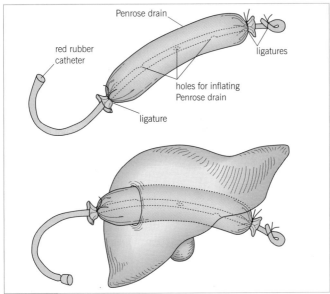

FIG. 23.4
Internal tamponade of penetrating liver injury using a red rubber catheter and Penrose drain. (From Morimoto RY, Birolini D, Junqueira AR Jr et al. Balloon tamponade for transfixing lesions of the liver. *Surg Gynecol Obstet* 1987; 164:87–88.)

K. **RETROHEPATIC INFERIOR VENA CAVA AND HEPATIC VEIN INJURIES.** Injuries to the retrohepatic IVC or hepatic veins are frequently lethal.

1. **If patients with these injuries are to survive**, it is critical that the injury is recognized early – prior to significant hemorrhage and coagulopathy.

2. **Techniques for repair** of these injuries require methods to decrease blood flow through this area and include total vascular isolation of the liver (clamping the supraceliac aorta, hepatoduodenal ligament, suprarenal IVC, and suprahepatic IVC sequentially) and the use of a transatrial chest tube or endotracheal tube shunts.

a. Vascular isolation of the liver can result in profound hypotension or cardiac arrest and is seldom used.

b. More often, a transatrial shunt (atriocaval) is used.

c. After a median sternotomy is performed, a 36F chest tube is passed through the right atrial appendage into the IVC with its distal end and side openings at the renal veins.

d. A side-hole made in the proximal end allows blood to flow from the shunt into the right atrium.

e. Rummel clamps are then tightened at the suprarenal and intrapericardial IVC.

3. **An alternative approach** utilizes an endotracheal tube as a shunt with a hole made in the proximal end in the right atrium (Figure 23.5).

a. This obviates the need to secure the suprarenal IVC since the balloon is inflated for occlusion.

b. An intracaval shunt can also be placed from below, thus eliminating the need to encircle the suprahepatic vena cava.

c. After the patient is shunted, the hepatic ligaments are taken down and the repair can be accomplished using standard vascular techniques.

4. **There is an occasional patient** who, after adequate mobilization of the liver, may be amenable to direct repair of the venous injury after a vascular clamp has been placed around the injury.

VIII. COMPLICATIONS

A. **RECURRENT BLEEDING.** This occurs in approximately 3% of all hepatic injuries but it increases to approximately 7% with complex (grade III or greater) injuries.

1. **If coagulopathy is excluded** and the patient's condition permits, reoperation and definitive control of specific bleeding is the procedure of choice.

2. **Perihepatic packing** can be used if the hemorrhage cannot be otherwise controlled.

3. **An alternative therapy**, especially with intrahepatic hemorrhage, is selective hepatic artery embolization in the angiogram suite.

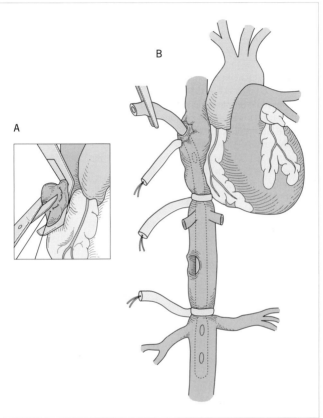

FIG. 23.5

Atriocaval shunt using a 36F chest tube. (From Pachter HL, Liang HG, Hofstetter SR. Liver and biliary tract trauma. In: Moore EE, Mattox KL, Feliciano DV, eds. *Trauma*, 2nd edn. East Norwalk: Appleton and Lange; 1991:450.)

B. **INTRA-ABDOMINAL ABSCESSES.** These abscesses occur in 2–10% of all cases of hepatic trauma and are related to the extent of hepatic injury, other associated injuries (especially colonic), the number of transfusions, and the type of drainage.

1. **If a perihepatic abscess does occur,** percutaneous CT-guided drainage is the treatment of choice with a success rate of >90%.

2. **If reoperation is necessary,** it is acceptable to perform the procedure through the previous incision to allow thorough exploration.

3. **An alternative method** is the extraperitoneal approach through the bed of the 12th rib thereby eliminating the need for a repeat celiotomy.

C. **BILIARY FISTULA.** This complication, as defined by >50mL of biliary drainage per day for 2 weeks, occurs in a small number of patients following hepatic injury (1–10%).

1. **Biliary fistula can most often be managed conservatively** with continued drainage and only rarely is there a need for reoperation.

2. **Endoscopic retrograde cholangiopancreatography (ERCP) and endoscopic drainage or stenting** may also be utilized in patients with persistent fistulae.

D. **HEMOBILIA.** This is another rare complication following hepatic trauma and usually presents after the patient has been released from hospital 4–30 days after injury.

1. **Approximately one-third of patients** present with the classic triad of right upper quadrant pain, gastrointestinal tract hemorrhage, and jaundice.

2. **Bleeding may be intermittent** and thus obtaining a history of trauma and high index of suspicion are key to making the diagnosis.

3. **The diagnosis is confirmed** by angiography and is treated by embolization of the offending artery. Surgical treatment is rarely required.

IX. GALLBLADDER INJURIES

A. **OCCURRENCE.** Injuries to the gallbladder are uncommon and are almost always associated with other intra-abdominal injuries.

B. **CLASSIFICATION.** Gallbladder injuries are classified into four categories:

1. Rupture.

2. Avulsion.

3. Contusion.

4. **Cholecystitis** (secondary to blood obstructing the cystic duct).

C. **TREATMENT.** The usual treatment for trauma is cholecystectomy; however, lesser procedures, such as cholecystostomy, may be desirable in the trauma patient with a coagulopathy or cirrhosis, or in the hemodynamically unstable patient where dissection of the gallbladder bed may lead to additional uncontrolled hemorrhage.

X. EXTRAHEPATIC BILE DUCT INJURY

A. **OCCURRENCE.** These injuries occur in 3–5% of patients with abdominal trauma.

1. **There is a high incidence** of associated intra-abdominal injury.

2. **The common bile duct** is injured most frequently followed by the right hepatic duct and then the left hepatic duct.

B. **MANAGEMENT.** Initial management begins as with any intra-abdominal injury.

1. **Control hemorrhage first**.
2. **Then obtain adequate exposure** if a bile duct injury is suspected. This usually involves performing a wide Kocher maneuver.

C. **DIAGNOSIS.** This is often facilitated by obtaining an intraoperative cholangiogram.

D. **CLASSIFICATION.** Injuries are categorized as simple (involving <50% of ductal wall) or complex (>50% of ductal wall or transection).

1. **Simple injuries** are usually managed by primary repair, placement of a T-tube, and drainage. T-tube placement may be difficult in a small normal bile duct.
2. **Complex injuries** generally require construction of roux-en-Y choledochojejunostomy (Figure 23.6) since primary repair is more often complicated by stricture formation.

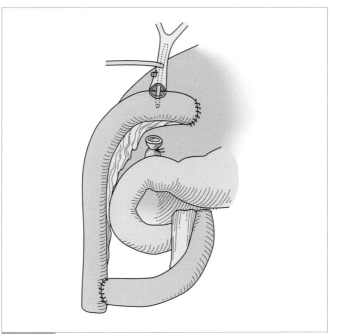

FIG. 23.6
Roux-en-Y choledochojejunostomy using one-layer anastomosis and T-tube decompression. (From Pachter HL, Liang HG, Hofstetter SR. Liver and biliary tract trauma. In: Moore EE, Mattox KL, Feliciano DV, eds. *Trauma,* 2nd edn. East Norwalk: Appleton and Lange; 1991:450.)

23

LIVER AND BILIARY TRACT TRAUMA

XI. PORTA HEPATIS INJURIES

A. **OCCURRENCE.** Porta hepatis injuries are rare and are usually associated with multiple intra-abdominal injuries.

1. **The portal vein** is the most commonly injured structure in the porta hepatis followed by the bile ducts and the hepatic artery.

2. **If the hepatic artery is injured** (and the portal vein is not) the most expedient solution is ligation.

B. **TREATMENT.** If the portal vein is also injured the artery or vein should be repaired.

1. **Portal vein injuries** are repaired with a lateral venorrhaphy if possible; however, if this is not possible then ligation of the vein is the preferred treatment.

2. **This will result in splanchnic sequestration** of blood and patients must have their fluid status monitored.

3. **On occasion it may be possible to place an interposition graft,** such as the left renal vein, in order to restore the portal circulation.

XII. PEARLS AND PITFALLS

1. **Upon first encountering a rapidly bleeding liver injury,** bimanual compression of the surrounding liver parenchyma can stop the hemorrhage and allow the anesthesia team to correct severe hypovolemia and shock.

2. **If hemorrhage continues after application of the Pringle maneuver,** then the patient must be considered to have a significant hepatic venous injury or an anomalous hepatic artery.

XIII. FURTHER READING

Delva E. Vascular occlusions for liver resections: operative management and tolerance to hepatic ischemia: 142 cases. *Ann Surg* 1989; 209:211.

Feliciano D. Management of 1000 consecutive cases of hepatic trauma (1979–1984). *Ann Surg* 1986; 204:438–445.

Huguet C, Nordlinger B, Bloch P. Tolerance of the human liver to prolonged normothermic ischemia. *Arch Surg* 1978; 113:1448.

Ivatury R, Stahl W. Liver trauma. *Adv Trauma* 1989; 4:193–210.

Pachter HL, Liang HG, Hofstetter SR. Liver and biliary tract trauma. In: Moore EE, Mattox KL, Feliciano, eds. *Trauma,* 3rd edn. Stamford: Appleton and Lange; 1996:487–523.

Weigelt, JA. The liver. In: Trunkey DD, Lewis FR, eds. *Current therapy of trauma,* 3rd edn. B.C. Decker: 1991:247–251.

23

LIVER AND BILIARY TRACT TRAUMA

SPLENIC TRAUMA

I. ANATOMY

A. **LOCALIZATION.** The spleen is found in the posterior left upper quadrant of the abdomen and is confined by the gastric fundus, left hemidiaphragm (at the level of the 9th–11th rib), left kidney, and splenic flexure of the colon.

B. **ATTACHMENTS.** The attachments include the splenophrenic, splenorenal, and splenocolic ligaments (relatively avascular, except for patients with portal hypertension), the gastrosplenic ligament (containing short gastric vessels), and attachments to the pancreas.

C. **PERITONEAL FOLDS.** The splenomental (often responsible for iatrogenic surgical injuries) and minor folds extend near the upper pole and the hilus.

D. **CAPSULE.** This consists of an external thin peritoneal layer and an internal fibroelastic layer, which is thicker and more elastic in children. In elderly and those with prior injuries it may be firm and thickly scarred.

E. **ACCESSORY SPLEENS.** These are present in 14–30% of patients.

F. **BLOOD SUPPLY.**

1. **The amount** is approximately 5% of the cardiac output.

2. **The arterial supply** is derived from the celiac artery (both the splenic artery and the short gastric arteries which are usually branches of the gastroepiploic or splenic arteries).

3. **Venous drainage.** The splenic vein is formed by a number of trunks arising at the hilus, receiving the left gastroepiploic, pancreatic, and often inferior mesenteric veins.

II. SPLENIC FUNCTION

A. **FILTRATIVE.** Mechanical filtration of particulate antigens, encapsulated microorganisms, and senescent or diseased cells, facilitated by lack of endothelium in the splenic cords.

B. **IMMUNOLOGIC.** Major reservoir of B lymphocytes, removal of bacteria and antibodies by immunocompetence cells, initiation of immune response, production of opsonin (properdin and tuftsin) and specific antibody, especially IgM.

C. **PITTING.** This is the excision of nuclear remnants (Howell–Jolly bodies) and other intraerythrocytic inclusions.

III. EPIDEMIOLOGY

A. **NONPENETRATING TRAUMA.** The spleen is the most commonly injured organ from blunt trauma to the abdomen or lower chest. Most frequent causes include automobile crashes, falls, and forces associated with contact sports.

B. **PENETRATING TRAUMA.** This is generally due to gunshot wounds or stab wounds to the lower chest or abdomen.

C. **INTRAOPERATIVE IATROGENIC TRAUMA.** This accounts for 20% of splenic injuries, usually as a result of excessive traction or mobilization of the stomach and colon.

D. **MORTALITY.** The overall rate is approximately 11.5%. Contributing factors include associated injury, mechanism of injury, presence of shock, and advanced age.

IV. MECHANISMS OF INJURY

1. **Blunt injury.**
2. **Deceleration** – usually produces capsular avulsions and tears in vascular collaterals, short gastric vessels, or hilar vessels.
3. **Blunt compression** – results either in a fracture according to segmental anatomy or in stellate fractures (when compression does not parallel segmental anatomy).
4. **Penetrating injuries** – gunshot wounds and stab wounds.
5. **Delayed rupture** – the interval between injury and rupture is called the latent 'period of Baudet'. This is a rare occurrence, which takes place days to weeks after initial injury, that results in subcapsular hematoma. The recognition of delayed rupture is decreased with the use of a CT scan.

V. DIAGNOSIS

A. **CLINICAL MANIFESTATIONS.**

1. **The history of the injury** may be seemingly slight, followed by nonspecific upper abdominal pain (30%), left shoulder pain (15-75%), or syncope.
2. **A physical examination** is accurate 65% of the time and includes left upper quadrant tenderness, referred left shoulder pain (Kehr's sign), fixed dullness to percussion on the left, and shifting dullness on the right (Ballance's sign).
3. **Clinical signs** include a slight to moderate reduction of the blood pressure, tachycardia, a reduction of hematocrit, and a moderate increase in the white blood cell count.

B. **PLAIN RADIOGRAPHS.** These are not a reliable diagnostic study but they may show left lower rib fractures (associated with splenic injury in 20% of patients), elevated left hemidiaphragm, left pleural effusion, intrathoracic gastric air bubble, an enlarged splenic shadow, or medial displacement of the gastric shadow.

C. **ULTRASOUND.**

1. **Can provide evidence of free fluid and pericapsular hematoma.** There is a high sensitivity for detection of free fluid in blunt trauma.
2. **Not useful for grading the degree of injury.**
3. **Used for follow-up of injuries** that are managed nonoperatively.

D. COMPUTED TOMOGRAPHY.
1. **The procedure of choice** for diagnosis and the estimation of the severity of splenic injury in the hemodynamically stable patient.
2. **CT contrast blush** (intraparenchymal hyperdense contrast collection) predicts failure of nonoperative management.
3. **Used for follow-up of the injuries** that are managed nonoperatively but it is generally not necessary unless there is a change in the clinical condition.

E. DIAGNOSTIC PERITONEAL LAVAGE.
1. **A safe, efficient, rapid, and inexpensive diagnostic study** but it is not organ specific.
2. **Recommended in the hemodynamically unstable patient.**
3. **Can lead to nontherapeutic laparotomy** rates of 6–25%.
4. **Positive** if >100,000 red cells/mm^3.

F. ANGIOGRAPHY.
1. **Rarely used in the diagnosis of this injury.**
2. **Primary indication** is selective splenic artery embolization in rare cases.

G. EXPLORATION.
1. **Mandatory in gunshot wounds to the abdomen**, or shock after blunt trauma.
2. **Low morbidity** associated with nontherapeutic procedures.

H. GRADING. The classification of splenic injury is given in Table 24.1.

VI. MANAGEMENT

A. NONOPERATIVE.
1. **Standard of care for low-grade** (mainly grade I–II and some grade III) isolated splenic injury in hemodynamically stable, nonintoxicated patients.
2. **Guidelines for nonoperative management of splenic injuries**:
a. Minimal or no abdominal findings.
b. Hemodynamic stability.
c. Minimal laboratory evidence of blood loss.
d. Low-energy trauma.
e. Isolated splenic injury on CT scan.
f. No hilar involvement or massive disruption on CT scan.
3. **Patient care** – hospital admission and monitoring is mandatory, preferably in the intensive care unit for the first day or two, with serial hematocrit determinations and constant availability of the operating room and surgeon.
4. **The recovery period** includes restricted activity (no contact sports, running, or similar stresses) for 1–3 months following injury, or until healing is documented.
5. **A blood transfusion** is used to keep the hematocrit >20–25%. This significantly increases the risk for perioperative infection and respiratory complication. If the transfusion requirement exceeds 2 units the patient should be seriously considered for surgery.

24

SPLENIC TRAUMA

TABLE 24.1

SPLENIC INJURY SCALE

Injury grade	Hematoma	Laceration
I	Subcapsular, nonexpanding, <10% surface, area	Capsular tear, nonbleeding, <1cm of parenchymal depth
II	Subcapsular, nonexpanding, 10–50% surface area; intraparenchymal <2cm in diameter	Capsular tear, active bleeding; 1–3cm parenchymal depth that does not involve A trabecular vessel
III	Subcapsular, >50% surface area or expanding; ruptured subcapsular hematoma with active bleeding; intraparenchymal >2cm or expanding	>3cm parenchymal depth or involving trabecular vessels
IV	Ruptured intraparenchymal hematoma with active bleeding	Involving segmental or hilar vessels producing major (>25% of spleen) devascularization
V	Major bleeding	Completely shattered or pulpified spleen with hilar disruption, devascularization, or avulsed fragments

6. **Conversion to surgical intervention** is taken at the first sign of hemodynamic instability, increased abdominal tenderness, inability to serially examine abdomen (e.g. intubation, operation for other injuries, head injury), and necessity of blood transfusions in the case of continuation of nonoperative management.

B. **OPERATIVE.**

1. **The indications include** hemodynamic instability, major splenic injury (grade IV–V), the failure of nonoperative management, and the presence of other intra-abdominal injuries.

2. **Incision and exposure** is made with a vertical midline celiotomy (from the xiphoid to below the umbilicus) with complete exposure of the spleen: gentle right retraction with the nondominant hand of the surgeon and countertraction of the left abdominal wall by assistant (Figures 24.1–24.3).

3. **The of operative management** include splenorrhaphy, partial splenectomy, and total splenectomy depending on the nature and extent of injury.

a. Factors contributing to operative splenic salvage are listed in Table 24.2.

b. Treatments for various degrees of injury are summarized in Table 24.3.

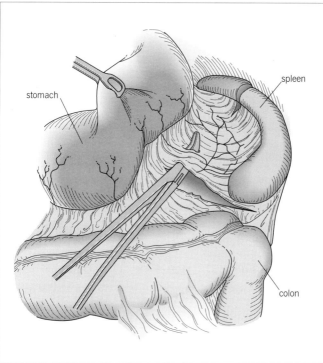

FIG. 24.1

The gastrolienal ligament is triangular, with its apex cephalad. Division of this ligament requires ligation of the short gastric vessels. (From Moore FA, Moore EE, Abernathy CM. Injury to the spleen. In: Moore EE, Mattox, KL, Feliciano DV, eds. *Trauma,* 2nd edn. East Norwalk: Appleton and Lange; 1991.)

TABLE 24.2

FACTORS CONTRIBUTING TO CHOICE OF OPERATIVE MANAGEMENT

Indication for operative splenic salvage	Indication for splenectomy
Blood loss <500mL (1/3 blood volume in pediatric patients)	Blood loss >1000mL
Minimal associated injuries	Significant associated injuries
No hilar involvement	Hilar involvement
Minimal or moderate degree of splenic injury	Massive splenic disruption
No coagulopathy	Coagulopathy

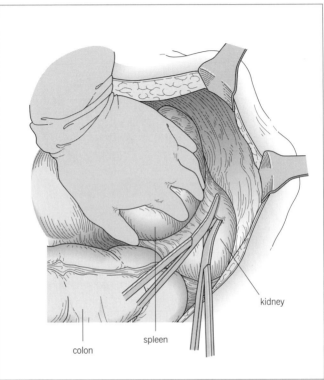

FIG. 24.2
Mobilization of the spleen is carried out by early division of the lienorenal ligament.
(From Moore FA, Moore EE, Abernathy CM. Injury to the spleen. In: Moore EE,
Mattox, KL, Feliciano DV, eds. *Trauma,* 2nd edn. East Norwalk: Appleton and Lange;
1991.)

TABLE 24.3

SUMMARY OF TREATMENTS FOR VARIOUS DEGREES OF SPLENIC INJURY

Grade	Treatment
I	Observation
II	Observation or splenorrhaphy
III	Débridement, evacuation of clot, suture ligation of bleeding vessels; splenorrhaphy in selected cases; splenectomy for indications in Table 24.2.
IV	Partial or total splenectomy
V	Splenectomy

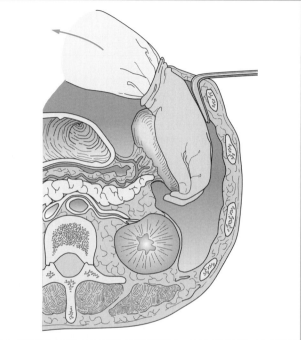

FIG. 24.3
Further blunt dissection is performed in the plane between the pancreas and retroperitoneal structures. (From Moore FA, Moore EE, Abernathy CM. Injury to the spleen. In: Moore EE, Mattox, KL, Feliciano DV, eds. *Trauma,* 2nd edn. East Norwalk: Appleton and Lange; 1991.)

4. **Splenorrhaphy.**
a. Applied mainly in grade II and III injuries.
b. The techniques include topical hemostatic agents (Avitene, gelatin sponge, topical thrombin, and absorbable knitted fabrics, e.g. Surgicel), electrocautery, argon laser, Vicryl or Dexon suture repair with or without Teflon pledgets, and absorbable mesh or omental wraps (Figures 24.4 and 24.5)
5. **Partial splenectomy.**
a. Used mainly in grade IV splenic injury.
b. Can be performed with stapler or with sharp dissection and suture approximation.
c. At least 30% of the spleen must be retained to obtain preservation of immune function.

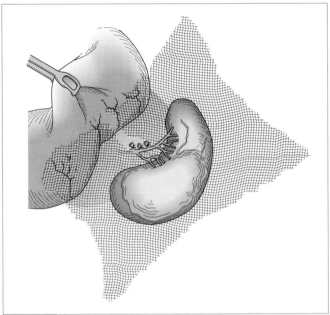

FIG. 24.4

With capsular loss, the spleen may be encased in a woven polyglycolic acid mesh. (From Moore FA, Moore EE, Abernathy CM. Injury to the spleen. In: Moore EE, Mattox, KL, Feliciano DV, eds. *Trauma,* 2nd edn. East Norwalk: Appleton and Lange; 1991.)

6. **Splenectomy** is indicated in massive irreparable injury, such as grade IV–V.
7. **Mobilization of the spleen** involves the division and ligation of all peritoneal folds and anterior attachments with their vessels followed by the division of the posterolateral attachments including the splenorenal ligament.
8. **Control of vasculature.**
a. Occlusion of the hilar vessels with the thumb and forefinger of the nondominant hand can be useful.
b. Controlled ligation and division of the segmental vessels is best performed posterior to the spleen.
c. Intrasplenic vessels are controlled by hemoclip or silk suture.
d. Residual sinusoidal ooze is eliminated by the application of microfibrillar collagen.

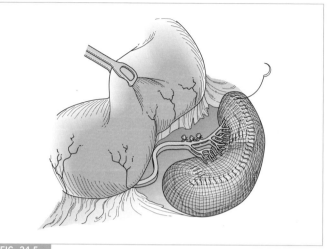

24

SPLENIC TRAUMA

FIG. 24.5

The mesh is sutured along the anterior surface of the spleen. (From Moore FA, Moore EE, Abernathy CM. Injury to the spleen. In: Moore EE, Mattox, KL, Feliciano DV, eds. *Trauma,* 2nd edn. East Norwalk: Appleton and Lange; 1991.)

9. **Replacement and drainage.**
a. Repaired or partially resected spleen is carefully repositioned in the upper left quadrant.
b. Intraperitoneal drainage for the splenic bed is not recommended unless there has been pancreatic injury or suspicion of such.

10. **Postoperative care.**
a. At least 24 hours in the intensive care unit.
b. Careful monitoring of clinical signs, hemoglobin, and hematocrit.

VII. POSTOPERATIVE COMPLICATIONS

A. **THE MOST COMMON** include atelectasis, left pleural effusion, and pneumonia.

B. **LEFT SUBPHRENIC HEMATOMA OR ABSCESS** have multiple causes, including pancreatic or gastric injury, inadequate hemostasis, use of drains in the splenic bed, and immunologic impairment.

C. **PANCREATIC OR GASTRIC INJURY.**

1. **Must be considered** in patients with postoperative sepsis. Injuries to pancreas may result in pancreatitis or fistula.

2. **Devascularization of the greater curvature of the stomach** with subsequent necrosis and perforation may sporadically occur.

3. **It is less likely to occur** with intraoperative decompression of the stomach.
D. POSTOPERATIVE BLEEDING.
1. **Requires re-exploration in 1.5% of patients.**
2. **Results from inadequate hemostasis** or from a coagulation disorder.
E. CHANGES IN BLOOD COMPOSITION.
1. **Thrombocytosis** (increase in platelet count $>400,000/cm^3$ that occurs 2–10 days after splenectomy) and leukocytosis are generally observed.
2. **In case of severe thrombocytosis** (platelets $>1,000,000$) aspirin and heparin are seriously considered for thrombosis prevention.
F. INFECTION.
1. **Asplenic patients** are subject to a variety of infections at a greater rate than that of the general population.
2. **Infections of most concern** include overwhelming postsplenectomy sepsis, fulminant bacteremia, pneumonia, and meningitis.
3. **Blood transfusions** increase the risk of infection.
G. OPERATIVE MORTALITY.
1. **For isolated penetrating injury** – $<1\%$.
2. **For isolated blunt trauma to the spleen,** 5–15%; with concomitant serious injuries, 15–40%.

VIII. OVERWHELMING POSTSPLENECTOMY SEPSIS

1. **Risk** – 0.6% in children and 0.3% in adults.
2. **Clinical features.**
a. Upper respiratory infection progressing to fulminant sepsis, associated with diffuse intravascular coagulation or adult respiratory distress syndrome, and adrenal insufficiency.
b. In most cases there is no identified site of infection.
3. **Symptoms** – abrupt onset of fever, chills, worsening headache, nausea, vomiting, diarrhea, and overwhelming weakness progressing to prostrate state.
4. **Laboratory studies** – hypoglycemia, acidosis, electrolyte imbalance.
5. **Blood culture** is tested mainly for encapsulated microorganisms including *Streptococcus pneumoniae* (in 50% of cases), *Haemophilus influenzae, Neisseria meningitidis, Escherichia coli,* staphylococcus and other streptococci.
6. **Mechanism** – failure of filtration of encapsulated organisms and defective function of reticuloendothelial system in clearing intravascular antigens, as well as decreased opsonization.
7. **Time of occurrence** is from weeks to many years after splenectomy in 50% of cases within the first 2 years.
8. **Mortality** is $>50\%$ of patients with overwhelming postsplenectomy sepsis.

IX. PREVENTATIVE MEASURES FOR OVERWHELMING POSTSPLENECTOMY SEPSIS

A. IMMUNOPROPHYLAXIS.

1. **Vaccination** with pneumococcus, meningococcus and *Haemophilus influenzae* type B as soon as possible after operation.
2. **Booster injections** every 5 years are recommended.
3. **Children <2 years of age** have a poor immune response to polysaccharide vaccine.
4. **Protein–polysaccharide vaccine** can be useful.

B. CHEMOPROPHYLAXIS.

1. **Oral penicillin or erythromycin** (250–500mg twice daily) for 1–2 years is controversial.
2. **Cefatriaxone** if fever develops in a patient taking penicillin.
3. **Upon cessation of penicillin prophylaxis**, amoxicillin should be immediately available to the patient in case of the onset of fever.
4. **Antibiotic prophylaxis** is usually not given to adults unless they develop a fever.

C. EDUCATION.
The patient should be informed about the risk of infection and advised to wear medical alert identification and seek immediate medical attention for any fever.

D. SPLENIC AUTOTRANSPLANTATION.
This technique is not used at Parkland Memorial Hospital.

X. FURTHER READING

Lucas CE. Splenic trauma. Choice of management. *Ann Surg* 1991; 213:98–112.

Morgenstern L. Splenic repair and partial splenectomy. In: Nyhus LM, Baker RJ. *Mastery of surgery.* Boston: Little Brown; 1992:1102–1109.

Sheldon GF, Croom RD III, Mayer AA. The spleen. In: Sabiston DC, ed. *Textbook of surgery*, 15th edn. Philadelphia: WB Saunders; 1997:1187–1214.

Shires GT, Thal ER, Jones RC, Shires GT III, Perry MO. Trauma. In: Schwartz SI, Shires GT, Spencer FC, eds. *Principles of surgery,* 6th edn. New York: McGraw–Hill; 1994:212–214.

Wisner DH, Blaisdell FW. When to save the ruptured spleen. *Surgery* 1992; 11:121–122.

COLON AND RECTAL TRAUMA

EPIDEMIOLOGY

A. **COLON INJURY OCCURRENCE.** Colon injuries occur in 15–39% of penetrating abdominal wounds.

1. **Large bowel trauma** tends to occur more often in association with injuries to other organs rather than as an isolated injury.
2. **The frequency of colon injuries** ranks second only to small bowel injuries from gunshot wounds and ranks third behind small bowel and liver injuries from abdominal stab wounds.
3. **Blunt trauma** to the colon is rare (<5%).
4. **The right colon** is the most common site of devascularizing injuries.
5. **A blowout injury** results from the sudden compression of air-filled bowel when seat belts tighten across the abdomen.
6. **Crush injuries** are associated with pelvic fractures.

B. **RECTAL INJURY OCCURRENCE.** Rectal injuries represent only 3–5% of the total injuries to the colon, but are considered to be the most serious of all intestinal injuries owing to the extraperitoneal location, and the rapid progression of perirectal infection throughout the pelvis and retroperitoneum. Causes of rectal injuries include:

1. **Surgical procedures** (obstetric, urologic, gynecologic).
2. **Perforation** from proctosigmoidoscopy or barium enemas.
3. **Ingestion** of foreign body.
4. **Blunt and penetrating trauma** to the perineum.
5. **Sexual assault.**
6. **Auto-eroticism.**
7. **Insertion** of enema nozzles and thermometers.
8. **Suicide attempt** by rectal administration of corrosives.
9. **Impalement** by foreign objects, which is most often due to falls and occurs most commonly in children.

II. EVALUATION

A. **PENETRATING COLORECTAL TRAUMA.**

1. **Chest and abdominal radiographs** are useful only to define the location of the missiles or the presence of a foreign body, such as a broken knife blade (anteroposterior and lateral views).
2. **Abdominal CT scans** are not sensitive enough to detect hollow viscus injuries accurately. Rectal contrast material may help identify colonic injuries.
3. **All patients with gunshot wounds to the abdomen** undergo exploratory celiotomy regardless of the physical examination findings at Parkland Memorial Hospital.

4. **Stab wounds to the abdomen** are difficult to evaluate: one-third do not penetrate the peritoneum; one-third penetrate the peritoneum but do not cause major damage; and one-third produce serious injury.
5. **Patients with abdominal stab wounds** are initially evaluated by physical examination. Peritonitis, evisceration, or intra-abdominal bleeding warrants exploratory celiotomy.
6. **In the absence of the above indications for celiotomy**, selective evaluation by local exploration and peritoneal lavage is performed.
a. Local exploration is positive if the end of the tract is seen to penetrate the posterior fascia or peritoneum.
b. Patients found to have a positive or equivocal local exploration undergo diagnostic peritoneal lavage unless there is a solid indication for operation.
c. This algorithm reduces the incidence of nontherapeutic celiotomies.
7. **Diagnostic laparoscopy** will accurately identify anterior abdominal peritoneal penetration but is rarely used at Parkland.
8. **Blood on rectal examination** may indicate colon or rectal injury. If either is suspected, proctosigmoidoscopy is performed.
9. **All patients with gunshot and stab wounds** who have stable normal vital signs and injuries in proximity to the rectum should undergo proctoscopy to 25cm prior to surgery.
10. **Diagnosis of extraperitoneal rectal injuries** by proctosigmoidoscopy is helpful in making intraoperative decisions. A retrograde cystourethrogram in men and a careful vaginal examination in women should be performed to exclude concomitant injuries to the urogenital system.
B. **BLUNT COLORECTAL TRAUMA.**
1. **Physical findings** of intra-abdominal bleeding or peritoneal irritation warrant exploration.
2. **Plain abdominal radiographs** are rarely of value in defining intra-abdominal injury, but air under the diaphragm helps diagnose a perforation.
3. **Abdominal sonography, diagnostic peritoneal lavage, or abdominal CT** may help identify an injury in hemodynamically stable patients without clinical evidence of intra-abdominal hemorrhage or peritonitis.
4. **The sensitivity of an abdominal CT scan** in defining bowel injuries is poor (50–70%).
5. **A high index of suspicion** for colorectal injury should be present when there are associated injuries, such as pelvic fractures, rectal foreign bodies, or crush injuries.
6. **The diagnosis** of most blunt colorectal injuries is made at operative exploration.
7. **Serosal tears** of the colon occur frequently but are rarely of clinical significance.

III. MANAGEMENT

A. NONOPERATIVE MANAGEMENT.

1. **Iatrogenic or accidental partial-thickness injuries** to the mechanically cleansed colon or rectum by endoscopy, enema tips, or thermometers can be cautiously observed.

2. **Patients are kept NPO** and i.v. antibiotics are administered; careful observation with serial abdominal examinations is usually sufficient.

a. Monitoring for signs and symptoms of sepsis needs to continue for a minimum of 48 hours.

b. Stab wounds of the abdomen can be safely observed in selective patients who are hemodynamically stable, alert, and cooperative.

c. Stab wounds of the flank or back may also be safely observed in stable patients with normal abdominal CT using the triple contrast technique.

d. If a perforation is caused by biopsy or fulgaration, the lesion is treated surgically as a stab wound and primarily repaired.

B. OPERATIVE MANAGEMENT – PENETRATING COLON INJURIES.

1. **Preoperative.**

a. Fluid resuscitation and stabilization.

b. Broad-spectrum i.v. antibiotics.

c. Define missile tract and identify any foreign bodies in vivo radiographically.

2. **Intraoperative.**

a. First control massive hemorrhage.

b. Control intestinal contamination (noncrushing bowel clamps or quick suturing of any perforations).

c. Careful, systematic inspection of the colon should be performed during all explorations. Retroperitoneal injuries of the large bowel are easily missed unless the colon is fully mobilized.

3. **Primary repair or colostomy?**

a. The anatomic, physiologic, and bacteriologic differences between the right and left colon do not determine the success of primary repair.

b. Injuries of all segments of the colon can usually be managed primarily.

c. The response of right-sided colon injuries to treatment does not differ from that of left-sided injuries despite anatomic, physiologic, and bacteriologic differences.

d. Criteria for primary repair:
   1) Hemodynamic stability.
   2) Wound involving less than one-third of the circumference of the bowel.
   3) No mesenteric involvement.
   4) Adequate blood supply.

    5) Injury less than 6–8 hours old.
    6) Minimal contamination.
    7) Treatment of associated injuries does not prolong the intraoperative course.
  e. Criteria for colostomy:
    1) Persistent hypotension.
    2) Severe hemorrhage – requiring >4 unit transfusion.
    3) Multiple injuries – >2 significant intra-abdominal injuries.
    4) Significant fecal contamination.
    5) Injury >8 hours old.
    6) Devitalized colonic tissue requiring resection on left side.

C. OPERATIVE MANAGEMENT – OPTIONS AND TECHNIQUES.

1. Primary repair.

a. Simple closure after adequate débridement of devitalized tissue to assure a good blood supply to the tension-free repair.

b. One- or two-layer closure techniques may be used.

c. Absorbable sutures are used for the inner layer (simple, running, or running-lock style) and permanent Lembert sutures (silk) are used for the outer layer.

d. A one-layer inverting closure using a Gambee stitch is also acceptable.

e. Criteria negatively affecting primary repair include the number of transfusions, the associated injuries, the degree of fecal contamination, the delay between injury and repair, and the severity of colon injury. Transient hypotension is not a contraindication to primary repair.

f. There is no consensus regarding the significance of these criteria determining the safety of primary repair of colon injuries, and the best analysis of the criteria for primary repair is the surgeon's intraoperative judgment for the specific patient.

2. Resection with primary anastomosis

a. Either a one-layer or two-layer closure is acceptable.

b. Stapled anastomosis may save time.

c. Indicated with extensive colon wall injury (>50% of bowel wall circumference) and when colon viability is in question.

d. Most frequently used with extensive wounds of the right colon.

e. Small bowel–colonic anastomoses tend to heal better than colon–colonic anastomoses.

3. Exteriorization of injury site with repair – this technique is not used at Parkland Memorial Hospital.

4. Colostomy.

a. Currently used in <30% of trauma patients with colon injuries, owing to the increased confidence in the safety of primary repair.

b. Indications:
   1) Rectal injuries.
   2) Left colon resection for extensive injury.
   3) Uncertainty about the quality of the colonic repair.
   4) Peritonitis.
c. When applicable, the mobile sigmoid or the right transverse colon is used to construct the colostomy.
d. The colostomy can be made at the site of the injured bowel. It can also be made proximal to the injury to protect a distal primary repair.
e. The right ascending colon and cecum are not used to construct colostomies.
   1) They are difficult to mobilize.
   2) The wall of the colon is thin and the lumen is large and difficult to fashion as a colostomy.
   3) The liquid stool is not substantially different from that found in the distal small bowel.
   4) Right colon injuries are best treated with primary repair or right hemicolectomy with ileocolonic anastomosis.
f. Loop colostomies are easily constructed and easily taken down.
   1) Questions regarding complete fecal diversion from the distal segment have been raised.
   2) Stapling of the distal segment of the loop colostomy prevents fecal spill into the distal limb.
g. Hartmann's procedure – proximal colostomy with sewn or stapled closure of the distal bowel – provides complete fecal diversion, but will require a celiotomy to close.
h. Double-barrel colostomy – proximal colostomy with distal mucous fistula.
   1) Provides complete fecal diversion.
   2) Easier to close the colostomy since the proximal end and distal mucous fistula share a common opening on the abdominal wall.
i. Contrary to popular opinion, colostomy is not always the safest way to manage a colon injury. Drawbacks include:
   1) Higher incidence of intraperitoneal and abdominal wound infection.
   2) Difficulty and additional cost of colostomy care.
   3) Prolonged hospitalization.
   4) Need for separate anesthetic, procedure, and hospitalization for colostomy closure.

5. Drains

a. Intraperitoneal drains are seldom indicated in patients with colonic injuries as infection rates are higher with their use.
b. When placed close to colonic suture lines, drains are thought to lead to an increased number of anastomotic leaks.

D. BLUNT COLON INJURIES.

1. **Operative management** is the same as outlined for penetrating injuries.
2. **Careful inspection** of subscrosal, pericolic, and mesenteric hematomas is essential to diagnosis and management.
3. **Blunt injuries** may not be amenable to simple repairs as often as penetrating injuries, owing to the associated involvement of the mesentery. Resection and primary anastomosis or resection of the injured segment with colostomy and mucous fistula are often necessary.

IV. POSTOPERATIVE CARE

1. **Skin incisions** are left open with almost all colon injuries having significant spill. They heal by secondary intention, or are managed by delayed primary closure at the bedside on the 4th or 5th postoperative day if the wound is clean and not infected.
2. **Oral feeding is** begun as soon as bowel function returns to normal: defined clinically as the presence of normal bowel sounds and the passage of flatus or stool.
3. **Colostomy closure** is usually performed 6–8 weeks postoperatively.
a. It is not necessary to obtain preoperative contrast studies of the colon in patients who have diversion after resection of a segment of colon.
b. If the diversion was done to protect a colon repair, barium enema examination of the distal segment should be performed to exclude leak or stricture at the site of the repair.
4. **All patients undergo bowel preparation** prior to colostomy closure. Systemic perioperative antibiotics are given as well.
5. **Although loop colostomies can be closed** without a formal celiotomy, resection and anastomosis is the practice at Parkland.
6. **In some cases the colostomy incision can be closed primarily**; however, it is safer to leave it open.
7. **Complications** include anastomotic leaks, small bowel obstructions, intra-abdominal abscess, wound infections, and anastomotic stricture.

V. MANAGEMENT OF RECTAL INJURIES

1. **Management of extraperitoneal rectal injuries** relies on the three Ds: diversion, débridement, and drainage.
2. **Sigmoid colostomy**, preferably a loop colostomy with a stapled distal end, is necessary for diversion of the fecal stream.
3. **Presacral drains** placed anterior to the coccyx are removed if no significant leak has occurred within 5 days postoperatively. Large Penrose drains or Jackson–Pratt suction drains are used.
4. **Repair of the injury is not necessary**, is potentially harmful, and should be attempted only if visualized and performed easily without extensive dissection.

5. **Distal washout** of the rectum with antibiotic solution, saline, or dilute povidone–iodine (Betadine) at the time of colostomy formation has been advocated by some, but is not practiced at Parkland.

6. **Foreign bodies.**

a. If the patient is stable and without abdominal tenderness, foreign bodies in the rectum are removed manually or by endoscopic maneuvers.

b. Celiotomy is reserved for patients with peritoneal signs and those patients with foreign bodies that cannot be removed from the rectum.

c. Celiotomy with primary repair is usually the preferred operative approach, but colostomy may be necessary if any of the aforementioned risk factors are present.

d. Transrectal removal of foreign bodies may be assisted by using a Foley balloon, obstetric forceps, plaster of Paris, or vacuum tractor.

VI. COMPLICATIONS OF COLORECTAL INJURIES

1. **Sepsis** accounts for the majority of the morbidity in these injuries. A penetrating abdominal trauma index score >25 is associated with an increased incidence of sepsis.

2. **Intra-abdominal abscess** occurs in 5–15% of patients and is the most lethal complication.

3. **Wound infection** rates are increased with advanced age, left colon injury, multiple blood transfusions, severe fecal spill, and associated organ injury.

4. **Enterocutaneous fistula** occurs in 1–4% of patients and is initially treated nonoperatively.

5. **Right colon injuries** – morbidity 32%; mortality 2%.

6. **Left colon injuries** – morbidity 33%; mortality 4%.

7. **Colorectal injuries** with associated multiple organ injuries have an increased mortality rate compared with a low mortality rate for isolated colorectal injuries.

8. **Anastomotic leak** – 7–9% of patients.

a. Typically occurs 4–7 days postoperatively.

b. Presents as subfascial wound infection and enterocutaneous fistula.

c. Treatment includes resection of the anastomosis with diverting colostomy and Hartmann's procedure.

VII. PEARLS AND PITFALLS

1. **Adequate mobilization of the retroperitoneal colon** will reduce the incidence of missed injuries.

2. **Fecal diversion or resection** is prudent in any instance where the viability of the colon is questionable.

VIII. FURTHER READING

Ivatury RR, Licata J, Gunduz Y et al. Management options in penetrating rectal injuries. *Am Surg* 57 1990; 1:50–55.

Smith LE. Traumatic injuries. In: Gordon PH, Nivatvongs S, eds. *Principles and practice of surgery for the colon, rectum, and anus*. St Louis: Quality Medical Publishing; 1992:957–980.

Stewart RM, Fabian TC, Croce MA et al. Is resection with primary anastomosis following destructive colon wounds always safe? *Am J Surg* 1994; 168:316–319.

Stone HH, Fabian TC. Management of penetrating colon trauma. *Ann Surg* 1990; 190:430.

Wilson RF, Walt AJ, Dulchavsky S. Injuries to the colon and rectum. In: Wilson RF, Walt AJ, eds. *Management of trauma: pitfalls and practice*, 2nd edn. Baltimore: William and Wilkins; 1996:534–553.

MANAGEMENT PRINCIPLES IN RENAL TRAUMA

I. EPIDEMIOLOGY

1. **Trauma to the upper urinary tract occurs in about 1%** of all injured patients.
2. **In 6–8% of patients with penetrating abdominal injuries** there is associated renal trauma.
3. **Blunt trauma accounts for nearly 90% of all renal injuries** while penetrating trauma (gunshot and stab wounds) account for the remaining 10%.
a. Blunt injuries to the kidney are associated with other intra-abdominal injuries in 44% of cases.
b. The incidence of associated intra-abdominal injuries with penetrating renal trauma ranges from 77% to 100%.

II. MECHANISM OF INJURY

1. **Penetrating trauma causes tissue disruption**. However, blast effect with high-velocity (>1100 feet per second) missile injuries must also be considered.
2. **Motor vehicle crashes, falls, and direct blows** to the flank lead to renal injuries as the kidney is thrust against the rib cage or vertebral column.
3. **Sudden deceleration injuries** may stretch the renal artery and produce an intimal tear or thrombosis. Children are prone to disruption of the ureteropelvic junction (UPJ) with rapid deceleration injuries, owing to the hyperextensibility of their spine.
4. **Fractured ribs and transverse processes of the lumbar spine** can cause laceration of the kidney.

III. CLASSIFICATION

A. **GRADE 1.** Contusion or contained subcapsular hematoma without parenchymal laceration.
B. **GRADE 2.** Nonexpanding, confined perirenal hematoma or superficial cortical laceration without urinary extravasation.
C. **GRADE 3.** Parenchymal laceration extending through the corticomedullary junction without extension into the collecting system.
D. **GRADE 4.** Parenchymal laceration extending through the corticomedullary junction with extension into the collecting system, or an isolated arterial or venous injury.
E. **GRADE 5.** Pedicle avulsion or shattered kidney.

IV. ANATOMY

1. **The kidney lies in the retroperitoneum** surrounded by perirenal fat, Gerota's fascia.
2. **The right kidney lies posterior to the liver** with the colon lying anterior and the duodenum anteromedially, and the left kidney lies inferior to the spleen and posterolateral to the pancreas.
3. **The tail of the pancreas** often lies in the hilar area of the kidney.

V. INITIAL EVALUATION

A. HISTORY.

1. Mechanism of injury - suspect renal injury with sudden deceleration events.
2. Ascertain type of weapon used.
3. Document presence or absence of hypotension in the field.

B. PHYSICAL FINDINGS SUGGESTIVE OF RENAL INJURY.

1. Flank or upper abdominal tenderness.
2. Flank contusion (ecchymosis).
3. Lower rib fractures.
4. Upper abdominal mass or fullness.
5. Crepitance over lower rib cage or lumbar area.
6. Site of gunshot wound entrance or stab wound penetration.

C. LABORATORY STUDIES.

1. **Microscopic hematuria.**
a. Patients with hematuria of any degree who are victims of penetrating injuries require further evaluation.
b. Those patients sustaining blunt trauma with a history of hypotension or associated injuries require radiographic evaluation.
2. **Gross hematuria.**
a. All patients with gross hematuria need radiographic evaluation.
b. Approximately 5–10% of patients with gross hematuria will have a significant renal injury, and half of that group will require surgical repair.
c. The degree of hematuria does not correlate with the severity of renal injury.
d. Up to 40% of renal pedicle injuries will not result in any hematuria.

D. RADIOLOGIC EVALUATION.

1. **Genitourinary trauma series.**
a. Will adequately stage 60–85% of renal injuries.
b. Significant findings include:
   1) Loss of the psoas shadow.
   2) Ground-glass appearance.
   3) Scoliosis away from the side of the injury.
   4) Extravasation of contrast.
   5) Nonvisualization or decreased visualization of the kidney.
c. When patients require immediate exploratory celiotomy an i.v. pyelogram (IVP) is performed intraoperatively.

d. The IVP is not performed if the patient is going to have an abdominal CT scan.

2. **CT scan.**

a. Spiral CT can be performed rapidly, has greater sensitivity and specificity than the IVP, and is useful in the diagnosis of other intra-abdominal injuries.

b. CT provides the most information about the traumatized kidney with minimal invasiveness when compared with all other modalities. It can be used in stable patients who have an equivocal trauma series.

c. It is the study of choice in the evaluation of pediatric patients who will require radiographic assessment of the kidneys.

d. Lacerations, contusions, subcapsular hemorrhage, vascular injuries, extravasation, and perirenal hematomas can be adequately staged with CT scan.

3. **Arteriography.**

a. Indicated in patients where there is nonvisualization of the kidney on the trauma series.

b. This modality can identify devascularized segments of the kidney which are at increased risk of delayed abscess formation.

c. Arteriography is used at Parkland Memorial Hospital as a second-tier study in patients with suspected renal vascular injury or unstable patients, mainly as a result of the time required to obtain this study.

VI. MANAGEMENT

A. **MINOR RENAL INJURIES.** Grade 1 and grade 2 account for 70% of all injuries and they do not require intervention.

B. **MAJOR RENAL INJURIES.**

1. **Grade 3 and 4 injuries** constitute 10–15% of all injuries. Their management depends on the clinical status of the patient and other associated injuries.

2. **Hemodynamically stable patients** without associated injuries that require exploration may be observed expectantly.

3. **When celiotomy is performed** for treatment of associated injuries, renal exploration and reconstruction is recommended. This reduces the rate of urologic complications, but may increase the nephrectomy rate.

4. **Nonoperative management of stab wounds** is acceptable after excluding associated trauma.

5. **If a large devascularized segment is noted**, partial or complete nephrectomy may be indicated.

6. **Grade 5 injuries** occur in 10–15% of patients with renal trauma. They almost always require immediate surgery to control life-threatening bleeding and often result in nephrectomy.

7. **Vascular injuries** identified by arteriogram should be surgically corrected. These injuries should be addressed as soon as possible and preferably no longer than 2–6 hours from the time of injury.

8. **The kidney may suffer warm ischemic damage** if diagnosis and repair is delayed beyond this duration.
9. **Selected vascular injuries** which can be managed without exploration include main arterial thrombosis and segmental arterial lacerations.
10. **Preservation of significant renal function** has been achieved in only 15–30% of revascularizations despite early diagnosis and repair of renal artery thrombosis.

C. ABSOLUTE INDICATIONS FOR EXPLORATION.
1. Persistent bleeding.
2. Expanding or pulsatile retroperitoneal hematoma.
3. Hemodynamic instability related to the renal injury.
4. Known grade 5 renal injury.

D. RELATIVE INDICATIONS FOR EXPLORATION.
1. Urinary extravasation.
a. If associated with a deep laceration with concomitant bleeding, the injury should be surgically repaired.
b. Recent literature supports the nonoperative management of extravasation due to renal injury and an attempt at endoscopic management (retrograde ureteral stenting) of persistent cases prior to renal exploration.
2. Devitalized segment.
a. Studies have confirmed the increased morbidity associated with devitalized fragments in the management of grade 3 and grade 4 renal injuries.
b. There is a two-fold increased incidence of urologic complications when devitalized fragments occur along with other intra-abdominal injuries.
c. These complications include urinoma formation, perinephric abscess, and sepsis.
3. Arterial thrombosis.
a. If discovered late, nephrectomy is usually necessary, but removal is not emergent.
b. Atrophy and hypertension will usually follow.

VII. OPERATIVE APPROACH TO THE KIDNEY

A. EARLY ISOLATION OF THE RENAL VESSELS.
1. **Incision of the retroperitoneum** over the aorta superior to the inferior mesenteric artery. With a large hematoma obscuring the view of the aorta, the incision should be made medial to the inferior mesenteric vein.
2. **Superior dissection** will reveal the left renal vein crossing the aorta anteriorly (3% of patients will have a retroaortic left renal vein). Both renal arteries should be easily seen at this time. All vessels are encircled with vessel loops.
3. **The kidney is now approached** by incising the retroperitoneum lateral to the colon. Simple lacerations may be closed after sharp débridement

with 2-0–4-0 chromic suture and drained with posterolaterally placed closed suction drains.

4. **Defects in the collecting system** should be closed in a watertight fashion with 4-0 chromic suture and drained as above. An indigo carmine injection into the pelvis with the ureter occluded helps define collecting-system defects.

5. **When possible, preserve the renal capsule** to close over with interrupted sutures. Large capsular defects may be covered with omentum or free grafts of peritoneum and drained.

6. **Wounds may be closed** over a bolster of Surgicel and gelfoam placed in the depths of the laceration.

7. **Nephrectomy may be necessary** if bleeding persists or if the patient becomes unstable secondary to continuing blood loss.

B. **POSTOPERATIVE CARE.**

1. **Postoperative hypertension** must always be investigated. Renal artery stenosis may accompany vascular repair at the time of the injury. Also, renal compression due to hematoma between the renal capsule and Gerota's fascia should be considered. This type of hypertension may necessitate nephrectomy if refractory to medical management.

2. **Observe for persistent hematuria.** Clot formation suggests a large amount of bleeding from the upper urinary tract. An arteriogram is strongly indicated in these patients. The possible causes are arteriovenous malformations or missed arterial bleeding at the time of celiotomy.

3. **Closed suction drains** can be removed when drainage becomes minimal, but be aware of the possibility of delayed urine leak.

4. **Hematocrits and creatinine** should be followed in the postoperative period.

5. **A follow-up IVP** is strongly recommended 2–3 weeks following discharge.

VIII. FURTHER READING

Carroll PR, McAninch JW. Staging of renal trauma. *Uro Clin North Am* 1989; 16(2):193–201.

Husmann DA, Morris JS. Attempted nonoperative management of blunt renal lacerations extending through the corticomedullary junction: the short-term and long-term sequelae. *J Urol* 1990; 143(4):682–684.

McAninch JW, Carroll PR. Renal exploration after renal trauma: indications and reconstructive techniques. *Urologic Clinics of North America* 1989, 16(2):203–212.

Mee SL, McAninch JW. Indications for radiographic assessment in suspected renal trauma. *Urol Clin North Am* 1989; 16(2):187–192.

Sagalowsky AI, Peters PC. Genito-urinary trauma. In: Walsh PC, Rebik AB, Vaughan ED Jr.,Wein AJ, eds. *Campbell's urology,* 6th edn. Philadelphia: WB Saunders; 1986:3085–3120.

27

RADIOLOGIC DIAGNOSIS AND MANAGEMENT OF INJURIES TO THE URETERS, BLADDER, AND URETHRA

I. RADIOGRAPHIC EVALUATION OF THE UROGENITAL TRACT IN TRAUMA

A. GENITOURINARY IMAGING.

1. **Indications.**
   a. Gross hematuria.
   b. Penetrating injuries and any degree of hematuria.
   c. Pediatric patients with any degree of hematuria.
   d. Microscopic hematuria and associated hypotension or history of hypotension (blood pressure <90mmHg systolic).
   e. Patients with significant injuries in proximity to urogenital structures (lower rib fractures, pelvic fractures, large flank hematoma, penetrating injuries with proximity to the genitourinary (GU) tract organs).
   f. Significant deceleration.

2. **Plain abdominal radiograph.**
   a. Usually part of the standard radiographic evaluation in the trauma patient with pelvic and abdominal trauma.
   b. Significant findings suggestive of a urogenic injury include:
      1) Rib fractures.
      2) Pelvic fractures.
      3) Foreign bodies.
      4) Missiles.
      5) Loss of psoas shadow.
      6) Vertebral fractures.

3. **Trauma series.**
   a. A scout plain abdominal radiograph.
   b. A 1-minute i.v. pyelogram (IVP) and static cystogram.
   c. A 5-minute IVP and drain film.

4. **Technique.**
   a. Intravenous access.
   b. Foley catheter.
   c. Intravesical and i.v. contrast.
   d. Adapter tubing for catheter.
   e. Radiographs obtained:
      1) Plain abdominal radiograph prior to instillation or injection of contrast.

    2) 1-minute film after instilling 300mL of contrast into the bladder through the catheter and injection of 1–2mL/kg i.v. contrast.

    3) 5–8-minute film after injection of the contrast with the contrast drained from the bladder.

5. **General considerations.**

a. Hypotensive or azotemic patients will have inferior quality pyelograms.

b. Look for prompt bilateral renal function, extravasation from the bladder (extraperitoneal – confined to pelvis; or intraperitoneal – diffuse extravasation into peritoneum), renal or ureteral extravasation, devitalized (nonexcreting) segments of kidney, and abnormal ureteral deviations.

6. **Causes of nonvisualization on IVP.**

a. Renal absence – congenital or surgical.

b. Renal ectopia.

c. Shock.

d. Renovascular spasm due to severe contusion.

e. Renal artery thrombosis.

f. Avulsion of renal pedicle.

g. High-grade obstruction.

B. CT SCAN OF ABDOMEN.

1. **CT provides greater sensitivity and specificity** than IVP in the detection and characterization of renal injuries.

2. **It is more sensitive** in detecting extravasation from the renal pelvis or the ureter.

3. **This technique is indicated** in patients with a suspected severe renal laceration, contusion, or crush injury from blunt trauma.

4. **A formal cystogram with intravesical contrast** is still required with postdrain films to rule out bladder injury. Clamping the Foley is not an acceptable alternative.

5. **Significant findings include:**

a. Renal laceration (low-density area).

b. Extravasation.

c. Crush.

d. Congenital abnormalities [i.e. ureteropelvic junction obstruction (UPJ)].

e. Perirenal hematoma.

f. Lack of function.

6. **This is the study of choice** in pediatric patients with trauma.

C. ARTERIOGRAM.

1. **This has largely been replaced** by the CT scan.

2. **This technique is indicated** if there is suspicion of a renovascular injury.

3. **If a nonfunctioning or slowly functioning kidney is noted** on IVP or CT scan, a renal pedicle injury must be considered. CT scans are very sensitive and may show only a small amount of contrast in the collecting system (cortical rim sign).

4. **Gross hematuria** that develops after abdominal trauma, (especially with a laceration of the kidney), may indicate the presence of an arteriovenous malformation. This would be best diagnosed by arteriography.

D. ULTRASOUND.

1. **This is of limited use** in the management of urogenital trauma.

2. **It can be used to diagnose testicular rupture.** (In a rupture of the testis a large fluid collection around the testes with a disruption in the tunica albuginea would be detected.)

3. **Resolution is generally poor,** but a ruptured kidney may be detected.

E. RETROGRADE URETHROGRAM.

1. Indications.

a. History of straddle injury.

b. History of major deceleration.

c. Blood at the meatus in an injured patient.

d. High-riding prostate on rectal examination.

e. Perineal 'butterfly' hematoma.

f. Scrotal or perineal crepitus suggestive of urine extravasation.

g. Inability to pass Foley catheter.

2. **Technique.**

a. Using a catheter-tip 60mL syringe, instill, in a retrograde fashion, 30mL of radiographic contrast into the meatus.

b. Obtain a radiograph with the patient in an oblique position while instilling contrast into the urethra with the penis on stretch.

3. **Significant positive findings.**

a. Disruption of the prostatomembranous urethra as evidenced by extravasation of contrast into the perineum.

b. Extravasation of the contrast from other parts of the urethra secondary to injury.

F. RADIONUCLIDE RENAL SCAN. This can be useful to document renal blood flow in patients with severe allergy to iodinated contrast.

II. URETERAL TRAUMA

A. EPIDEMIOLOGY AND MECHANISM OF INJURY.

1. **Injury to the renal pelvis and ureter** is a rare occurrence.

a. Penetrating trauma accounts for >80% of ureteral injuries.

b. Incidence is 2.2–5% in abdominal gunshot wounds.

c. Often associated with colon or bowel injuries.

d. 70–100% of penetrating ureteral injuries are associated with other injuries in the abdomen.

2. **Blunt trauma** usually causes avulsion of the ureter at the UPJ.

3. **Children are prone to this type of injury** owing to the hyperextensibility of the spine, which exerts tension on the upper ureter and UPJ when stretched.

4. **Stab wounds or bullet injuries** lead to either severe contusion (blast effect), partial or complete transection, or laceration.

5. **Iatrogenic injuries** often occur as a result of ligation, laceration, or avulsion.

B. **ANATOMY.**

1. **The blood supply** lies immediately adjacent to the ureter in the adventitial sheath.

2. **The ureteral blood supply** is derived from branches of the renal artery, aorta, umbilical or superior vesical arteries, internal spermatic artery, and internal iliac vessels.

3. **The blood supply is usually from multiple vessels**.

C. **INITIAL EVALUATION.**

1. **History and physical examination.**

a. Clinical suspicion is the key to diagnosis. Injuries may be silent, making recognition and prompt intervention difficult.

b. Be suspicious in patients with a gunshot or stab wound to the flank.

c. With delayed presentation, the patient may have:
   1) An unexplained fever.
   2) An abdominal mass.
   3) A prolonged ileus.
   4) Hematuria.
   5) An elevated serum creatinine.

2. **Laboratory.**

a. Do not count on the presence of hematuria to exclude ureteral injury.

b. 20–40% of ureteral injuries are not associated with either gross or microscopic hematuria.

c. UPJ avulsion has the lowest incidence of hematuria.

3. **Radiographic evaluation** (see section I).

a. IVP is 95% accurate in diagnosing ureteral injuries.

b. Findings suspicious for ureteral injury include:
   1) Hydronephrosis.
   2) Extravasation - the *sine qua non* of ureteral injuries.
   3) Incomplete visualization of the upper urinary tract.
   4) Loss of the psoas shadow.
   5) Extravasation may appear as a small fluid collection at the level of the injury on the CT scan.

4. **Operative evaluation.**

a. Intraoperatively, the diagnosis can be made with i.v. indigo carmine or methylene blue (indigo carmine is preferred as methylene blue effects pulse-oximeter readings).

b. Extravasation can be seen in the retroperitoneum as a blue-green staining.

c. Direct injection of indigo carmine into the renal pelvis or proximal ureter should identify any full-thickness injury to the ureter.

D. **MANAGEMENT.**

1. **General principles.**

a. Débridement of ureter back to bleeding viable tissue.

b. Tension-free anastomosis.
c. Adequate drainage of repair. A Penrose-type drain is preferable to closed-suction drains for large repairs as it causes less negative pressure on the suture line.
d. Double-J stents or nephrostomy tubes are recommended in all repairs.
e. Exclusion of the repair from adjacent associated injuries.
f. If the patient is unstable or secondary repair is indicated, cutaneous ureterostomy or ligation of the ureter with percutaneous nephrostomy drainage are viable temporizing options.
g. Injuries to the ureter are classified according to anatomic location as this has an impact on the technique of repair.

2. **Proximal ureter** – renal pelvis and UPJ.
a. Usually can perform uretero-ureterostomy in this section of the ureter.
b. If the ureter is avulsed from the UPJ, ureteropyelostomy or dismembered pyeloplasty can be performed over a ureteral stent, with or without a percutaneous nephrostomy tube.
c. After debridement the ureter should be spatulated 1cm and repaired in a watertight fashion with interrupted fine 4-0 or 5-0 chromic suture over a double-J stent.
d. If a large gap needs to be bridged, mobilization and fixation (pexy) of the kidney can provide 1–3 cm of ureteral length.
e. Transureteroureterostomy is an option if primary reanastomosis cannot be performed. A 1–2 cm incision is made in the medial border of the contralateral ureter and the spatulated ipsilateral ureter is anastomosed over a stent, again with fine interrupted sutures.
f. Penrose or closed-suction drainage of the injury site is essential.

3. **Midureter** – abdominal ureter from the UPJ to the iliac vessels.
a. Management of choice is ureteroureterostomy.
b. If further mobilization is necessary, a Boari flap may be considered. This involves creation of a bladder flap which is tubularized superiorly to the level of the ureter. The bladder is secured to the psoas minor tendon with 3–4 nonabsorbable sutures with care taken not to place the sutures through the bladder epithelium. The ureter is reimplanted into this flap over a stent.
c. Transureteroureterostomy may also be performed if a large defect is created by the injury.

4. **Distal ureter** – iliac vessels to the ureterovesical junction.
a. Injury to the ureter below the level of the vessels jeopardizes the ureteral blood supply, therefore primary repair is not recommended.
b. Management of choice is ureteroneocystostomy.
   1) The Politano–Ledbetter method of reimplantation of the ureter is preferred.
   2) A 5:1 submucosal length to ureteral diameter will most often prevent vesicoureteral reflux.

      3) Mucosa-to-mucosa anastomosis with 4-0 chromic sutures is important.
      4) A psoas hitch may be helpful in bridging a gap in ureteral length.

E. POSTOPERATIVE CARE.

1. **The stent can be removed** at approximately 4–6 weeks.
2. **Oral antibiotics** are required only for the initial 5–7 days after stent placement.
3. **IVP after stent removal** is necessary to rule out stricture.
4. **Patients may have prolonged drainage** from the Penrose or closed-suction drain. The drains should be left in place until the drainage subsides, to prevent urinoma formation.
5. **Fever, prolonged ileus, abdominal mass, or an increase in blood urea nitrogen or creatinine** is suggestive of urinoma formation.

F. COMPLICATIONS.

1. **Prolonged drainage** requires continued Jackson–Pratt drainage or placement of a percutaneous nephrostomy tube with antegrade stent placement.
2. **Fistula formation** can occur with the colon, duodenum, or other portions of the small bowel. This can be managed initially with percutaneous nephrostomy diversion, but eventually will require surgical excision of the fistulous tract.
3. **Strictures** may be treated endoscopically (balloon dilatation or incision with cutting electrode) or surgically (open repair). Stricture formation varies widely (incidence is poorly documented).
4. **Ureteral reconstruction**, when necessary, should be delayed for 6 months until all inflammation resolves.
5. **Urinoma formation** can be treated with percutaneous drainage by CT guidance and urinary diversion with a percutaneous nephrostomy tube.

III. URINARY BLADDER TRAUMA

A. CLASSIFICATION OF BLADDER TRAUMA.

1. **Bladder contusion (BC).**
a. May include bladder wall hematoma or mucosal disruption without loss of wall continuity or extravasation.
b. Clinical diagnosis is based on:
      1) Mechanism.
      2) Hematuria.
      3) Negative diagnostic evaluation for bladder rupture or upper tract trauma.

2. **Extraperitoneal bladder rupture (EBR).**
a. Complete disruption of bladder wall into extraperitoneal space usually occurring at lateral bladder or base.
b. Incidence is around 50% and it is more common than intraperitoneal bladder rupture (IBR).

3. **IBR** rupture is the complete disruption of the bladder wall, usually at the dome of bladder, with extravasation of urine into peritoneal cavity.
4. **Combined IBR and EBR (CBR)** accounts for 10% of bladder injuries.

B. **ANATOMIC CONSIDERATIONS.**
1. **Adult bladder.**
   a. Extraperitoneal organ deep within pelvis.
   b. Protected by bony pelvis, pelvic floor musculature, and rectum.
   c. Normal capacity 300–400mL.
2. **Pediatric bladder.**
   a. Bulk of bladder intraperitoneal.
   b. Capacity determined by the formula: 2 + age in years = capacity in ounces. (One ounce is approximately 30mL.)

C. **EPIDEMIOLOGY.**
1. **>85% of patients with bladder rupture** have other serious associated injuries with a mortality rate of 22–60%.
2. **85% have pelvic fractures.**
3. **Hemodynamic instability** is rarely due to an isolated bladder injury (<3% at Parkland Memorial Hospital).
4. **95% of EBRs** are associated with pelvic fractures while only 5–10% of pelvic fractures are associated with EBR.

D. **MECHANISM.**
1. **May be due to blunt or penetrating trauma**.
2. **Common blunt etiologies** include motor vehicle collisions, falls, and abdominal blows.
3. **Common penetrating etiologies include:**
   a. Gunshot wounds.
   b. Stab wounds.
   c. Iatrogenic injuries.
   d. Self-instrumentation injuries.
4. **Blunt trauma** accounts for 75–85% of bladder injuries.
5. **The type of bladder injury varies** with the volume of urine present at time of trauma.
6. **Blunt anteroposterior trauma** imposed on a full bladder disperses force equally such that disruption occurs at the bladder dome, causing IBR. This is common in restrained occupants involved in motor vehicle collisions.
7. **EBR is associated with pelvic fracture** and intravesical penetration by a bony spicule or a shearing of the bladder from the pelvic side-wall.

E. **DIAGNOSIS.**
1. **History and physical examination.**
   a. Considerations:
      1) 98% of patients with bladder rupture present with gross hematuria.

    2) Presenting complaints may include inability to urinate or suprapubic pain.

    3) A normal bladder may be compromised by prior surgery, irradiation, malignancy, or pregnancy.

b. Examination of abdomen may include:

    1) Tenderness.

    2) Ecchymosis.

    3) Edema.

    4) Pelvic instability or deformity.

c. Examination of the external genitalia may include:

    1) Ecchymosis.

    2) Edema.

    3) Blood at the urethral meatus.

d. Examination of the perineum may include:

    1) 'Butterfly' hematoma.

    2) Crepitus.

e. Examination of the rectum may include:

    1) Bleeding.

    2) High-riding prostate.

f. A speculum examination is essential in females to rule out concomitant vaginal or urethral injury.

g. Laboratory.

    1) Diagnostic peritoneal lavage may be positive with isolated IBR.

    2) Electrolyte screen may reveal acidosis or azotemia due to reabsorption of organic acids, creatinine, and urea, especially if diagnosis is delayed.

    3) Laboratory values are usually not helpful in the acute setting.

h. Uroradiographic evaluation.

    1) Perform initial retrograde urethrography if a catheter cannot be passed or an obviously high-riding prostate is palpated, blood is present at the urethral meatus, or perineal ecchymosis is noted on physical examination.

    2) An IVP is necessary to rule out upper tract injury.

    3) Obtain a plain abdominal radiograph and cystogram with 300mL of iodinated contrast (in adults) followed by a drain film.

    4) A plain abdominal radiograph is obtained to assess possible pelvic fracture, loss of psoas shadow, missile position, subcutaneous air, or pelvic fluid density which may accompany bladder injury.

    5) The cystography drain view is most sensitive for subtle submucosal tears and minor degrees of extraperitoneal extravasation.

    6) IBR will fill the peritoneum to outline the bowel loops and solid viscera.

7) EBR appears as a wisp of contrast usually confined to the pelvis but occasionally extending high into the retroperitoneum.

8) Compressed 'tear drop' or high-riding 'pie-in-the-sky' bladder may be seen due to pelvic hematoma.

9) Cystography is the recommended evaluation for bladder injury.

F. MANAGEMENT.

1. **Small EBR or contusions with submucosal extravasation.**

a. Catheter drainage for 7–10 days.

b. Vesicostomy in young children may be performed to avoid prolonged catheterization.

2. **Large EBR or EBR with an associated intravesical pelvic bony fragment.**

a. Exploration, cystostomy, débridement, and primary repair of injury.

b. Large-bore (24–30F) suprapubic tube cystostomy tube is placed for drainage.

c. A urethral catheter is optional unless the bladder neck is in need of repair.

3. **IBR or CBR.**

a. Celiotomy and intraperitoneal irrigation with primary repair of bladder.

b. Large-bore suprapubic tube cystostomy tube or possibly vesicostomy in child.

G. PENETRATING INJURIES.

1. **All penetrating injuries** should be explored, owing to the likelihood of associated injuries.

2. **In all cases requiring exploration**, an ampule of i.v. indigo carmine should be used to assess lower ureteral patency and the bladder neck should be inspected to rule out injury.

3. **Extravesical suction or Penrose drains** should be placed adjacent to, but not abutting, the repair to prevent delayed healing or fistulae.

4. **Closure** should always be in 1–2 layers and watertight using 3-0 or 4-0 chromic gut or polyglycolic acid suture to prevent encrustation or bladder calculus formation.

H. POSTOPERATIVE CARE.

1. **Immediate.**

a. Intravenous antibiotic prophylaxis.

b. Maintain extravesical drainage until the output is <30mL per day.

c. Rule out urinary leakage by assessment of the drain fluid creatinine (Cr) if outputs remain high.

1) Normal drain fluid Cr = serum Cr.

2) With leakage, drain fluid Cr > serum Cr, and usually by at least 3–4-fold.

d. Maintain extravesical drainage as long as leak persists.

e. Persistent unexplained fever should be worked up with pelvic sonography or CT to rule out urinoma or abscess.

f. If fluid collection is present or an abscess is discovered, sonographically or CT-guided aspiration or drainage may be performed unless loculated or persistent, when open drainage may be required.
g. Maintain catheter or suprapubic drainage for 7–10 days.
2. Delayed.
a. Prior to catheter removal, lack of extravasation must be confirmed cystographically.
b. Follow-up urinalysis to rule out persistent hematuria or infection.
3. Complications.
a. Pelvic, retroperitoneal, or intra-abdominal abscess.
b. Vesicoperitoneal, enteric, retroperitoneal, or cutaneous fistulae.
c. Incontinence or impotence due to bladder neck injury or pelvic fracture.
d. Bladder outlet obstruction and bladder neck contracture.

IV. URETHRAL TRAUMA

A. CLASSIFICATION OF URETHRAL TRAUMA.
1. By mechanism.
a. Blunt.
    1) Posterior urethral disruption (prostatic and membranous urethra).
    2) Anterior urethral injury, usually a straddle injury (bulbous and penile urethra).
b. Penetrating.
c. Iatrogenic.
2. By degree of injury.
a. Type I – stretching and elongation without rupture.
b. Type II – partial or complete rupture of prostatomembranous urethra.
c. Type III – partial or complete rupture of prostatomembranous urethra with injury to the urogenital diaphragm and bulbous urethra.
B. EPIDEMIOLOGY.
1. **Urethral injury** occurs in approximately 10% of pelvic fractures and only a minority of these are complex.
2. **Total transection** occurs more frequently than partial, approximately 65% vs 35%, respectively.
3. **Iatrogenic injuries** are thought to occur in <5% of transurethral procedures.
4. **Anterior urethral injuries** are more common than posterior injuries.
C. MECHANISM.
1. **Prostatomembranous urethral disruption (PMD).**
a. Usually occurs at the superior leaf of the genito-urinary diaphragm as the prostatic urethra is sheared from the pelvic floor.
b. 90% of these are associated with pelvic fractures.
c. Generally occur with violent deceleration such as motor vehicle collisions or falls. Women usually have associated vaginal injury.

2. **Bulbous urethral straddle injuries.**

a. Occur when the bulbous urethra is impinged against the inferior edge of the symphysis pubis.

b. No strong association with pelvic fracture.

c. Usually due to motorcycle crashes, horseriding injuries, bicycle crashes, or a kick to the external genitalia.

3. **Penetrating injuries.**

a. Usually secondary to:
   1) Gunshot wound.
   2) Stab wound.
   3) Therapeutic or self-instrumentation.
   4) Catheterization.

b. Most commonly occur in pendulous urethra and less frequently in the bulb although bulbous injury is more commonly due to instrumentation.

c. May see perineal impalement after falls.

D. **ANATOMY.**

1. **Posterior urethra (male).**

a. Composed of prostatic and membranous urethra.

b. Neurovascular erectile mechanism runs posterolateral and adjacent to the posterior urethra.

c. Voluntary continence rests in the striated external sphincter within the membranous urethra.

2. **Anterior urethra (male).**

a. Composed of bulbar and penile or pendulous urethra along with glanular urethra including fossa navicularis and meatus.

b. Most narrow portion of a normal urethra is at the meatus.

c. Surrounded by corpus spongiosum with corpora cavernosa superiorly.

3. **Buck's fascia.**

a. Surrounds the anterior urethra and corporal bodies – a sleeve of the penis.

b. Ecchymosis secondary to urethral disruption is confined to the penis if Buck's fascia is intact.

4. **Colles' fascia.**

a. If Buck's fascia is disrupted, urine and blood can extravasate along this fascial plane which is contiguous with Scarpa's fascia on the abdominal wall.

b. Ecchymosis may extend on to the abdominal wall, but not on to the thigh or buttocks.

c. Boundaries:
   1) Coracoclavicular ligaments.
   2) Fascia lata of thigh.
   3) Triangular fascia of the perineum.

E. DIAGNOSIS.

1. **History and physical examination.**

a. Classic triad includes:

   1) Blood at the urethral meatus.
   2) Inability to void.
   3) Distended, palpable urinary bladder.

b. Rectal examination may reveal a high-riding prostate, and perineal 'butterfly' hematoma may be present.

c. Catheterization should not be attempted and is usually unsuccessful.

d. May see discoloration within Buck's or Colles' fascial boundaries.

e. Mechanism of injury is probably the most important component of the history.

2. **Laboratory.**

a. Delayed presentation with urinary tract obstruction may lead to resorptive azotemia or acidosis.

b. If pelvic fracture present, hematocrit may be decreased.

c. No consistent laboratory findings in the acute setting.

3. **Uroradiologic evaluation** – see section I.

a. Retrograde urethrography (RGUG) should be performed if any of the classic triad symptoms are seen.

b. Cystography:

   1) May be performed via small-bore punch cystostomy or be omitted if immediate exploration and suprapubic tube cystostomy planned.
   2) 'Pie-in-the-sky' bladder if an elevating pelvic hematoma disrupts the prostatomembranous urethra and bladder.

F. MANAGEMENT.

1. **Iatrogenic or self-manipulation injury** or contusion with minimal extravasation.

a. Usually the result of attempted catheter placement and creation of a false passage.

b. Often patient has underlying urethral stricture disease or an enlarged prostate.

c. Best managed with urethral catheter drainage for 4–7 days to allow mucosal healing. Late stricture rate unknown if urethra left unstented.

2. **Major penetrating urethral injury.**

a. Débridement and spatulated primary repair with absorbable suture over a silastic catheter.

b. Débridement with exteriorization and later-staged closure if inadequate tissue available for primary closure.

c. Suture repair of associated corporal injury.

3. **Type I injuries** can be managed with simple urethral catheter drainage for 3–5 days.

4. **Type II and III injuries to the posterior urethra.**

a. Goal of initial therapy is urinary diversion in an attempt to prevent the most common long-term complications of stricture, incontinence, and erectile dysfunction.

b. Minor urethral disruptions can often be managed by gently placing a urethral catheter for 10–14 days.
   1) With careful placement a partial urethral disruption is unlikely to be converted to a complete urethral disruption.
   2) If any difficulty is encountered the attempt should be aborted and a suprapubic tube placed.
c. Owing to recent advances in endoscopic techniques, primary realignment at the time of the injury utilizing flexible cystoscopy and placement of a catheter across the disruption is being examined. Stricture rates and the need for future formal urethroplasty are almost halved.
d. Endoscopic techniques are also being used as the definitive delayed management of urethral strictures.
   1) Most successful with strictures <3cm.
   2) Involves retrograde or antegrade approach to the stricture with cold knife, laser, or electrical incision.
   3) Long-term success under investigation, but most patients have required periodic visual internal urethrotomy (VIU) or urethral dilatation to maintain patency.

5. **Anterior urethral injuries.**
a. Usually the result of straddle injuries, or a direct blow.
b. Pelvic fracture is an uncommon cause of urethral injury.
c. Can produce partial or complete disruption of the urethra and surrounding investing fascia.
d. Most injuries will require surgical exploration, débridement, and repair with 4-0 or 5-0 absorbable suture over a urethral catheter left in place for 10–14 days.

G. **POSTOPERATIVE CARE.**

1. **Immediate.**
a. Intravenous antibiotic prophylaxis with Gram-negative coverage.
b. Highest stricture rate in the postoperative period is associated with a urinary tract infection.
c. Suprapubic catheter:
   1) Maintained until the urethra is cleared of injury or stricture.
   2) May be left in place for months if delayed repair is deemed necessary.
   3) Necessitates monthly change of each catheter until repair successfully completed.

2. **Delayed studies.**
a. Assess via RGUG performed alongside a urethral catheter prior to its discontinuation to rule out extravasation.
b. Perform voiding cystourethrogram and concomitant RGUG to assess for presence and length of stricture after straddle injury.
c. Retain suprapubic tube if stricture or extravasation present.
d. Reimage on a weekly basis or until definitive management performed.

3. **Long-term complications.**
a. Incontinence.
b. Impotence.
c. The incidence of impotence and incontinence is not improved with either early or late repair.
d. Obstruction:
   1) Impassable strictures develop in 95% of patients managed with suprapubic tube alone vs 53% of those managed with primary realignment, although the vast majority of the latter group do require further therapy with prolonged follow-up.
   2) This entails either VIU for impassable strictures or progressive urethral dilatation using filiforms and followers.
   3) Both usually require patient self-dilatation for an extended period to maintain patency of the urethra.

V. FURTHER READING

Bright TC, Peter PC. Ureteral injuries due to external violence: 10 years experience with 59 cases. *J Trauma* 1977; 17(8):616–620.

Guerriero WG. Ureteral injury. *Urol Clin North Am* 1989; 16(2):237–238.

Herschorn S, Thijssen A, Radomski SB. The value of immediate or early catheterization of the traumatized posterior urethra. *J Urol* 1992; 148:1162–1165.

Mee SL, McAninch JW. Indications for radiographic assessment in suspected renal trauma. *Urol Clin North Am* 1989; 16(2):187–192.

Sagalowsky AI, Peters PC. Genito-urinary trauma. In: Walsh PC, Retik AB, Vaughan ED Jr, Wein AJ, eds. *Campbell's urology*, 7th edn. Philadelphia: WB Saunders; 1998:3085–3120.

Peterson NE, Pitts JC. Penetrating injuries of the ureter. *J Urol* 1981; 126(5):587–590.

Pierce JM. Disruptions of the anterior urethra. *Urol Clin North Am* 1989; 16(2):329–334.

Quint HJ, Stanisic TH. Above and below delayed endoscopic treatment of traumatic posterior urethral disruptions. *J Urol* 1993; 149:484–487.

Sandler CM, Corriere JN. Ureterography in the diagnosis of acute urethral injuries. *Urol Clin North Am* 1989; 16(2):283–289.

Webster GD. Perineal repair of membranous urethral stricture. *Urol Clin North Am* 1989; 16(2):303–312.

Wessells H, McAninch J. *Update on upper urinary tract trauma*. AUA Update Series. Houston: American Urologic Association Inc. Office of Education; 1996; 15:lesson 14.

GENITAL AND PERINEAL TRAUMA

I. PENILE TRAUMA

A. PENILE FRACTURE
(TRAUMATIC RUPTURE OF CORPUS CAVERNOSUM).

1. **Occurrence.**
   a. Rare injury – 1 in 175,000 admissions.
   b. Occurs in the erect penis usually during coitus, but occasionally with other blunt trauma.
   c. History of vigorous intercourse with bending of the penis accompanied by cracking sound and immediate pain, swelling, and rapid loss of erection.
   d. Involves disruption of the tunica albuginea of the corpus cavernosa: usually only one corpus is affected, but more severe trauma may injure both.
   e. Tear in tunica albuginea is usually transversely oriented.
   f. Concomitant urethral injury is present in 20% of cases. In the absence of urethral injury, the ability to void is usually preserved.

2. **Physical examination.**
   a. Deviation of the penis away from the injured side.
   b. Marked swelling.
   c. Ecchymosis.

3. **Diagnosis.**
   a. Primarily a clinical diagnosis.
   b. Magnetic resonance imaging (MRI) is diagnostic, but expensive and rarely needed.
   c. Sonography and cavernosography may be helpful, but are less sensitive.
   d. Retrograde urethrogram should be performed to evaluate the urethra.

4. **Management.**
   a. Surgical exploration with evacuation of the hematoma.
   b. Débridement and repair of the injury to the tunica albuginea via a circumcising or overlying incision.
   c. Primary repair of urethral injury over a catheter should be attempted since urethral injury is usually minor.

5. **Long-term prognosis usually good.**

B. PENILE AMPUTATION.

1. **Occurrence.**
   a. Rare injury, usually due to self-emasculation in a psychotic patient or in an assault.
   b. Very rarely may occur with neonatal circumcision.

2.   **Management.**

a.   Severed penile segment should be immediately cooled and kept moist.

b.   Control bleeding with compression, not a tourniquet as this may compensate viability of remaining penile tissue.

c.   Reconstruction should be attempted early, preferably with microvascular reanastomosis.

d.   Reapproximation of the corporal tunics, spongy tissue, and urethra is frequently successful.

e.   Distal amputations should be debrided and the corpora closed.

f.   The urethra can be spatulated and imbricated to a button-holed dorsal skin flap to achieve a highly functional phallus.

g.   If reanastomosis is unsuccessful, a phallus may be constructed using a radial forearm free graft or tubularized abdominal pedicle graft.

C.   **DEGLOVING OF PENILE OR SCROTAL SKIN (POWER TAKE-OFF INJURY).**

1.   **Occurrence.**

a.   Avulsion of penile skin may be complete or partial and frequently is accompanied by scrotal avulsion.

b.   Mechanism usually involves farm or industrial equipment in which the patient's clothes become caught.

2.   **Management.**

a.   Reconstruction should be delayed 12–24 hours and local care with moist soaks applied to the penis before débridement.

b.   A thick split-thickness skin graft is later used for coverage.

c.   Partial avulsions with remaining distal penile skin should be converted to complete avulsions by débridement to prevent distal penile edema.

d.   After scrotal avulsion, the testes should be kept moist and then implanted into the thigh pouches. The thigh pouches may then be mobilized as cutaneous flaps and used for later scrotal reconstruction.

3.   **Long-term prognosis is good.**

D.   **PENILE STRANGULATION.**

1.   **Occurrence** – usually due to twine, condoms, or metal rings.

2.   **Management.**

a.   Strangulating material should be removed immediately and may require operative anesthesia or metal-cutting equipment.

b.   Even though the distal penis may initially appear nonviable, satisfactory outcomes are usually obtained with conservative therapy.

E.   **PENETRATING PENILE TRAUMA.**

1.   **Management.**

a.   Requires radiographic evaluation of urethra especially with entrance or exit wounds in close proximity.

b.   Exploration required with corporal and urethral repair as needed.

F. HUMAN BITE, ZIPPER INJURY, OR PREPUTIAL FRENULA TEAR.

1. **Management.**

a. Respond well to local care.

b. Antibiotic prophylaxis is necessary, owing to high incidence of post-traumatic cellulitis.

c. Rarely may require circumcision.

d. Frenula injury is usually related to coitus and must be differentiated from meatal bleeding in uncircumcised patients. The foreskin must be everted to differentiate these conditions as these patients are almost always uncircumcised.

II. SCROTAL AND TESTICULAR TRAUMA.

A. SCROTUM.

1. **Blunt injuries.**

a. Rare, owing to the scrotum's protected position and mobility.

b. Must rule out testicular torsion and epididymitis.

c. Urinalysis may demonstrate pyuria with epididymitis while testicular radionuclide scanning may be necessary to exclude torsion.

d. Scrotal ultrasound may show diffuse hematoma in the scrotal layers.

e. Treatment is conservative with bed rest, analgesia, and scrotal elevation.

2. **Penetrating injuries.**

a. Simple skin lacerations may be debrided and closed primarily.

b. If dartos fascia is lacerated, it should be closed separately to prevent hematoma formation. Scrotal exploration is also required in this circumstance to rule out testicular injury or penetration of tunica vaginalis.

c. Sonography may be helpful preoperatively, particularly with regard to diagnosis of testicular trauma in questionable cases.

3. **Scrotal avulsion** necessitates testicular transposition into the thigh pouches and later reconstruction (see section I).

B. TESTES.

1. **Testicular laceration or disruption.**

a. In the presence of penetrating trauma, usually a gunshot or stab wound, exploration is indicated.

b. Following blunt trauma, usually a kick or a direct blow, scrotal ecchymosis, acute hematocele, loss of palpable testicular contour, and marked pain and tenderness are present.

2. **Diagnosis.**

a. Sonography (7.5MHz transducer) will demonstrate:
   1) Acute hematocele.
   2) Laceration of the tunica albuginea testis.
   3) Loss of normal contour.
   4) Extrusion of parenchymal tissue.

b. A normal sonogram does not rule out a testicular disruption.

28

GENITAL AND PERINEAL TRAUMA

c. The diagnostic accuracy of ultrasound in the detection of traumatic testis rupture has:
    1) Specificity 75%.
    2) Sensitivity 64%.
    3) Positive predictive value 78%.
    4) Negative predictive value 60%.
d. If clinical suspicion is high, exploration is mandated.
e. In all cases with antecedent trauma, testicular torsion should be excluded (usually in men <30 years old; however, occasionally it is seen in older men).
f. Acute epididymitis can be detected sonographically and is usually accompanied by pyuria.

3. Management.
a. Surgical exploration of the affected testis.
b. Débridement.
c. Reapproximation of the tunica albuginea.
d. Scrotal drainage (generally Penrose type).
e. The spermatic cord should be examined and any obvious bleeding controlled prior to scrotal closure.
f. Drainage is maintained for a minimum of 24 hours or until drain output is minimal.
g. Follow-up sonography may be used to document healing; serum testosterone and luteinizing hormone levels are monitored if parenchymal loss has been significant.

III. PERINEAL TRAUMA AND LACERATION

1. **The mechanism** is generally either impalement after a fall, motor vehicle or pedestrian collision, or avulsion of perineal skin due to power take-off injury.
2. **These injuries are frequently associated** with pelvic fracture and concurrent genitourinary or rectal injuries.
3. **Treatment** may require a temporary diverting colostomy or a urinary diversion with a suprapubic tube to prevent contamination prior to closure or skin grafting. A gracilis muscle flap may be required for definitive coverage.

IV. CHEMICAL, ELECTRICAL, AND THERMAL INJURY TO THE GENITALIA AND PERINEUM

A. **THERMAL INJURIES.** The treatment is similar to that of other skin burns and utilizes topical antimicrobial agents and sterile dressings. A cautious approach to débridement should be used.
B. **CHEMICAL BURNS.** These are usually superficial and, after flushing the area copiously, the chemical burn is treated as a thermal injury.

C. **ELECTRICAL BURNS.** The innocent appearance of an electrical burn can be misleading. Despite minimal skin injury, the current is dissipated through the vessels causing extensive destruction of deep structures. After 24 hours of conservative management, the limits of destruction should be determined and then the tissue debrided.

V. FURTHER READING

Jordan GH, Gilbert DA. Management of amputation injuries of the male genitalia. *Urol Clin North Am* 1989; 16(2):359–367.

McAninch JW. Management of genital skin loss. *Urol Clin North Am* 1989; 16(2):387–397.

Sagalowsky AI, Peters PC. Genito-urinary trauma. In: Walsh PC, Retik AB, Vaughan ED Jr., Wein AJ, eds. *Campbell's urology,* 6th edn. Philadelphia: WB Saunders; 1998:3085–3120.

28

GENITAL AND PERINEAL TRAUMA

EXTREMITY VASCULAR TRAUMA

I. EPIDEMIOLOGY
1. **Upper extremities** are involved in 18–26% of civilian injuries and 32% of military injuries (United States only).
2. **Lower extremities** are involved in 20% of civilian injuries and in 62% of military injuries (United States only).
3. **Up to 80% of patients with arterial injury** have other associated injuries.
4. **Motor vehicle crashes are the most common cause** of blunt vascular injury.

II. MECHANISM OF INJURY
1. **Approximately 80% of peripheral vascular trauma** occurs as a result of gunshot wounds, shotgun wounds, stab wounds, or slash wounds.
2. **Blunt injuries are most common** following dislocations, especially of the knee, shoulder, and elbow, as well as fractures.
3. **Iatrogenic injuries**, which have increased in incidence, are usually due to catheterizations.

III. EVALUATION
A. HISTORY.
1. **A careful history of the amount and nature of the bleeding** at the scene of the injury, associated motor or neurologic deficits, and the exact mechanism of injury must be determined if possible.
2. **A history of pulsatile bleeding** strongly supports an arterial injury.
B. PHYSICAL EXAMINATION.
1. **The physical examination must be meticulous** and include pulse character, caliber, ankle–brachial indices (ABIs) for lower extremities, and a complete neurologic evaluation of the injured extremity.
2. **An assessment** of bone and joint integrity, temperature, capillary refill, and venous insufficiency must be evaluated (Table 29.1).
3. **Pulse changes** in relation to orthopedic maneuvers must be noted.
4. **Local evaluation of the area of injury** including auscultation for the presence of a bruit or palpation of a thrill, as well as characterization of any hematoma and assessment of proximity to known major vascular structures.
5. **The six Ps** – pulselessness, pallor, pain, paresthesia, paralysis, and poikilothermia – are key clinical features to assess when evaluating a patient for possible arterial injury.
C. ULTRASONIC FLOW DETECTION.
1. **Patients with extremity trauma** and no clinical evidence of arterial injury should be screened with Doppler arterial-pressure measurements.

TABLE 29.1

SIGNS OF ARTERIAL INJURY

Hard signs	Soft signs
Circulatory deficit	Small, stable hematoma
Ischemia	Adjacent nerve injury
Pulse deficit	Shock (otherwise unexplained)
Bruit	Proximity to major vascular structures, <1cm from anatomic position of vessel
Expanding or pulsatile hematoma	Difference in ankle–branchial indices >0.15 injured extremity
Arterial bleeding	

2. **Patients with normal Doppler studies** (ABI >0.9) may be followed up with serial noninvasive examinations. Arteriography (or operation) is reserved for those patients with abnormal Doppler results (ABI <0.9).

3. **Segmental pressure determinations** (ABIs) are useful in identifying obstructing lesions as suggested by a low-pitched monophasic signal.

4. **The limitations of Doppler examination** include its inaccuracy for venous injuries, for damage to nonaxial vessels, such as the profunda femoris artery, and for nonocclusive arterial injuries, such as pseudoaneurysms.

5. **Proximal injuries** (axillosubclavian and iliac arteries) continue to require arteriography as a primary screening examination.

D. **DUPLEX SCANNING.** Duplex ultrasonography, though highly sensitive in screening for vascular injury, has limited use secondary to its requirement for expensive instrumentation and skilled operation and interpretation, which may not always be immediately available when evaluating the injured patient.

E. **ARTERIOGRAPHY.**

1. **Arteriograms are usually obtained** for one of three reasons in the management of patients with suspected major arterial injuries.

a. To detect injuries that might otherwise not be apparent despite a careful history and physical examination.

b. To plan the operative management of complex injuries:

c. To exclude the need for surgical exploration in patients who have no other indication for operation.

2. **Arteriography is frequently obtained** in patients who sustain shotgun wounds unless immediate exploration is indicated because of exsanguinating hemorrhage or threatened viability of the extremity.

3. **Positive signs on angiography** include obstruction, extravasation, early venous filling or arteriovenous fistula (AVF), wall irregularity, filling defect or intimal flap, and pseudoaneurysm.

4. **Angiographic embolization in acute trauma** may be considered for distal false aneurysms or AVFs in unstable patients, or in those who have no other injury if the vessel is a small muscular branch.
5. **The role of venography** is not clearly determined, but it may be helpful in selected cases. This may be performed intraoperatively.

IV. MANAGEMENT

A. PREOPERATIVE PREPARATION.

1. **Intravenous antibiotics** to cover Gram-positive cocci are begun preoperatively.
2. **The prepared area** should include the entire injured extremity. The chest is included for proximal upper extremity injuries.
3. **The lower extremity** should be prepared from toe to groin, and as a source of donor site for autologous vein graft.

B. OPERATIVE TECHNIQUE.

1. **A generous incision** is used to allow proximal and distal control to be obtained prior to direct exploration of the suspected injury.
2. **Following proximal and distal control of the vessel** with vessel loops, the artery is carefully dissected, taking care to preserve all collateral branches if possible.
a. Proximal and distal embolectomy is routinely performed with Fogarty catheters.
b. Vessels are then flushed with 1:1000 heparinized saline solution both proximally and distally and clamped with a Heifetz clip or a vascular clamp.
3. **Simple lacerations** are repaired by lateral arteriorrhaphy using fine monofilament suture of 5-0–7-0 Prolene (polypropylene).
4. **Following débridement**, repair is attempted by primary end-to-end anastomosis if adequate vessel length can be achieved. This generally requires 4–5cm of vessel mobilization for each 1cm of lost vessel length.
5. **The vessels are spatulated**, then anastomosed with a running monofilament suture if larger than 4–5 mm or interrupted monofilament if smaller. Occasionally spatulation can be omitted if the vessel is large enough in caliber or if length is restricted (Figure 29.1).
6. **If a tension-free anastomosis cannot be achieved** because of significant loss of vessel length, then repair is performed by an interposition graft.
a. The primary choice of graft conduit at Parkland Memorial Hospital is autologous reversed saphenous vein if it is available and of adequate caliber.
b. Foot or ankle saphenous vein is used for forearm and infrapopliteal vessels, while saphenous vein from the groin is preferred for axillary, brachial, femoral, and popliteal repair.

29

EXTREMITY VASCULAR TRAUMA

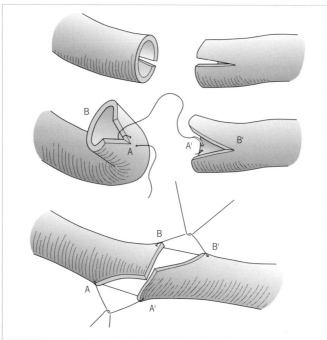

FIG. 29.1
Spatulation technique for small-vessel anastomoses. The vessel ends are slit longitudinally and fashioned into a cobra-head shape.

c. If no satisfactory autologous tissue is available, a prosthetic interposition graft may be used. The preferred option at Parkland is 6-mm expanded polytetrafluoroethylene (PTFE).

V. VENOUS INJURY

A. **CONCOMITANT VENOUS INJURIES.** These injuries are repaired if a primary repair can be achieved; otherwise they are ligated. The exception is the popliteal vein, where a complex repair even requiring vein or prosthetic interposition is recommended.

B. **EXTREMITY WITHOUT DISTAL BLOOD FLOW.** If an extensive débridement or interposition graft is required in an extremity which is without distal blood flow following thrombectomy and systemic anticoagulation, an appropriate-sized vascular shunt is used at Parkland to restore distal perfusion as quickly as possible.

C. **VASCULAR SHUNTS.** Placement of temporary vascular shunts (Javid or Argyle) allows time for the initial repair of venous injury to improve outflow prior to arterial repair as well as allowing time to harvest a saphenous vein. This also allows time for orthopedic stabilization in the presence of severe, unstable orthopedic trauma.

D. **CONCOMITANT FRACTURES.** The management of concomitant fractures is dependent on both the distal perfusion status and the degree of orthopedic instability.

1. **For unstable fractures without distal perfusion,** vascular exploration with placement of an arterial and, if necessary, a venous shunt is performed initially, followed by orthopedic stabilization. This allows for definitive vascular repair to be completed without anastomotic disruption secondary to fracture motion during reduction and fixation.

2. **When distal perfusion is preserved** as documented by Doppler examination, fractures may be addressed prior to exploration and repair. This can also be accomplished if fracture reduction can be done expediently.

3. **Distal pulse status** is frequently assessed during all orthopedic manipulation and stabilization procedures.

E. **NEUROLOGIC INJURY.** Associated neurologic injury is managed according to the discretion of the neurologic, orthopedic, or plastic consulting surgeon.

1. **Generally, contused nerves and continuity nerves are managed conservatively.**

2. **Sharply transected nerves** are repaired under magnification by group fascicular approximation with fine monofilament suture, and nerves transected by gunshot wounds or avulsion are tagged with permanent suture and repaired electively at a later time.

F. **FASCIOTOMY.** This technique is used liberally according to the indications described in Chapter 33. Fasciotomy is performed at Parkland prior to any repair where ischemia has been present, or will be present, for a significant period of time.

G. **CLOSURE.** Exposed vascular repairs are covered with myocutaneous flaps or heterografts at the initial procedure regardless of the amount of débridement required, or if subsequent débridement will be required.

29

EXTREMITY VASCULAR TRAUMA

ABDOMINAL VASCULAR INJURY

30

I. EPIDEMIOLOGY

1. **Abdominal vascular injury (AVI)** occurs in 5–10% of patients with blunt trauma and in 15–20% of patients with penetrating trauma.
2. **Abdominal vascular trauma** accounts for 20–30% of all reported vascular trauma, 18% of all arterial injuries, and 48% of all venous injuries.
3. **In >75% of all cases of penetrating vascular injuries,** patients will present in shock.

II. MECHANISM OF INJURY

A. BLUNT TRAUMA.

1. **Avulsion injuries** of small branches of major vessels.
2. **Intimal tear with secondary thrombosis** (e.g. in renal artery, caused by a seat belt).
3. **Majority of hepatic vein injuries** and one-third of renal artery injuries are secondary to blunt trauma.

B. PENETRATING TRAUMA.

1. **Blast effect** may cause intimal flaps and secondary thrombosis.
2. **Lateral wall defects** may be caused by stab wounds or bullets.
3. **May cause transection** with either free bleeding or thrombosis.
4. **Bullet embolization** is seen on rare occasions.

III. EVALUATION

A. EMERGENCY ROOM RESUSCITATION should follow the Advanced Trauma Life Support (ATLS) protocol.

B. PERTINENT FINDINGS ON PHYSICAL EXAMINATION. The following should be noted:

1. **Presence or absence of pulses.**
2. **Presence of thrills and bruits.**
3. **The number and locations of all penetrating wounds.**

C. STAB WOUNDS.

1. **Patients with stab wounds** anterior to the anterior axillary line and below the costal margin undergo local exploration if physical examination does not indicate the need for an operation (Chapter 9).
2. **If the local exploration is negative** – end of tract visualized or posterior fascia not violated – the wound can be closed and the patient discharged home.
3. **If the local exploration is positive** or equivocal – posterior fascia violated – a diagnostic peritoneal lavage (DPL) is performed and the decision to operate is based on the DPL results.

D. GUNSHOT AND SHOTGUN WOUNDS.

1. **All patients** at Parkland Memorial Hospital undergo celiotomy following abdominal gunshot wounds.
2. **Upper extremity vascular access is desirable**, especially if suspicion of inferior vena caval injury is high. Lower extremity access is acceptable.
3. **Plain abdominal radiographs** are obtained with radiopaque markers on the entrance and exit wounds to visualize missiles in the hemodynamically stable patient.
4. **A one-shot i.v. pyelogram (IVP)** is often obtained to evaluate renal function.
5. **Unstable patients** require resuscitation en route to the operating room.

E. BLUNT ABDOMINAL INJURIES.

1. **Diagnostic modalities** include CT scans in stable patients and DPL in unstable patients.
2. **Gross hematuria is evaluated** with an IVP and cystourethrography unless a CT scan is obtained. The CT scan will give good evaluation of the genitourinary (GU) tract; however, a cystogram is generally obtained as well.
3. **Microscopic hematuria** in the presence of a high index of suspicion, flank hematoma, transverse lumbar fracture, hypotension, or pelvic fracture will also require urologic evaluation.
4. **The absence of renal enhancement** or presence of the cortical rim sign on abdominal CT is highly suggestive of renal artery thrombosis and mandates early surgical exploration for the salvage of the kidney.
5. **Arteriography of the iliac arteries** may occasionally be required in the setting of a pelvic fracture.

IV. OPERATIVE MANAGEMENT

A. OPERATIVE PRINCIPLES.

1. **Assure availability of blood**, an autotransfusion apparatus, an aortic compressor, vascular instruments, sponge sticks, and vascular suture.
2. **Prep the patient while still awake**.
3. **Prep from the chin down to and including both knees**. If there is a high suspicion of iliac injury or abnormal pulses on that extremity the entire leg should be prepped.
4. **Keep the patient warm** – warming blanket, warm humidified oxygen, warm fluids.
5. **Perioperative broad-spectrum antibiotics** are given.
6. **Exposure is expeditiously achieved** via a midline incision from the xiphoid to the pubis.
7. **Evacuation of clots** is the first priority.
8. **Identify and control bleeding sources**.
9. **If the patient has persistent hemorrhage** despite packing, direct aortic compression with an aortic compressor or a large Richardson retractor should be attempted.

10. **Venous bleeding** can usually be controlled with a sponge stick.
11. **Following control of hemorrhage** other abdominal injuries can be addressed. Hollow viscus spillage is controlled with Babcock clamps, suture, or a stapling device.
12. **Remove packs systematically** starting in areas of least suspicion first.

B. **INTRA-ABDOMINAL HEMATOMA.**

1. **The retroperitoneum** encompasses three zones, which reflect the contents of each and provides guidelines for surgical therapy.

a. Zone I – central hematoma.
   1) Area extending from the diaphragm down to the level of the bifurcation of the common iliacs with its lateral boundaries encompassing bilateral renal pedicles.
   2) Includes aorta and inferior vena cava (IVC) along with their associated branches.

b. Zone II – lateral hematoma.
   1) Encompasses area to the left and right of zone I.
   2) Inferior border is at the bifurcation of the common iliacs.

c. Zone III – pelvic hematoma.
   1) Superior boundary is at the level of the bifurcation of the common iliac arteries.
   2) The inferior boundary is the cul-de-sac.

2. **All hematomas secondary** to penetrating injuries need to be explored.

3. **All zone I hematomas** require surgical exploration.

4. **Blunt injuries** causing a nonexpanding hematoma in zones II and III are generally not explored.

5. **An expanding hematoma** requires exploration.

6. **If the previous urologic evaluation showed nonvisualization** of a kidney or possible urine leak the hematoma should be explored.

C. **INTRAOPERATIVE EXPOSURE.**

1. **Abdominal vascular injuries** generally occur in one of five locations:
a. Midline supramesocolic.
b. Midline inframesocolic.
c. Lateral perirenal.
d. Lateral pelvic.
e. Portal.

2. **For the purpose of discussing vascular exposure**, these locations can further be grouped into four separate abdominal areas.
a. Area I:
   1) Midline supramesocolic – left lateral perirenal hematomas include suprarenal aorta, celiac axis, superior mesenteric artery (SMA), superior mesenteric vein (SMV), and left renal artery and vein.
   2) In the presence of active hemorrhage, proximal supraceliac aortic control is required, using manual aortic compression or application of a large vascular clamp.

3) If active hemorrhage is not present this area is best exposed with left medial visceral rotation (Mattox maneuver). The left colon, kidney, spleen, and tail of the pancreas can be reflected medially (Figure 30.1). The left kidney can be left posteriorly by dividing the splenic renal ligaments. Additional exposure is obtained by dividing the left crus at the 2 o'clock position.

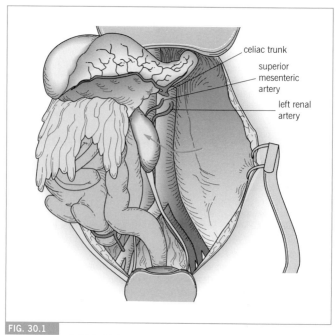

celiac trunk

superior mesenteric artery

left renal artery

FIG. 30.1

Medial rotation of all left-sided intra-abdominal viscera (Mattox maneuver) allows for visualization of the entire abdominal aorta from the hiatus to the aortic bifurcation. (Copyright Baylor College of Medicine 1981.) (From Mattox KL, Moore EE, Feliciano DV, eds. *Trauma*. East Norwalk: Appleton and Lange; 1987).

4) Left medial visceral rotation allows complete exposure of the aorta. The disadvantage is the time required and the possibility of iatrogenic injury to the spleen or pancreas.
5) For isolated splenic vessel injury, control may be obtained at the base of transverse mesocolon, through the gastrocolic ligament, or by performing a splenectomy.

b. Area II:
   1) Midline supramesocolic – right perirenal and portal hematomas include right renal artery, right-side SMA, SMV, common hepatic artery, IVC, and portal vein.
   2) Exposure here is obtained by a right medial visceral rotation (Cattell–Brausch maneuver).
   3) The right colon and hepatic flexure are mobilized and an extensive Kocher maneuver of the duodenal C-loop and head of the pancreas is performed.
c. Area III:
   1) Midline inframesocolic hematoma includes infrarenal aorta and proximal iliac vessels.
   2) Retract the transverse mesocolon cephalad, eviscerate the small bowel towards the patient's right upper quadrant, and then open the midline peritoneum (Figure 30.2).
   3) Divide the ligament of Treitz and identify the left renal vein. On rare occasions, exposure of the bifurcation of the IVC will require transection of the right common iliac artery with lateral rotation of the aorta (Figure 30.3). Once the venous injury has been controlled or repaired, the right common iliac artery can be primarily repaired.
d. Area IV:
   1) Lateral pelvic hematoma includes distal common iliac and external and internal iliac vessels.
   2) No visceral mobilization is required.
   3) On the right, the ileocecal valve usually lies over the right iliac bifurcation. To expose the right iliac system the cecum is mobilized cephalad.
   4) On the left, the bifurcation of the iliac artery is covered by the mesentery of the sigmoid colon: reflect the sigmoid colon and distal descending colon medially, and dissect the peritoneum overlying the vessels. The ureter crosses over the iliac bifurcation; therefore one must be conscious of associated urologic injuries in this region (Figure 30.4)

V. MANAGEMENT
A. GENERAL PRINCIPLES.
1. **Obtain proximal and distal control** before entering a hematoma.
2. **In the presence of contamination**, autologous tissue is preferred.
3. **Occasionally a synthetic conduit may be required**, as with extensive injuries or blast effect to the supraceliac aorta.
4. **If using a synthetic conduit** it is important to pack away any injured bowel and change gloves before performing the anastomoses.
5. **If venous ligation needs to be performed**, it is best to ligate the vein just cephalad to a major branch to avoid forming a large cul-de-sac which predisposes to clot formation.

30

ABDOMINAL VASCULAR INJURY

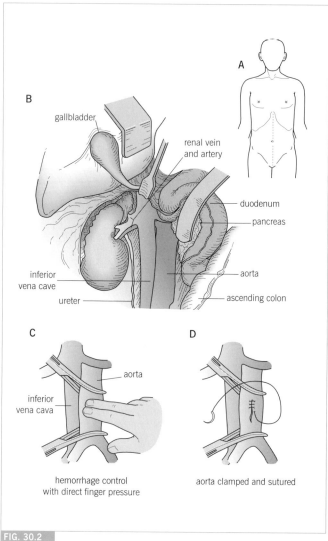

FIG. 30.2

(A,B) Adequate exposure of the abdominal aorta is rapidly obtained through an adequate midline incision. (C) Digital compression of the laceration will control hemorrhage prior to repair, which is frequently possible by suture of the laceration (D). Additional exposure can be obtained as illustrated from the right side. (From Rich NM, Spencer FC, eds. *Vascular trauma*. Philadelphia: WB Saunders; 1978:453.)

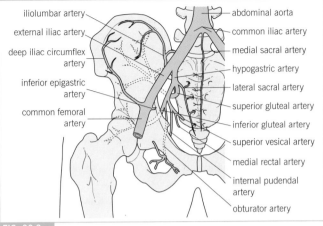

FIG. 30.3
The common iliac arteries arise at the bifurcation of the abdominal aorta. The two major divisions are the external and internal (hypogastric) iliac arteries. The major branches are also shown. (From Rich NM, Spencer FC, eds. *Vascular trauma.* Philadelphia: WB Saunders; 1978:477.)

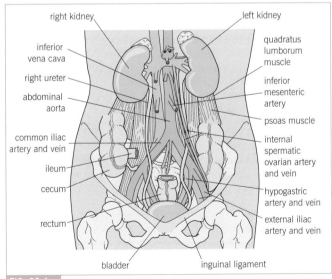

FIG. 30.4
Illustration emphasizing the close proximity of the ureters, the iliac veins, and the intestine to the iliac arteries. (From Rich NM, Spencer FC, eds. *Vascular trauma.* Philadelphia: WB Saunders; 1978:478.)

6. **The left gastric artery and splenic artery** can be safely ligated.
a. Ligation of the splenic artery does not necessitate splenectomy.
b. Ligation of the splenic vein usually requires splenectomy because of resultant congestive splenomegaly and thrombocytopenia.
7. **Ligation of the common hepatic artery** proximal to the gastroduodenal artery is acceptable because of the extensive collateral flow.
8. **Injuries distal to the gastroduodenal artery** should be repaired when feasible.
9. **In the unstable patient**, without a concomitant portal vein injury, the hepatic artery can be ligated.
a. This may result in an increased incidence of liver abscesses.
b. If ligation is performed a cholecystectomy should also be done.
10. **If the entire celiac axis is injured**, it is best to ligate all three vessels.
11. **Because of the small size of the SMA**, repair usually requires autologous bypass.

B. **FULLEN CLASSIFICATION OF SUPERIOR MESENTERIC ARTERY INJURIES.**

1. **Zone I** – injury to the SMA beneath the pancreas.
a. Ligation at this level would jeopardize the small bowel, the ascending colon, two-thirds of the transverse colon, and the pancreas.
b. May require transection of the pancreas at the neck for exposure and repair.
2. **Zone II** – injury to the SMA at the base of the transverse colon. Ligation at this location would affect all of the above except the pancreas.
3. **Zone III** – injury beyond the middle colic and right colic artery. Ligation would affect a variable extent of the small bowel.
4. **Zone IV** – injury to the vasa recta and the distal arcades. Ligation affects segments of the small or large bowel.
5. **Zone I and II injuries** may be ligated on rare occasions if the collateral flow is adequate.
a. Bowel viability must be accessed by either direct visualization, Doppler examination, or, occasionally, by giving 1g of fluoroscein and observing with a Wood's lamp.
b. If the patient is hypotensive, the collateral flow may not be adequate owing to vasoconstriction and a saphenous vein bypass may be required.
6. **Zone III injuries** require repair since the injury is beyond the collateral flow.
7. **Zone IV injuries** require segmental resection of bowel.
8. **If bowel viability is a question**, a second-look operation is required within 24–48 hours. This decision is made in the operating room at the time of the first operation.

C. **PERIRENAL HEMATOMA (AREAS I AND II).**

1. **A perirenal hematoma**, secondary to blunt trauma, that is not expanding or pulsatile with a normal IVP or CT scan need not be explored.

2. **All perirenal hematomas**, secondary to penetrating trauma, require exploration.
3. **The renal artery** is small and repair usually requires an interposition graft from the aorta or hepatic artery to the right renal artery or splenic artery to the left renal artery.
4. **When considering revascularization vs nephrectomy** the following must be considered:
a. Hemodynamic stability and magnitude of associated injuries.
b. Extent of vascular, ureteral, and renal parenchymal damage.
c. Results of IVP (i.e. functioning contralateral kidney).
d. Duration of ischemia: the interval between the time of trauma and operation is critical.
e. Thrombosis secondary to blunt trauma.
f. Consideration should be given to autotransplantation in the iliac fossa.
5. **One-third of patients with an unsuccessful repair** will develop subsequent hypertension requiring delayed nephrectomy.
D. LATERAL PELVIC HEMATOMA (AREA IV).
1. **Penetrating iliac artery and vein injuries.**
2. **About 80% will be hypotensive on arrival.**
3. **The clinical triad:**
a. Hypotension.
b. Peritoneal signs.
c. Entrance wound below umbilicus.
4. **Mortality** is usually secondary to hemorrhage, coagulopathy, or irreversible shock. Combined arterial and venous injuries have a mortality of 47%.
5. **Individuals who respond clinically to resuscitation** have a good prognosis.
6. **Mortality is affected by** absence of retroperitoneal tamponade (i.e. freely bleeding intra-abdominally – 46% die), difficult exposure in pelvis, and high incidence of associated injuries.
7. **A normal peripheral vascular examination** does not exclude injury.

VI. OPERATIVE APPROACH
A. ILIAC ARTERY AND VEIN.
1. **If necessary, the inguinal ligament can be divided** to expose and clamp the femoral vessels.
2. **In combined arterial and venous injuries** the venous injury is repaired first unless viability is threatened. In those circumstances, it may be necessary to shunt the artery while repairing the vein.
3. **Iliac vein injuries** may require division of the internal iliac artery for exposure. This artery does not need to be repaired.
4. **If the venous injury can be repaired easily** (i.e. lateral venorrhaphy) it should be repaired with 5-0 or 6-0 nonabsorbable suture (Prolene).

5. **If the patient is unstable**, with multiple associated injuries or has multiple venous injuries, the vein should be ligated.

a. Sequential compression devices and leg elevation postoperatively will reduce the incidence of severe leg swelling.

b. Transient extremity edema occurs in one-third of patients but usually resolves within 12 weeks.

c. Pulmonary embolus postligation is rare. The reported incidence is <2% with no statistical difference between repair and ligation.

6. **Fasciotomy (4 compartment) is performed if clinically indicated:**

a. More than 6 hours from time of injury to repair.

b. Elevated compartment pressures.

c. Combined arterial and venous injury.

B. **INFERIOR VENA CAVA.**

1. **Extensive injuries to the IVC** can usually be controlled with sponge-stick compression or Satinsky vascular clamps. Backbleeding from large lumbar veins can usually be controlled with large Debakey aortic clamps.

2. **Injury at the confluence of the common iliac veins** may be exposed by dividing the right common iliac artery and reflecting the aorta to the left. The right common iliac artery is repaired after the venous repair.

3. **Perforations at the level of the renal veins** can be controlled temporarily with sponge sticks.

4. **Control of the infrahepatic IVC**, renal veins, and infrarenal vena cava can then be obtained with umbilical tape (Figure 30.5).

5. **Medial mobilization of the right kidney** is helpful for exposure of posterior perforations of the suprarenal vena cava.

6. **Control of hemorrhage from the IVC** may also be obtained with the use of a 30mL balloon catheter by placing the catheter either proximally or distally through the injury site.

7. **Anterior perforations** are best repaired in a transverse fashion.

8. **Posterior perforations** can usually be visualized and repaired from inside the vena cava.

9. **If the patient is exsanguinating** and extensive repair is necessary, ligation is performed. Most young trauma patients will tolerate this as long as the circulating volume is aggressively maintained in the postoperative period.

10. **Elastic compression wraps** are applied to both lower extremities for 5–7 days.

11. **At time of discharge**, the patient is instructed to wear full-length custom support hose.

12. **Injuries to the suprarenal vena cava** need to be repaired in order to prevent postoperative renal failure.

13. **If autogenous vein is not available,** polytetrafluoroethylene (PTFE) may be considered.

14. **Retrohepatic caval injuries** are discussed in Chapter 23.

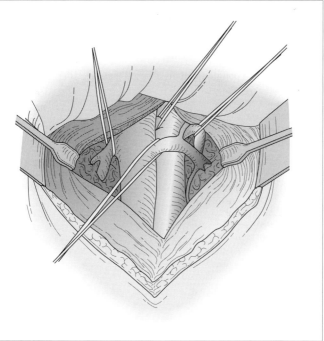

FIG. 30.5

Before any perirenal hematoma is entered, proximal vascular control is attained by looping the respective artery and vein with umbilical tapes. (Copyright Baylor College of Medicine 1980.) (From Mattox KL, Moore EE, Feliciano DV, eds. *Trauma*. East Norwalk: Appleton and Lange; 1988).

C. **PORTAL VEIN AND ITS TRIBUTARIES (AREA II).**
1. **When a hematoma involves the portal triad** in right upper quadrant, the proximal hepatoduodenal ligament should be looped with an umbilical tape or noncrushing vascular clamp (Pringle maneuver) before the hematoma is entered.
2. **Selective ligation of the hepatic artery and portal vein branches** to one lobe of the liver will likely lead to necrosis of that lobe.
3. **Selective ligation of the right hepatic artery alone** will generally require a cholecystectomy.
4. **The inferior mesenteric vein** can be ligated with no untoward effects.
5. **Aggressive attempts to repair the SMV** should be made: if necessary the SMV may be ligated. In this situation aggressive resuscitation is needed to avoid bowel ischemia.

6. **Division of the neck of the pancreas**, on rare occasions, is necessary to visualize perforations of the retropancreatic portal vein.
7. **Lateral venorrhaphy**, end-to-end anastomosis, or insertion of an interposition graft (e.g. left renal vein) are all acceptable methods of repair.
8. **Ligation of the portal vein** in the absence of hepatic artery injury is compatible with survival.
a. On rare occasions it may be associated with portal hypertension and encephalopathy.
b. If ligation is performed, aggressive resuscitation must be undertaken to compensate for splanchnic hypervolemia.

VII. MORBIDITY AND MORTALITY

A. MORBIDITY.
1. Infection.
2. Aortoenteric fistulae.
3. Thrombosis.
4. False aneurysm.
5. **Coagulopathy** – usually the result of hypothermia, multiple transfusions or acidosis.

B. MORTALITY. This is affected by a number of factors.
1. **Location of the injury.**
a. Supraceliac – 50%.
b. Suprarenal – 80–90%.
c. Infrarenal – 50%.
2. **Mechanism of the injury.**
a. Shotgun – 80%.
b. Gunshot – 60%.
c. Blunt – 50%.
d. Stab – 20%.
3. **Presentation of the patient.**
a. Hypotensive vs normotensive.
b. Number of associated visceral injuries.
c. Number of associated vascular injuries.
d. The presence of coagulopathy, hypothermia, and metabolic acidosis accounts for 80% of deaths.

THERMAL BURNS, CHEMICAL BURNS, AND COLD INJURIES

I. BURN INJURY

1. **Approximately 100,000 patients per year require hospitalization** for thermal injuries in the United States and result in a 10% overall mortality.
2. **Severe burns require triage** to regional burn centers.
3. **Morbidity and mortality of burns** are a function of burn depth, size, and location as well as patient's age and pre-existing conditions (Tables 31.1 and 31.2).
4. **The terminology** of first-, second-, and third-degree burns (Table 31.3) has been replaced with partial-thickness burns which will heal within 14–21 days, without much scar formation, and generally do not require grafting.

TABLE 31.1

AMERICAN BURN ASSOCIATION BURN SEVERITY CATEGORIZATION

Burn classification	Characteristics	Implications for treatment
Minor burn injury	1° burns	These patients may qualify for outpatient therapy
	2° burn <15% BSA in adults	
	2° burn <5% in children or aged	
	3° burn <2% BSA	
Moderate burn injury	2° burn 15–25% BSA in adults	Hospitalization is required
	2° burn 10–20% BSA in children or aged	Given adequate staff and facilities, a community hospital may suffice
	3° burn <10% BSA	
Major burn injury	2° burn >25% BSA in adults	Care in a specialized burn center is indicated
	2° burn >20% BSA in children or aged	
	3° burn >10% BSA	
	Burns involving hands, face, eyes, ears, feet, or perineum	
	Most patients with inhalation injury, electrical injury, concomitant major trauma, or significant pre-existing diseases	

(From Trunkey DD, Lewis FR. *Current therapy of trauma*. Philadelphia: BC Decker; 1984–1985.)
BSA, body surface area.

TABLE 31.2

PREDICTED MORTALITY FOLLOWING BURN INJURY

Age (years)	% BSA burned									
	10	20	30	40	50	60	70	80	90	100
10	0	4	14	37	60	78	91	97	99	100
20	0	3	13	35	59	77	90	97	99	100
30	0	4	16	39	62	79	92	97	99	100
40	1	7	22	47	69	84	94	98	100	
50	3	13	35	59	77	90	96	99	100	
60	9	27	53	72	87	96	99	100		
70	24	49	70	85	95	99	100			
80	51	71	86	95	99	100				
90	75	89	97	99	100					

(From Trunkey DD, Lewis FR. *Current therapy of trauma*. Philadelphia: BC Decker; 1984–85.)

TABLE 31.3

CHARACTERISTICS OF FIRST-, SECOND-, AND THIRD- DEGREE BURNS

	First	Second	Third
Cause	Sunlight or minor flash	Scald, flash, some chemical agents	Flame, chemical agents, electrical
Color	Light pink or slight darkening	Pink or mottled red	Pearly white, translucent, deep red in infants
Texture	Dry or small blisters	Blisters or wet surface	Dry, thrombosis of superficial vessels: spongy necrosis with alkali
Sensation	Painful	Painful	Anesthetic
Healing	3–6 days	10–21 days	Requires grafting

5. **Full-thickness burns involve** deep dermal structures, heal poorly or not at all, and will frequently require grafting.

II. EVALUATION

A. PREHOSPITAL.

1. **The goal** is to prevent additional injury and limit microbial contamination.

2. **Clean bed sheets or a large absorbent dressing** should be used to protect the burn wound.
3. **The application of cool water** on partial-thickness burns in the first 10–15 minutes may reduce residual heat in the wound, thereby preventing extension of tissue damage.
4. **The practice at Parkland Memorial Hospital** is to apply agents that are easily removed and do not cause further damage, such as shaving foam.
5. **The protection of a compromised airway** and initiation of i.v. fluid resuscitation should be considered depending on time of transport.
B. EMERGENCY DEPARTMENT.
1. **Evaluation is performed,** as in all trauma patients, using the ABC algorithm of the primary survey (Table 31.4).
2. **Patients with facial or neck burns,** and those suspected of having sustained inhalation injuries (burns in an enclosed space), must be evaluated for airway compromise.
3. **Prophylactic intubation** is frequently performed prior to airway compromise, which may occur with fluid resuscitation of large burns.
4. **Patients who require intubation are sedated,** without paralysis, to the point where they tolerate nasotracheal or orotracheal intubation.
a. Incremental doses of morphine (2mg) and diazepam (2–5mg) are used at Parkland while ventilating the patient with a bag-valve mask device until they can tolerate intubation.
b. Pharmacologic paralysis is used only when intubation is unsuccessful using the above method.
5. **In addition to ensuring adequate spontaneous or mechanical ventilation,** all patients receive 100% oxygen to cover the possibility of carbon monoxide intoxication.

TABLE 31.4

SYSTEMIC MANIFESTATIONS OF BURN INJURY

Cardiovascular	Increased capillary permeability
	Decreased cardiac output
	Increased peripheral vascular resistance
Pulmonary	Hyperventilation
Renal	Decreased glomerular filtration rate
Gastrointestinal	Ileus (burns ≥ 30% total body surface area)
	Gastritis, duodenitis
Metabolic	Increased oxygen consumption
Hematologic	Early depression of platelet and fibrinogen correlations with subsequent rebound and leukocytosis
	Immediate red cell destruction proportional to burn extent
Immunologic	Impaired cellular and humoral immunity
Integument	Increased insensible water losses (up to 200mL/m^2/h)
	Increased evaporative water losses

31

THERMAL BURNS, CHEMICAL BURNS, AND COLD INJURIES

6. **Two large-bore i.v. catheters are inserted**, preferably through unburned skin. However, these can be placed through burned skin, if necessary, without significant morbidity.
7. **The circulation is assessed** by noting the vital signs and urine output.
8. **The secondary survey** will identify associated injuries and other pertinent issues that may need to be addressed.
9. **The extent of the burn is assessed** using the rule of 9s (upper limbs 9% each, lower limbs 18% each, anterior and posterior trunk 18% each, head and neck 9%) (Figure 31.1).

III. RESUSCITATION

A. **THE PARKLAND FORMULA.** This formula (Table 31.5) is used for resuscitation of burns >10% total body surface area (TBSA) in pediatric and geriatric patients and for burns >20% TBSA in adults.
1. **The Parkland formula consists of** 4mL/kg per % TBSA Ringer's lactate (RL) for the first 24 hours and colloid and D5W maintenance fluid for the second 24 hours given as described below:
a. 2mL/kg per %TBSA over first 8 hours postburn.
b. 1mL/kg per %TBSA over second 8 hours postburn.
c. 1mL/kg per %TBSA over third 8 hours postburn.
d. 0.5mL/kg per %TBSA 5% albumin over first 4 hours of the second day.
e. 1mL/kg per %TBSA D5W per day maintenance fluid.
2. **This formula is used as a guide** and the patient must be continually reassessed for adequate vital signs and a urine output of 0.5–1mL/kg per hour (up to 50mL per hour).
3. **Peripheral i.v. access is preferable** to a central venous catheter and is adequate for resuscitating the majority of burn patients.
4. **Central access** for CVP monitoring and pulmonary artery catheters are reserved for patients that do not appropriately respond to resuscitation or have known compromised cardiac function.
5. **Colloid solutions are administered** in the second 24 hours postburn after the burn-induced capillary leak begins to resolve.

TABLE 31.5

PARKLAND FORMULA FOR RESUSCITATION

Parkland formula	4mL Ringer's lactate/kg/% TBSA in 24 hours post burn
First 8 hours	Ringer's lactate 2mL/kg/% TBSA
Second 8 hours	Ringer's lactate 1mL/kg/% TBSA
Third 8 hours	Ringer's lactate 1mL/kg/% TBSA
Next 4 hours	Fresh frozen plasma 0.5mL/kg/% TBSA
Maintain	D5W 1mL/kg/% TBSA per day

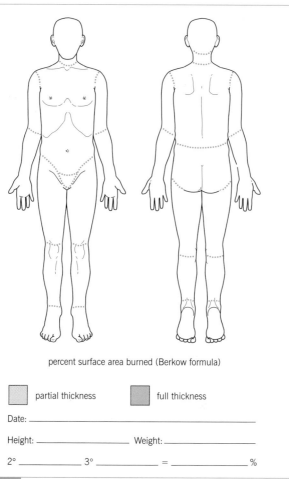

percent surface area burned (Berkow formula)

partial thickness   full thickness

Date: _____

Height: _____ Weight: _____

2° _____ 3° _____ = _____ %

FIG. 31.1

Burn record, Dallas County Hospital District, Dallas.

6. **Maintenance fluids are replaced** with D5W.
7. **Packed red blood cells should be transfused** to support oxygen delivery and in anticipation of surgical blood loss.
8. **The patient is given both active and passive tetanus prophylaxis** in opposite shoulders while in the emergency department.

   a. The dose of tetanus immune globulin (Hypertet) is 4 units/kg.

   b. Tetanus prophylaxis is the only medication that should be administered intramuscularly to the burn patient as these patients have poor skin and muscle perfusion.

9. **A nasogastric tube should be inserted** to prevent gastric dilatation, vomiting, and aspiration in patients with burns exceeding 25% TBSA. These patients have a tendency to develop an ileus.

10. **Antacids are used** to prevent stress ulceration. Maintenance of gastric pH >5 with antacids is as effective as the use of H2 blockers.

11. **Prophylactic antibiotics are not administered;** however, patients at Parkland receive prophylactic nystatin 450,000 units postoperatively twice daily as swish-and-swallow since they are at risk for immunosuppresssion and subsequent fungal infection.

B. **ESCHAROTOMY.**

1. **Escharotomy is performed for circumferential burns** of the extremities when there is evidence of vascular compromise.

2. **Restriction of chest wall motion by edema** to the point where ventilatory exchange is impaired (elevated peak airway pressure) is an indication for chest-wall escharotomy.

3. **Electrocautery is used** to incise the eschar on a circumferentially burned limb. The incision is made along the midlateral and midmedial line and extends the entire length of the burned area. It is carried down through the eschar and superficial fascia to a depth sufficient to allow the cut edges of the eschar to separate.

4. **Fasciotomies are required** when the edema extends beneath the investing fascia. This occurs in patients with high-voltage electrical injury or those associated with significant soft tissue, long bone, or vascular injury.

5. **Escharotomies can be performed** in the emergency department or intensive care unit with sedation.

6. **Fasciotomy is usually painful** and requires a general anesthetic.

IV. BURN WOUND CARE

A. **INITIAL CARE.** All burn wounds should be dealt with as follows:

1. Cleansed with a mild antiseptic solution.

2. Debrided of nonviable skin.

3. Have hair shaved from the burned areas.

4. Have a topical antibiotic agent applied.

5. Have the wound bandaged.

6. **Daily wound care** as outlined above with reassessment of burn depth and monitoring for invasive infection.

B. **MANAGEMENT.** Partial-thickness burn wounds are managed with topical antimicrobial agents and gauze dressings.

1. **Neomycin ointment** is used without a dressing for partial-thickness facial burns.
2. **Silver sulfasalazine or Sulfamylon** is used with a gauze dressing for other partial-thickness burns. Silver sulfasalazine is bacteriostatic on the surface of the wound and is poorly absorbed through an intact eschar. Silver sulfasalazine (Silvadene):
a. Is painless.
b. Is easy to apply.
c. Has a broad antibacterial spectrum.
d. Can cause a self-limiting neutropenia which does not predispose the patient to increased risk of infection.
3. **Mafenide acetate** (Sulfamylon)
a. Has excellent tissue and eschar penetration.
b. Is primarily effective against Gram-negative organisms.
c. Is associated with significant patient pain.
d. Causes carbonic anhydrase inhibition resulting in a metabolic acidosis.
e. Indicated for burn wounds with invasive infection, pseudomonas growth, and ear burns because of the good penetration into the cartilage tissue.

V. OPERATIVE MANAGEMENT
A. EXCISION.
1. **Full-thickness burn wounds** require early excision and coverage with autograft or a biologic dressing.
2. **Excision of full-thickness burns** is considered as soon as the patient has recovered from resuscitation.
3. **Early excision reduces the length of stay** in the intensive care unit and hospital, blunts the stress response, and improves the cosmetic appearance by reducing wound contracture.
4. **Because of the large blood loss associated with tangential excisions**, the extent of each operation is limited to approximately 20% of the body surface area.
5. **Burn wounds are excised** by either tangential excision (the sequential shaving of nonviable tissue until a uniformly viable wound bed is obtained) or fascial excision.
6. **The disadvantage of tangential excision** is massive blood loss.
7. **Blood loss can be decreased** by subcutaneous infiltration (clysis) with epinephrine and extremity tourniquets.
8. **Excision of the burn wound to fascia** with electrocautery minimizes blood loss but results in an inferior cosmetic result.
B. DRESSINGS.
1. **Freshly excised and grafted areas** are dressed with neomycin ointment and fine mesh gauze.

2. **Human allograft, porcine xenograft, or one of the synthetic biologic dressings** can be used for wound coverage after excision when autograft is not available.
3. **Operative dressings are changed**, except for the fine mesh gauze, on postoperative day 2–3. The wound continues to be covered with neomycin-impregnated fine mesh gauze until epithelialization is complete.

C. EXERCISE.

1. **Joints are exercised** on postoperative day number 5.
2. **Ambulation is restricted** in those patients who have wounds that are grafted above the knee until postoperative day 3–5 and in patients with grafts below the knee ambulation is restricted until postoperative day 5–10.

VI. NUTRITION

A. METABOLISM.

1. **The metabolic rate rises** in proportion to the extent of the injury and may reach levels twice those of normal individuals.
2. **Postburn hypermetabolism** is manifested by increased oxygen consumption, elevated cardiac output and minute ventilation, increased core temperature, wasting of body mass, and increased urinary nitrogen excretion.

B. REQUIREMENTS.

1. **Nutritional requirements are calculated** at 1.5g of protein/kg per day.
2. **The required ratio for nonprotein calories** to grams of nitrogen is 150:1.
3. **Alternative methods of calculating nutrition requirements** are obtained either from the measured energy expenditure or the estimated energy expenditure (EEE) formula using the Harris–Benedict equation.
4. **Recommended nutritional needs** are derived by multiplying the EEE by 1.5.
5. **Nutritional support** is begun immediately after resuscitation.
6. **Enteral feedings are used** for all patients with a functional gastrointestinal tract.

VII. COMPLICATIONS OF BURN INJURY

A. PNEUMONIA.

1. **Pneumonia is now the most common infection** in the burn patient and is often preceded by atelectasis. It is commonly seen several days after an inhalation lung injury.
2. **Diagnosis is challenging** as patients often demonstrate signs and symptoms in the absence of pulmonary infection.
3. **Diagnosis is made on the basis** of the development of new infiltrates on chest radiography, leukocytosis, and increased tracheal secretions.

4. **Sputum cultures and cultures of broncho-alveolar lavage aspirates** will identify the organisms and direct antimicrobial therapy.
5. **The infection is usually caused by a mixed flora.** A study from the burn unit at Parkland Memorial Hospital demonstrated streptococcus as a common cause, infection occurring within 48–72 hours of admission.
6. **Treatment** consists of ventilatory support, pulmonary toilet, and broad-spectrum antibiotics that are adjusted to the results of the patient's sputum culture and sensitivity.
7. **Prophylactic antibiotics and steroids are not indicated.**
B. BURN WOUND INFECTION.
1. **Bacterial infections** cause a spectrum of complications (Table 31.6).
2. **All burn wounds became colonized**; some become locally infected causing cellulitis and few cause systemic infections and overt sepsis.
3. **The use of topical antimicrobial agents and early excision** reduce the complications of bacterial invasion.
4. **The signs of the burn wound sepsis** are enumerated in Table 31.6.
5. **Quantitative wound cultures** differentiate between colonization and infection.
6. **Cultures yielding** 1×10^5 or more organisms per gram of tissue are suggestive of burn wound infection.
7. **Treatment** includes a change to topical Sulfamylon and systemic broad-spectrum antibiotics.
C. GASTROINTESTINAL ULCERATION.
1. **Curling's ulcers** are acute ulcerations of the upper gastro-intestinal tract.
2. **They present as** either diffuse gastritis or as punctate, well-demarcated superficial lesions in either the gastric and duodenal mucosa.
3. **The incidence** is directly related to the burn size and the presence of septic complications.
4. **When the gastric pH is maintained** at ≥ 5, using either antacids or H2 antagonists, the incidence of gastrointestinal hemorrhage is <1% at Parkland Memorial Hospital.

TABLE 31.6

LOCAL SIGNS OF BURN WOUND INFECTION

1. Conversion of partial-thickness burn to full-thickness burn
2. Hemorrhage discoloration of subeschar tissue
3. Accelerated eschar separation
4. Dark, violaceous discoloration of burn wound, either local or generalized
5. Erythematous nodular lesions, often with central necrosis, in unburned skin erythrema gangrenosum
6. Edema and violaceous discoloration of unburned skin at margins of burn wound
7. Degeneration of granulation tissue and subsequent formation of neoeschar
8. Vesicles in healing partial-thickness burns (herpes infection)

5. **Sucralfate is also effective** and may decrease associated aspiration pneumonia.

D. **ILEUS.**

1. **Patients with large burns** frequently develop intestinal dysmotility which generally resolves spontaneously.

2. **Other causes,** such as sepsis, pancreatitis, colonic pseudo-obstruction, diabetes, acute mesenteric ischemia, intra-abdominal sepsis, and electrolyte abnormalities, must be considered.

3. **Prolonged cases are managed by decompression** with a nasogastric or gastrostomy tube and the use of prokinetic agents.

E. **WOUND.**

1. **Hyperpigmentation and hypopigmentation** are common following burn injury.

2. **Hyperpigmentation can be reduced** by reducing exposure to sunlight during the first year following the burn.

3. **Hypertrophic scars** require compression dressings, while keloids might benefit from steroid injection.

4. **Prolonged treatment of wound complications** is accomplished in consultation with the plastic surgeons and rehabilitation specialists.

5. **Joint contractures are common** where the scars cross joint surfaces.

6. **These are initially managed nonoperatively** by aggressive physical therapy, including active and passive motion exercises.

7. **When this fails,** operative tissue releases, with or without skin grafting, may improve the outcome.

8. **Chronic burn wounds** may develop squamous cancers; thus nonhealing ulcers should undergo punch biopsy.

VIII. ELECTRICAL BURNS

A. **CHARACTERIZATION.** Electrical burns are characterized by both cutaneous burns and deep muscle damage.

1. **Mortality** is dependent on TBSA and associated trauma.

2. **Appearance of the contact wounds** may be deceptively benign while extensive subfascial tissue damage may be present.

B. **CARDIAC ABNORMALITIES.** These are evident either on admission to the emergency department or within several hours.

1. **Most arrhythmias** are transient and therapy is unnecessary in the absence of hemodynamic instability.

2. **Observation** in a telemetry or intensive care unit is mandatory when arrhythmias are noted.

C. 10% of patients with electrical injuries have associated traumatic injuries requiring treatment.

D. **FLUID RESUSCITATION.** This is of primary importance in all patients with thermal injury.

1. **Additional fluid is required** in electrical injuries because of the muscle damage.

2. **The minimum fluid requirement** for electrical injury is based on the size of the cutaneous injury (4mL/kg per % burn).

E. **URINE OUTPUT.** This must be maintained between 50 and 100mL per hour.

1. **If pigment (myoglobin or hemoglobin) is present**, the urine output should be increased to 100–150mL per hour until all gross pigment clears.

2. **Prompt diuresis** can be initiated by giving 12.5g of mannitol i.v.

3. **One ampule of sodium bicarbonate** may be given to alkalinize the urine.

4. **The presence of pigment in the urine** should cause suspicion of underlying muscle damage.

F. **THE TECHNETIUM STANNOUS PYROPHOSPHATE 99 MUSCLE SCAN.** This sensitive scan is used to locate and determine the extent of deep muscle damage.

G. **ANTIMICROBIAL AGENT.**

1. **Sulfamylon** is the topical antimicrobial agent of choice as a result of its broad antimicrobial spectrum and penetration of the dense eschar of the electrical burn.

2. **An i.v. antimicrobial agent** effective against anaerobes and aerobes is given to patients suspected of having underlying devitalized muscle.

H. **ANTIBIOTICS** are discontinued after all nonviable muscles are debrided.

I. **EARLY EXCISION** and aggressive surgical débridement is performed to decrease the incidence of bacterial complications associated with retained nonviable muscle.

J. **NEUROLOGIC DAMAGE.** Acute and chronic neurological sequelae are often associated with high-voltage electrical injuries.

1. **Repeat neurologic examinations** should be performed to detect early or late neuropathology.

2. **Early spinal cord deficits** may be transient; however, those that appear late in the postinjury course are generally permanent.

K. **REGIONAL ANESTHESIA** should be avoided.

L. **FUNDOSCOPIC AND SLIP LAMP EXAMINATION** of the eyes is essential since electrical injury can cause both immediate and delayed changes in the lenses (cataracts).

M. **LIGHTNING INJURIES.** The site of entry and exit, as well as positioning and grounding of the victim, determine the extent of injury.

1. **Cutaneous thermal injuries** caused by lightning have unique serpiginous or arborizing patterns caused by the spread of the current in the skin.

2. **Following a lightning strike**, death may be caused by either cardiac stand-still or apnea.

3. **Cardiopulmonary resuscitation** should be promptly instituted.

4. **Further care of the burn injuries** is accomplished in the same manner as for those who have a high-voltage electrical injury.

5. **Rarely is a significant burn or deep tissue injury present**.

IX. CHEMICAL BURNS

A. ONE OF THE MAJOR PROBLEMS with chemical burns is the failure to appreciate ongoing destruction of tissue.

B. THE MOST IMPORTANT FACTOR in the initial management is dilution by copious amounts of tap water.

C. NEUTRALIZATION OF THE CHEMICAL is not indicated as the exothermic chemical reaction might cause further tissue loss.

D. TREATMENT.

1. **Treatment is best facilitated** by removal of all clothing and immediate copious water lavage for at least 15 minutes, which is continued in the emergency department for a total of 2 hours using mild soap and running tap water.

2. **In the case of strong alkaline injury**, in which rapid tissue penetration occurs, irrigation of even longer duration may be necessary.

3. **Hydrogen fluoride** (HF) is an industrial solvent that can cause severe covert chemical burns.

a. HF binds avidly to calcium in the tissues.

b. HF is neutralized with calcium carbonate used topically, infused locally, or given systemically depending on the extent of burn.

X. COLD INJURY

A. CHARACTERIZATION.

1. **Freezing injuries** (frostbite).

2. **Nonfreezing injuries** (immersion foot, trench foot, and chilblain).

3. **Generalized hypothermia**.

B. FROST BITE. This results in the freezing of tissues with the formation of ice crystals.

1. **First-degree frostbite** causes hyperemia and edema of the skin without necrosis.

2. **Second-degree frostbite** causes hyperemia and vesicle formation with partial-thickness necrosis of the skin.

3. **Third-degree frostbite** results in necrosis of the entire skin thickness and extends to a variable degree to the underlying subcutaneous tissue.

4. **Fourth-degree frostbite** causes necrosis of the full skin thickness and all underlying structures.

5. **Prediction of tissue loss** is usually not possible for weeks following frostbite injury.

C. TREATMENT.

1. **Treatment of frostbite** should begin as soon as is feasible.

2. **Rewarming of the frozen part** is the single most therapeutic maneuver for preserving potential viable tissue.

3. **The frozen part is placed in water at 40°C.**

4. **Narcotics** are required for pain control.

5. **The patient is placed at bed rest** with all injured extremities elevated and wounds exposed to the air.
6. **Since the assessment of tissue viability is difficult** and often inaccurate, surgical intervention must be delayed until clear demarcation of dead tissue has occurred.

XI. PEDIATRIC BURNS

A. INCIDENCE.
1. **Approximately one-third of burn unit admissions** include children under the age of 15 years.
2. **One-third of all burn deaths** involve children.
3. **About 10% of pediatric burn injuries** are a result of deliberate abuse by adults and another 10–20% are the result of negligence.
B. SKIN in children is thinner and more delicate than that in adults. Additionally the smaller the patient the greater the surface area relative to body mass.
C. MAINTENANCE FLUIDS. In young children, especially those <2 years of age, nonburned maintenance fluids are 5–10 times those of an adult (per kg body weight).
1. **These nonburned fluids** must be added to most patients' i.v. resuscitation.
2. **Calculated fluid volume** may be given as D5RL.
3. **Endogenous glucose production** is poor in children. Management requires frequent monitoring of serum glucose and mandatory use of sugar-containing i.v. fluids.
4. **After the first day,** children are also sensitive to changes in sodium concentration, especially hyponatremia (seizure activity may occur at levels of 130 mEq/dL).
5. **The best maintenance fluid** is D5/one-quarter normal saline (1mL/kg per %TBSA plus nonburn maintenance).
6. **Careful evaluation of hypotonic oral intake** must be made and appropriate restrictions applied.
7. **Burn size and depth estimations** must be formally reviewed and updated on the second postburn day.
8. **If abuse is suspected,** skull radiographs and a long-bone series should obtained.
9. **All infants and children** with burns >20% TBSA must have body temperature carefully monitored and maintained.
10. **The most common cause of acute bradycardia** in a burn patient is hypoxia.
11. **When indicated, nasotracheal intubation** is the method of choice.
a. Pediatric endotracheal and tracheostomy tubes have no cuff until the internal diameter reaches 5mm.

THERMAL BURNS, CHEMICAL BURNS, AND COLD INJURIES

31

b. The general rule is that the size of the tube is the same as the tip of the patient's fifth finger.
c. The small internal diameter of the endotracheal tubes increases the risk of obstruction by secretions.
d. Tracheostomy in a child is often considered earlier than in an adult.

12. **Hypertension**, which is usually asymptomatic, is an idiopathic response to a large burn (40% TBSA). This has been reported in up to 20% of children. Treatment is with hydralazine, reserpine, or α-methyldopa.

PRINCIPLES OF TREATMENT OF FRACTURES AND DISLOCATIONS

32

I. CLINICAL FEATURES OF FRACTURES AND DISLOCATIONS

1. Pain.
2. Deformity, angulation, shortening, rotation.
3. Swelling.
4. Diminished range of motion, or pain and crepitus on motion.
5. Abnormal vascular or neurologic examination.
6. Lacerations, or other soft tissue injury.

II. RADIOGRAPHIC EXAMINATION OF FRACTURES AND DISLOCATIONS

A. **ANTEROPOSTERIOR (AP) AND LATERAL VIEWS.** Both these views of the injured site should be obtained and they should include the joints above and below the injury.
B. **OBLIQUE RADIOGRAPHS.** These define fractures at joints (e.g. at the acetabulum or tibial plateau).
C. **'DYNAMIC', OR 'STRESS' STUDIES.** These studies reveal ligamentous injury by showing abnormal bony translation (e.g. flexion and extension views of the cervical spine for cervical instability, or clenched-fist views for scapholunate instability).
D. **CT SCANS.** These scans can be invaluable in defining fractures in areas that are not well seen radiographically (e.g. the posterior wall of the acetabulum, depressed articular fractures of the tibial plateau, compression fractures of the sacro-iliac joint).
E. **MAGNETIC RESONANCE IMAGING (MRI).**
1. Superior visualization of soft tissues.
2. Aids in the diagnosis of ligament or tendon rupture.
3. The spinal cord and intervertebral disks can be evaluated.
4. Magnetic resonance venography (MRV) is used to aid in the diagnosis of deep venous thrombosis, especially in the pelvic veins.

III. INITIAL MANAGEMENT OF FRACTURES

A. **PHYSICAL EXAMINATION.** A physical examination of the patient, including a neurologic and vascular examination, is mandatory.
1. **Extremity injuries are sometimes overlooked** in the emergency department, especially in multiply injured patients.
2. **A thorough musculoskeletal examination must be done** on each trauma patient to ensure that injuries are not missed.
B. **OPEN FRACTURE WOUNDS.** These should be cleaned.
1. **All gross contaminants should be removed,** and the wound covered with a sterile dressing.

2. 'Second looks' at the open wound should be avoided.

C. PROVISIONAL REDUCTION OF THE FRACTURE. This should be done in the emergency department as it reduces the risk of skin necrosis and diminishes pressure on nerves and vessels.

D. SPLINTING OF THE INJURED EXTREMITY. Splinting prevents further soft tissue injury and alleviates pain; it also allows for transportation of the patient.

IV. DEFINITIVE MANAGEMENT OF FRACTURES AND DISLOCATIONS

A. THE GOAL should be the rapid return of normal function with a minimum of morbidity.

B. REDUCTION. The restoration of normal alignment of bone and joint, or reduction, can be accomplished by either closed or open methods.

1. **Closed reduction** is the manipulation of a bone or joint to restore normal alignment without opening the skin.

2. **Open reduction** is the manipulation of a bone or joint through an incision to restore normal alignment.

3. **Immobilization maintains reduction** and allows healing.

C. TRACTION AND BED REST.

1. **Traction can be applied** through pins placed directly into the bone ('skeletal traction') or through tapes applied to the skin ('skin traction').

2. **The advantages of traction include:**

a. Ease of application.

b. Avoidance of a surgical procedure.

3. **The disadvantages include:**

a. Inability to maintain reduction.

b. Difficulty correcting rotational, length or angular deformity.

c. Prolonged bed rest causes deconditioning, decubitus ulcers, contractures, and increases the risk of deep venous thrombosis and pulmonary complications.

D. SPLINTS 'HALF-CASTS'.

1. **Reduction is maintained** while allowing for the swelling around the fracture to subside.

2. **The splints prevent** compartment syndrome.

3. **The splints are normally used** as a temporary form of immobilization.

E. CASTS.

1. **Circumferential casts** are made of plaster or fiberglass.

2. **They are a reliable way to maintain reduction** in some fractures. Complications of their use include:

a. Loss of reduction.

b. Pressure necrosis.

3. CASTS ARE USUALLY APPLIED, at Parkland Memorial Hospital, after a period of splinting, usually 1–2 weeks, to allow for swelling to subside.

F. CAST BRACES. These 'hinged casts' allow for motion at a joint while maintaining reduction. They are commonly used in conjunction with limited internal fixation of articular fractures.

G. EXTERNAL FIXATION.

1. **Pins placed into the bone** proximal and distal to the fracture are attached to external bars, which span the fracture and maintain reduction.

2. **The advantages include**:

a. Rapid application.

b. No manipulation of the fracture site.

c. Allows access to surrounding soft tissue injuries.

d. Allows stabilization of fractures where internal fixation is precluded because of soft tissue loss.

3. **The disadvantages include:**

a. Pin tract infections.

b. Osteomyelitis at the pin sites.

c. Loss of reduction due to instability of the external fixator.

H. INTERNAL FIXATION.

1. **Any implanted device used to maintain reduction** is a form of internal fixation. Pins, screws, plates, rods, and bioabsorbable implants are all forms of internal fixation.

2. **The advantages include:**

a. Accurate, stable restoration of normal anatomy, especially in articular fractures.

b. Early mobilization.

c. Limits the need for external immobilization.

3. **The disadvantages include:**

a. Risk of infection.

b. Implant failure.

c. Injury to the surrounding soft tissues caused by the surgical dissection.

4. **Periosteal stripping during internal fixation** can delay fracture healing and increase the risk of avascular necrosis of bone.

I. COLONIZATION OF HARDWARE. This is a potential problem and recent studies done at Parkland Memorial Hospital demonstrate that asymptomatic hardware is often colonized with bacteria. Conceivably, such colonization could complicate procedures such as total joint replacement, if the joint replacement was performed immediately after hardware removal.

V. OPEN FRACTURES

A. GENERAL PRINCIPLES.

1. **An open fracture** is one in which a communication exists between the fracture and the external environment. This communication is usually a skin laceration or degloving injury which exposes the fracture.

2. **If no communication exists**, the fracture is termed closed.
3. **Open injuries have the potential to become infected** by bacterial contamination of the exposed fracture site.
4. **Soft tissue complications**, such as skin and muscle necrosis, are more common in open fractures.

B. **CLASSIFICATION OF OPEN FRACTURES.** The most widely used classification of open fractures is that described by Gustilo et al.[1]; however, the interobserver agreement with use of this classification is poor.

1. **Grade I open fractures.**
   a. Skin opening <1cm in length.
   b. These fractures are simple or minimally comminuted.
   c. There is minimal soft tissue injury.
2. **Grade II open fractures.**
   a. Wounds which are between 1 and 10cm in length.
   b. Moderate amount of soft tissue injury and bony comminution.
3. **Grade III open fractures.**
   a. Wounds >10cm in length.
   b. Soft tissue injury and bony comminution are more severe.
   c. These have been subclassified by Gustilo et al.[1], as follows:
      1) Grade IIIA open fractures have extensive bony comminution and lacerations, but there is adequate soft tissue for coverage of the bone.
      2) Grade IIIB open fractures have extensive soft tissue loss and require some sort of procedure to cover the bone, such as a rotational flap or free flap.
      3) Grade IIIC open fractures have an associated vascular injury requiring vascular repair. The amputation rate with injuries such as this can be as high as 50% and the limb loss is usually due to arterial insufficiency or infection.
   d. In addition, any open fracture with the following characteristics should be considered a Grade III fracture:
      1) Gross wound contamination.
      2) Segmental fracture.
      3) Soil contamination.
      4) Farm injuries.
      5) Lawnmower injuries.
      6) Tornado injuries.
      7) Close-range shotgun wounds.
4. **The infection rate** is related to the severity of the bony and soft tissue injury.
   a. Grade I – 0–2%.
   b. Grade II – 2–7%.
   c. Grade III – 10–50%.

5. **To prevent infection**, the surgeon must strictly adhere to the principles of irrigation and débridement of all open fractures. Following these principles will minimize the risk of infection.

C. TREATMENT OF OPEN FRACTURES.

1. Initial treatment.
a. A detailed examination is mandatory.
b. Documentation of neurovascular status is essential.
c. A good description or drawing of the open wound is useful.
d. Serial examination is important to assure compartment syndrome does not occur.

2. Initial cleansing.
a. In the emergency room, gross debris should be removed and a sterile dressing should be applied to the wound.
b. Gross displacement of fractures should be reduced and splinted.
c. Perfect alignment of the fracture is not essential, since all open-fracture patients should be taken emergently to the operating room for definitive treatment.
d. All open fractures should be considered 'limb-threatening' injuries.

3. Intravenous antibiotics.
a. Should be given immediately.
b. A first-generation cephalosporin (cefazolin) is given to open-fracture patients every 8 hours for the first 48 hours of hospital stay.
c. Penicillin is added if soil contamination is present.
d. After the first 48 hours, i.v. cephazolin is given for 24 hours after each successive surgical irrigation and débridement.

4. **Tetanus prophylaxis** should be given to all open-fracture patients, according to standard guidelines.

D. SURGICAL TREATMENT.

1. **Irrigation and débridement is mandatory** in all open fractures. This is done in the operating room under sterile conditions.
2. **The open wound should be extended** to allow complete visualization of the fracture ends and injured soft tissues.
3. **Any necrotic or devitalized tissue should be removed**. Any loose bone stripped of its soft tissues should be removed.
4. **The wound should be copiously irrigated** with a pulsed-lavage system (at least 10L of fluid).
5. **Wounds should be left open** and covered with saline-soaked gauze (although surgical incisions used to extend the wound can be closed).
6. **Stabilization of the fracture** will prevent further soft tissue injury and makes wound care easier.
7. **Internal fixation can be used** after irrigation and débridement in many open fractures, as long as soft tissue coverage of the implant is possible.
a. Intramedullary nailing of some types of open tibia and femur fractures has given results equal or superior to those seen with other methods.

PRINCIPLES OF FRACTURES AND DISLOCATIONS   32

b. Articular fractures often require internal fixation for anatomic reduction.
8. External fixation has many advantages in the treatment of open fractures.
a. Can be placed out of the zone of the injury.
b. Does not require additional dissection.
c. Allows access to the wound for further surgery.
d. The disadvantages include:
   1) Many fractures are not amenable to treatment with external fixation.
   2) Pin sites may become infected.
   3) The nonunion rate is higher than with internal fixation, owing to the lesser stability of external fixation.
9. **Repeat irrigation and débridement** should be done every 48 hours after the initial surgery. Necrotic tissue will be more clearly defined with time.
10. **Delayed primary closure of the wound** should be performed when the wound is clean, usually at 3–7 days after injury.
a. Rotation-flap or free-flap coverage may be necessary.
b. This should be done within 1 week of injury for best results.
11. **Primary amputation of an injured limb** is sometimes indicated.
a. Many scoring systems have been devised to help define which limbs are ultimately salvageable.
b. Whether a limb can be saved is not the same question as whether it should be saved.
c. The goal in treating these injuries is a functional, viable extremity. If this cannot reasonably be achieved, or if the surgery required would place the patient's life at risk, amputation is a good option.

VI. REFERENCE

1. Gustilo RB, Mendoza RM, Williams DN. Problems in the management of type III (severe) open fractures: a new classification of type III open fractures. *J Trauma* 1984; 24:742–746.

VII. FURTHER READING

Brumback RJ. Open tibial fractures: current orthopedic management. In: *Volume 41, Instructional Course Lectures.* American Academy of Orthopedic Surgeons; 1992:101–107.

Brumback RJ, Jones AL. Interobserver agreement in the classification of open fractures of the tibia. *J Bone Joint Surg* 1994; 76A:1162.

Gustilo RB, Anderson JT. Prevention of infection in the treatment of 1025 open fractures of long bones. *J Bone Joint Surg* 1976; 58.

COMPLICATIONS OF MUSCULOSKELETAL TRAUMA

I. THROMBOEMBOLIC DISEASE

A. **THROMBOEMBOLIC DISEASE** is a common complication in general surgical (20%) and trauma (50%) patients in general, and in fracture patients in particular. Risk of pulmonary embolism in trauma patients is 1%.

B. **RISK FACTORS FOR THROMBOEMBOLIC DISEASE.**

1. Trauma patients are at high risk of deep venous thrombosis.
2. Patients with multiple injuries.
3. Patients with age >40 years.
4. Patients with spinal cord injury.
5. Obesity.
6. Immobilization.
7. Prior thromboembolic disease.

C. **PREVENTION OF DEEP VENOUS THROMBOSIS (DVT).**

1. **The majority of pulmonary emboli in trauma patients** occur within the first week following injury; hence, all trauma patients should receive some form of prophylaxis.
2. **Pneumatic compression devices** (thigh-length or calf-length, or foot pumps) are used. Foot pumps are currently the device of choice, owing to their effectiveness and ease of application.
3. **Minidose heparin is used in most patients.** The current regimen is 5000 units s.c. three times per day. Clotting parameters are not followed.
4. **Active mobilization.**
5. **Thigh ultrasound and magnetic resonance venography** (MRV) is done in all pelvic and acetabular fracture patients.

D. **DIAGNOSIS OF DVT.**

1. **Clinical signs are notoriously unreliable.**
   a. <10% of patients with proximal vein thrombosis have clinical signs of DVT.
   b. Symptoms can include calf pain, swelling tachycardia, and fever.
2. **Ultrasound is useful** in detecting thigh, or 'proximal' vein thrombosis.
   a. It has an accuracy rate of about 90%.
   b. It is not as useful in detecting calf thrombi.
3. **Venography** is still considered the 'gold standard' for DVT detection.
   a. It is highly accurate, but carries the risk of allergic reaction to the contrast agent and a small risk of thrombosis at the injection site.
   b. It also requires the presence of a skilled radiologist to perform the test. It is not commonly used at Parkland Memorial Hospital.
   c. MRV is possibly more accurate than venography in the detection of pelvic vein thrombi.

d. MRV can be used to evaluate the thigh and calf veins. It is currently used at Parkland in acetabular and pelvic fracture patients, who are considered to be at high risk for DVT.

E. DIAGNOSIS OF PULMONARY EMBOLUS.

1. **The clinical symptoms**, as listed below, are often nonspecific:
a. Dyspnea.
b. Chest pain 'tightness'.
c. Tachycardia.

2. **EKG**, such as right axis deviation, S1Q3T3 (10%), T-wave inversion (40%), and right bundle-branch block (20%) are sometimes present.

3. **Chest radiograph** showing atelectasis or patches of consolidation.

4. **Arterial blood gases** reveal a Pao_2 <80mmHg on room air in >90% of patients with pulmonary embolism.

5. **Ventilation and perfusion scans**. However, a scan that is read as 'moderate probability for pulmonary embolism' implies a 15–85% chance of pulmonary embolism.

6. **Pulmonary arteriography** is the test of choice in a patient who has a considerable risk of pulmonary embolism.

F. TREATMENT OF THROMBOEMBOLIC DISEASE.

1. **DVT.**
a. Intravenous heparin [10,000 unit loading dose followed by 1000 units per hour infusion, with the rate adjusted to keep partial thromboplastin time (PTT) 1.5–2 times normal] and oral coumarin.
b. After 3–4 days, the coumarin will have adequately elevated the international normalized ratio (INR) to 1.5–2 times normal. The heparin is then stopped and the coumarin continued for 3–6 months. Patients with pulmonary embolism will require 6 months of anticoagulation, while those with hypercoagulable states or multiple recurrent pulmonary embolus require lifelong anticoagulation with warfarin.
c. If the patient requires further surgery, or if there is some contraindication to anticoagulation, an inferior vena cava filter is placed.
d. If no contraindication to anticoagulation exists, heparin is continued after inferior vena cava filter placement, and then stopped about 6 hours prior to the surgery. This allows normalization of the PTT.
e. Anticoagulation with heparin and coumarin is then resumed after surgery.

2. **Pulmonary embolus.**
a. Anticoagulation as above.
b. Ventilatory support may be required.
c. Surgical removal of massive emboli has been successful in isolated cases at Parkland.

3. **Inferior vena cava filter.**
a. Indications:
    1). Contraindication to anticoagulation, i.e., concomitant neurologic injury.
    2) Recurrent pulmonary embolus during anticoagulation.
    3) Free-floating iliac or inferior vena cava thrombus.

b. Complications of filter placement:
   1) Post-thrombotic syndrome – 33%.
   2) Recurrent DVT – 30%.
   3) Venous insufficiency – 30%.
   4) Venous ulcers – 10%.
   5) Filter migration – 30–50%.
   6) Inferior vena cava obstruction – 5%.
   7) Mortality – 0.12%.

II. COMPARTMENT SYNDROME

A. COMPARTMENT SYNDROME is a condition that arises when the pressure within a closed compartment becomes high enough to compromise cellular function inside that compartment.

B. NECROSIS of nerves, muscles, vessels, and all other tissues will ensue if the pressure is not corrected.

C. CAUSES OF COMPARTMENT SYNDROME.

1. Fractures (tibia most common in adults, supracondylar humerus in children).
2. Arterial injury.
3. Crush injury to soft tissues.
4. Circumferential burns.
5. Prolonged compression of a limb (as can occur after a drug overdose).

D. DIAGNOSIS OF COMPARTMENT SYNDROME.

1. Pain is the earliest and most reliable symptom. Pain on passive stretch of muscles or pain out of proportion to the injury are hallmarks.
2. Paresthesias.
3. Paralysis – late finding.
4. Pallor – late finding.
5. Pulselessness – late finding.
6. Compartment pressure monitors can be used in patients who have altered mental status (Figure 33.1).

E. TREATMENT OF COMPARTMENT SYNDROME.

1. Immediate fasciotomy.
2. If compartment pressure monitors show pressures of 30–40mmHg, or pressures within 20–30mmHg of diastolic blood pressure, fasciotomies should be done.
3. Compartment syndrome should be considered a limb-threatening emergency.
4. Technique: lower leg.
a. The anterior and lateral compartments are released through a 15cm incision midway between the tibial crest and fibula (Figure 33.2).
   1) The septum between the anterior and lateral compartments is identified and the fascia comprising the two compartments is incised using Metzenbaum scissors.

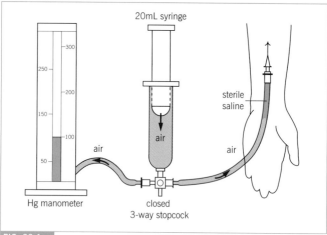

FIG. 33.1

Whitesides' method of measuring tissue pressures. The three-way stopcock is open to the 20mL syringe and to both extension tubes. The pressure within the closed compartment is overcome by injecting a minute quantity of saline, and the pressure required to do this is read on the mercury manometer. (From Green DP. *Operative hand surgery*, 2nd edn. New York: Churchill Livingstone; 1988.)

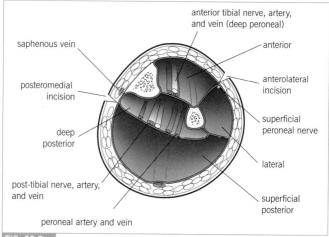

FIG. 33.2

Fascial compartments of leg. (From Snyder WH III, Thal ER, Perry MO. Vascular injuries of the extremities. In: Rutherford RB (ed.) *Vascular surgery*, 3rd edn. Philadelphia: WB Saunders; 1989.)

2)   The superficial peroneal nerve crosses through the lateral compartment's fascia at the junction of the middle and distal third of the leg, and must be protected.

b.   The deep and superficial posterior compartments are approached through a 15cm incision about 3cm posterior to the tibia's posteromedial edge (Figure 33.3).

1)   The saphenous nerve and vein are protected while the superficial compartment's fascia is incised.

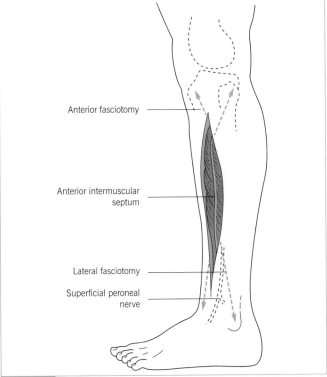

FIG. 33.3A

An anterolateral skin incision is used to approach the anterior or lateral compartments. The incision is made halfway between the fibular shaft and the tibial crest. This is approximately over the anterior intermuscular septum, dividing the anterior and lateral compartments, and allows easy access to both. The length of the skin incision should extend the length of the compartments of the leg, unless intracompartmental pressures are monitored intraoperatively, in which case a small skin incision can be used. (From Mubarak SJ, Owen CA. Double incision fasciotomy of the leg for decompression in compartment syndrome. *J Bone Joint Surg* 1977, 59A:184.)

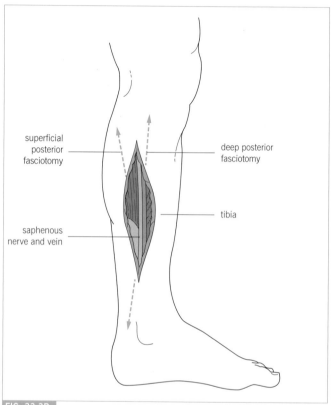

FIG. 33.3B

A posteromedial incision is used for an approach to the superficial or deep posterior compartments. The incision is slightly distal to the previous incision and 2cm posterior to the posterior tibial margin. By making the incision at this location, injury to the saphenous nerve and vein, which run along the posterior margin of the tibia in this area, is avoided. (From Mubarak SJ, Owen CA. Double incision fasciotomy of the leg for decompression in compartment syndrome. *J Bone Joint Surg* 1977; **59**A:184.

2) The deep posterior compartment is approached in the distal portion of the incision.

3) The tendon of the flexor digitorum longus can be seen lying anterior to the belly of the soleus and can be used as a guide to reach the compartment.

5. Technique: forearm.

a. A volar incision should be made, beginning 2cm proximal to the medial epicondyle and coursing obliquely across the antecubital fossa to the radial side of the forearm (Figure 33.4).

   1) The incision should be carried distally.

   2) The fascia of the forearm's flexor compartment should be incised longitudinally using scissors.

   3) The wrist should be crossed obliquely, and a flap of skin should be left to cover the median nerve after carpal tunnel release (Figure 33.5).

   4) The mobile wad can usually be released through the volar incision.

b. A dorsal incision should be made straight down the middle of the dorsal compartment of the forearm, and the underlying fascia incised in line with the skin incision (Figures 33.6 and 33.7).

6. **The muscle should be assessed** at the fasciotomy site.

a. Muscle that appears viable (contracts when squeezed with a forcep, is pink, etc.) should be left.

b. Necrotic muscle should be debrided.

c. The wounds should be packed with moist gauze and closed in a delayed fashion after 3–5 days.

d. Skin grafting is occasionally necessary to cover fasciotomy wounds.

III. FAT EMBOLISM SYNDROME

A. FAT EMBOLISM is the deposition of fatty elements from the marrow of an injured bone into the lung capillaries, causing increased pulmonary capillary permeability and respiratory compromise.

B. CEREBRAL MANIFESTATIONS may also occur.

C. THE PATHOGENESIS of the disorder is still poorly understood, but it is felt to be an important cause of respiratory insufficiency in multiply injured patients.

D. DIAGNOSIS.

1. **Fat embolism is a diagnosis of exclusion**. Other causes of respiratory compromise must first be ruled out. The symptoms are often nonspecific.

a. Shortness of breath – arterial hypoxemia.

b. Restlessness.

c. Confusion, disorientation, and occasionally frank coma.

d. Fever to 39°C.

e. Tachycardia.

f. Petechiae on the chest, axilla, neck, and conjunctivae. This usually fades rapidly.

2. **Chest radiographs** show 'snowstorm' pulmonary infiltrates, which worsen as the patient's condition worsens.

33

COMPLICATIONS OF MUSCULOSKELETAL TRAUMA

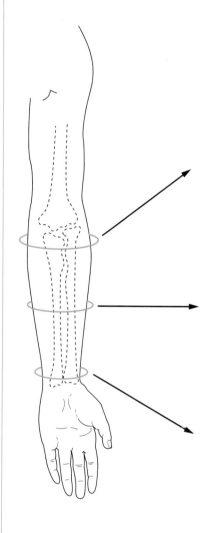

Forearm compartments: transverse sections through the left forearm at various levels. (From Mubarak SJ, Hargens AR. *Compartment syndromes and Volkmann's contracture*. Philadelphia: WB Saunders; 1981.)

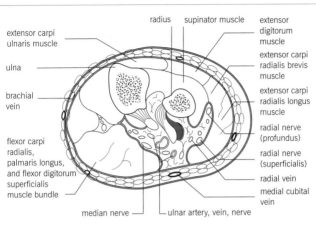

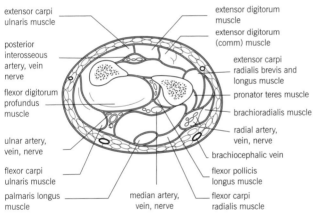

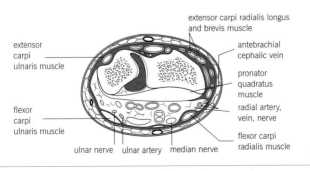

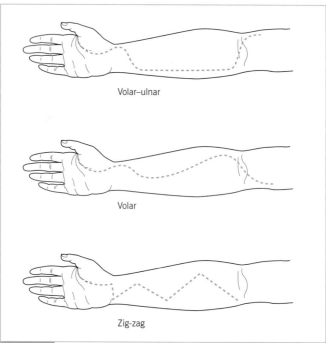

FIG. 33.5
Various skin incisions used for performing a volar forearm fasciotomy. (From Green DP. *Operative hand surgery*, 2nd edn. New York: Churchill Livingstone; 1988.)

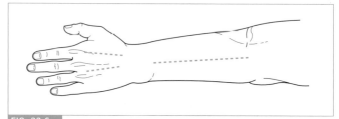

FIG. 33.6
To decompress the dorsal and mobile wad compartments, the author prefers straight incisions because fewer veins will be damaged. (From Green DP. *Operative hand surgery*, 2nd edn. New York: Churchill Livingstone; 1988.)

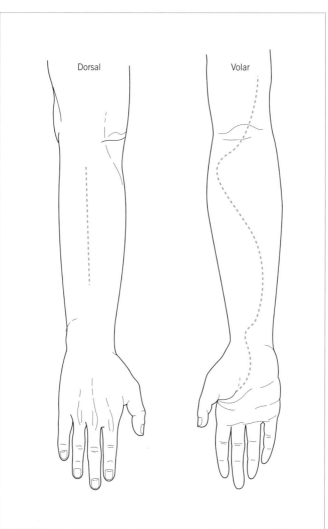

FIG. 33.7
The dorsal and curvilinear volar incisions used for forearm decompression. The curvilinear volar incision is preferred because of the exposure afforded to major nerves, brachial artery, and mobile wad. (Modified from Gelberman RH et al. Decompression of forearm compartment syndromes. *Clin Orthop* 1978; 134:225–229.)

E. TREATMENT.
1. Treatment is generally supportive.
2. Oxygen should be administered immediately.
3. Intubation and mechanical ventilation may be necessary.
4. **Ethanol, heparin, hypertonic glucose, and corticosteroids** have all been described in the treatment of fat embolism syndrome but are not currently used.
F. PREVENTION.
1. **It has consistently been shown that early (≤ 24 hours) stabilization** of long bone fractures in multiply injured patients prevents pulmonary complications, including fat embolism syndrome.
2. **Prevention through early stabilization** remains the primary method of combating fat embolism at Parkland.

IV. FURTHER READING

Geerts WH, Code KI, Jay RM et al. A prospective study of venous thrombo-embolism after major trauma. *N Engl J Med* 1994; 331:1601–1606.

Heeg M, Oostvegel HJM, Klasen HJ. Conservative treatment of acetabular fractures: the role of the weight-bearing dome and anatomic reduction in the ultimate results. *J Trauma* 1987; 27:555–559.

Montgomery K, Potter HG, Helfet DL. Magnetic resonance venography to evaluate the deep venous system of the pelvis in patients who have acetabular fractures. *J Bone Joint Surg* 1995; 77A:1639–1649.

Rockwood CA, Green DP, Bucholz RW. *Fractures,* 3rd edn. Philadelphia: Lippincott; 1991.

Tipton WW, D'Ambrosia RD, Ryle GP. Nonoperative management of central fracture dislocations of the hip. *J Bone Joint Surg* 1975; 57A:888–893.

A. ANATOMY.

1. Musculoskeletal anatomy.

a. The pelvis is a ring, comprising the two innominate bones and the sacrum.

b. Anteriorly, the symphysis pubis holds the two hemipelves together. The symphysis is composed of superior and inferior ligaments, with a disk-like fibrocartilage center.

c. Posteriorly, the sacro-iliac (SI) ligaments support the SI joints. The posterior SI ligaments are up to 1 inch thick and very strong, while the anterior SI ligaments are less strong.

d. The strong sacrotuberous and sacrospinous ligaments prevent rotation of the innominate bone away from the sacrum.

2. Soft tissue anatomy.

a. Vascular structures:

    1) The internal iliac artery bifurcates at the pelvic brim into anterior and posterior branches.

    2) The anterior division gives off the obturator and internal pudendal arteries.

    3) The posterior division gives off the superior and inferior gluteal arteries.

    4) Owing to their positions these arteries, and the veins that run with them, are at risk if the SI joint is disrupted.

    5) These vessels can be the source of significant bleeding in pelvic fractures.

b. Neurologic structures:

    1) The lumbosacral plexus lies anterior to the SI joint.

    2) Its components, particularly the dorsal sacral nerve roots that make up the peroneal portion of the sciatic nerve, can be injured if the SI joint is disrupted.

c. Urologic structures: the urethra and bladder are occasionally injured in pelvic fracture patients.

B. EVALUATION.

1. Physical examination.

a. Forceful stressing of the pelvis to assess stability should be avoided.

b. Pain at the symphseal region and at the sacrum should be noted.

c. Blood at the urethral meatus or a high-riding prostate are indicators of urologic trauma.

d. Rectal tears or perineal lacerations are indicators of an open pelvic fracture.

e. Neurologic deficits in the legs must be ruled out.

f. Ongoing hemodynamic status of the patient must be evaluated.

2. Radiologic studies.

a. An anteroposterior (AP) view of the pelvis should be included in the initial evaluation of all trauma patients.

    1) If the AP film shows any abnormality, inlet and outlet films are obtained.

    2) The inlet view shows the ring of the true pelvis, and reveals the presence of injury to the SI joints.

    3) The inlet view also reveals posterior displacement of the hemipelvis.

    4) The outlet view reveals cephalad displacement of the hemipelvis and offers good visualization of the sacral foramina.

b. CT scans are obtained on all pelvic fracture patients.

    1) The CT confirms fractures seen on plain films and gives better information about the posterior pelvic ring.

    2) Sacral foraminal and SI joint injuries are well delineated on CT.

    3) Iliac wing fractures, which can be subtle on plain film, are well defined on CT.

3. Urologic studies – urethrograms or cystograms are performed if the following conditions exist:

a. Gross hematuria.

b. Urinary obstruction.

c. High-riding or nonpalpable prostate gland.

C. **CLASSIFICATION OF PELVIC FRACTURES.** The Young and Burgess classification is used at Parkland Memorial Hospital. This system is useful because it aids in treating the pelvic fracture and in identifying associated injuries.

1. Lateral compression (LC) injuries.

a. Associated with injuries to the head, thorax, and abdomen.

b. Not typically associated with the ongoing hemorrhage as seen with anteroposterior compression (APC) injuries.

c. The SI joints or iliac wing are compressed, not blown open.

d. However, LC III, the 'windswept' pelvis, does have an open SI joint component, and can result in massive blood loss.

2. APC injuries.

a. Associated with injury to the lumbosacral plexus and the pelvic vessels due to disruption of the SI joint.

b. These patients can have high transfusion requirements.

c. APC III is the most morbid type injury.

3. Vertical shear injuries – these patients show elements of more than one injury pattern.

a. Associated with vessel and nerve injury due to disruption of the SI joint.

b. Can have high transfusion requirements.

c. Combined mechanical injuries.

D. TREATMENT. The methods of stabilizing pelvic fractures currently in use at Parkland Memorial Hospital are as follows:

1. **External fixation.**

a. An anterior frame applied to the pelvis can be used to 'close the book' of the pelvis in hemodynamically unstable patients.

b. This reduces pelvic volume, and can tamponade bleeding from pelvic vessels.

c. External fixators can be applied rapidly.

d. Fluoroscopic imaging of the pelvis to place an anterior external fixator is easy, and can be accomplished emergently in most trauma centers.

e. Stabilizing the anterior ring and reducing pelvic volume are often all that is necessary to restore hemodynamic stability in the immediate post-injury period.

f. The external fixation pins can be used to manipulate fracture fragments during reduction of SI joint injuries during later placement of iliosacral screws.

2. **Iliosacral screws.**

a. Large (6.5–7.3mm) cannulated screws are placed percutaneously to stabilize SI joint disruptions or sacral fractures after reduction has been obtained.

b. Safe placement of these screws requires expertise, both by the surgeon and by the fluoroscopy technician.

c. Iliosacral screws are usually placed electively, so that all members of the surgical team are available.

d. Two screws are usually placed in the bodies of S1 and S2.

3. **Symphyseal plating.**

a. Used to stabilize symphysis pubis disruptions.

b. Open dissection can disturb fracture hematoma and result in massive bleeding.

c. Symphysis plating is usually delayed for 3 days after injury.

d. If anterior stabilization is required to stop bleeding, an external fixator is placed instead.

e. If emergent celiotomy is to be done, the plate can be placed through the celiotomy incision.

4. **Percutaneous screws.**

a. These large fragment, cannulated screws can stabilize iliac wing fractures, pubic ramus fractures, and anterior and posterior column fractures of the acetabulum.

b. Percutaneous placement limits blood loss and soft tissue stripping.

c. As with iliosacral screws, safe placement requires expertise.

5. **Open plating.**

a. Can stabilize iliac wing fractures, ramus fractures, and fractures of the sacrum or SI joint.

b. Open dissection permits direct, anatomic reduction of these injuries, but must be balanced against the risk of bleeding from pelvic hematoma and the possibility of infection.

c. As with symphyseal plating, this is normally delayed for several days after injury.

6. Skeletal traction.

a. Can be used preoperatively to prevent proximal migration of an unstable hemipelvis.

b. This modality is used only temporarily. Every effort is made to stabilize pelvic fractures and mobilize the patient to prevent the complications of bed rest.

E. MANAGEMENT OF SPECIFIC FRACTURE TYPES.

1. Lateral compression fractures.

a. LC I – these injuries are stable and usually require no treatment other than limited weight bearing on the affected side for pain relief.

b. LC II.

1) If hemodynamically stable, these can be treated with bed rest followed by delayed open reduction internal fixation (ORIF) or percutaneous fixation after 3–5 days.

2) If hemodynamically unstable, these can be managed with an acute anterior pelvic external fixator, followed by later surgery on the posterior ring injury.

c. LC III.

1) Often hemodynamically unstable.

2) If unstable, they should be managed with an anterior external fixation frame.

3) If they are to undergo emergent celiotomy for other injuries, either an anterior external fixator or open plating of the symphysis or rami can be performed.

4) Later, the SI joint injury can be addressed with iliosacral screws, while the iliac fracture can be treated with percutaneous screws or open plating.

2. Anteroposterior compression fractures.

a. APC I.

1) These injuries are rare – <2cm widening of the symphysis pubis, and simple stretch of the anterior SI ligaments.

2) They are stable, and require no surgical treatment.

3) Hemodynamic instability is rare.

b. APC II.

1) If hemodynamically unstable, these can be treated with an anterior external fixation frame.

2) If hemodynamically stable, they can be treated with anterior symphysis plating 3–5 days after injury.

   3) SI joint partial disruption is usually treated with percutaneous iliosacral screws, often on the day after injury, or at the time of symphyseal plating.
c. APC III.
   1) Often hemodynamically unstable.
   2) If unstable, they should be treated with an emergent anterior external fixation frame.
   3) If stable, they can be kept at bedrest for 3–5 days followed by symphyseal plating.
   4) The SI joint disruption should be stabilized using iliosacral screws.

3. Vertical shear (VS) injuries.
a. These are treated much like the APC III types.
b. Reduction often requires placement of Schanz pins into the ilium to aid in reduction.

4. Combined mechanical type injuries must be treated according to the particular injury pattern found.

F. SPECIAL SITUATIONS.

1. Hemorrhage.
a. Hemorrhage in pelvic fractures can arise from fractured ends of bone; small, torn arteries or veins; or from large, named arteries.
b. Significant bleeding is most likely to occur with APC, LC III, or VS-type injuries.
c. Initial treatment to control this hemorrhage should be some form of closure of the 'open pelvic book' to tamponade the bleeding.
d. In prehospital transport, this can be done with military antishock trousers (MAST).
e. Control of hemorrhage.
   1) Close the pelvic book in hemodynamically unstable patients with an external fixation frame.
   2) If the patient's hemodynamic status does not improve after external fixation, arteriography and embolization of bleeding arteries can sometimes be of benefit.
   3) Direct exploration and ligation of bleeding arteries is fraught with complications.
   4) Disturbance of the pelvic hematoma should be avoided if exploratory celiotomy is being done.

2. Urologic injury.
a. About 16% of pelvic fracture patients will have some form of urologic injury.
b. Bladder ruptures and urethral tears are not uncommon.
c. Urologists will manage most of these injuries with an indwelling Foley catheter, or a suprapubic tube.
d. A suprapubic tube increases the risk of infection of hardware placed on the anterior pelvic ring (e.g. symphyseal plates).

e. In some centers, a suprapubic tube is felt to be a contraindication to anterior hardware, so external fixation is used instead.

3. **Open pelvic fractures.**

a. These have increased risk of hemorrhage, infection, wound complications, and mortality.

b. The mortality with open pelvic fractures is about 25% in recent series.

c. They are divided into anterior and posterior types according to the position of the open wound.

d. Anterior type:
    1) Have lacerations on the thigh or flank, and do not communicate with the perineum, scrotum, vagina, or rectum.
    2) These usually involve only lacerations of muscle tissue.
    3) They should be considered high-energy injuries, and be debrided aggressively.
    4) All such wounds should be left open, and should undergo serial débridement.

e. Posterior type:
    1) Involve lacerations of the rectum or anus, and can involve the distal urologic structures.
    2) Injuries in this area should be aggressively debrided and treated with early fecal diversion by a colostomy.
    3) The wounds should be left open, and should undergo serial débridement.
    4) Hardware has to be used judiciously in these patients, owing to the markedly increased risk of infection.

II. ACETABULAR FRACTURES

A. ANATOMY.

1. **The acetabulum** is made up of contributions from the ischium, ilium, and pubis.

2. **The arrangement of these three bones** forming the acetabular cup is best seen in the immature skeleton, prior to closure of the triradiate cartilage

3. **In the adult**, the acetabulum is best thought of as an inverted 'Y', with anterior and posterior columns.

4. **There are also anterior and posterior walls**, which form the boundaries defining the acetabular cup.

5. **The involvement of these four structures** determines the classification of each particular acetabular fracture.

a. Anterior and posterior columns.

b. Anterior and posterior walls (Figures 34.1 and 34.2).

6. **By convention**, the 90° arc at the top of the acetabular dome is termed the weight-bearing dome.

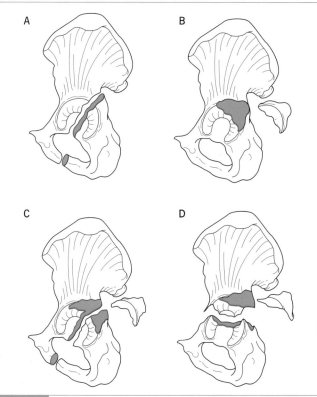

FIG. 34.1
Type I acetabular fracture: (A) posterior column; (B) posterior wall; (C) associated with posterior wall; (D) associated with transverse fractures. (From Kozin SH, Berlet AC. *Handbook of common orthopedic fractures*. Westchester: Medical Surveillance; 1989.)

B. EVALUATION.
1. **Each acetabular fracture is evaluated** using an anteroposterior radiograph of the pelvis, coupled with iliac oblique and obturator oblique views. (These oblique views are termed Judet views in honor of Robert Judet who pioneered their use.)
2. **A CT scan is obtained**, with 5mm sections through the iliac wings, and 2mm sections through the acetabulum itself.

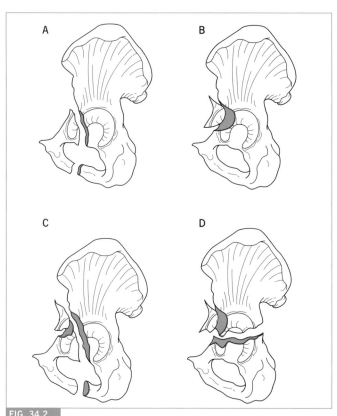

FIG. 34.2
Type II acetabular fracture: (A) anterior column; (B) anterior wall; (C and D) associated with anterior column, or transverse fractures. (From Kozin SH, Berlet AC. *Handbook of common orthopedic fractures*. Westchester: Medical Surveillance; 1989.)

3. **The CT is invaluable** in demonstrating the extent of marginal impaction of fractures, especially at the posterior wall.
4. **The CT reveals** minimally displaced fractures and intra-articular bone fragments.
C. **CLASSIFICATION.**
1. **Emile Letournel's classification system** comprises five elementary fracture types and five associated fracture types.
2. **The associated types are complex**, and include combinations of the elementary types.

D. TREATMENT.

1. **The principles of acetabular fracture treatment** are the same as those for other articular fractures.

a. Any articular incongruity greater than 2mm in the weight-bearing dome of the acetabulum should be treated with open reduction and internal fixation.

b. Unwell, elderly patients are not good candidates for acetabular fracture surgery, which can often be lengthy and is associated with significant blood loss.

2. **Surgical approaches.** The approach used is determined by the fracture class.

a. Kocher–Langenbeck – this approach is familiar to many orthopedic surgeons owing to its use in total hip arthroplasty. It is used for fractures of the posterior column and posterior wall.

b. Ilio-inguinal – this approach is used for fractures of the anterior column, anterior wall, and iliac wing.

c. Extensile – the 'Big T' approach, as described by Reinert, et al.[1], is used for transverse fractures, both column and T-type fractures, and anterior column with posterior hemitransverse fractures. This approach offers visualization of the entire acetabulum, iliac wing, and quadrilateral plate.

E. PERIOPERATIVE MANAGEMENT.

1. **Surgery should be delayed** 3–5 days after injury to avoid excessive bleeding.

2. **Skeletal traction should be used** to maintain reduction if the hip was dislocated.

3. **Traction will prevent impaction and scuffing** of the femoral head on the fracture.

4. **Preoperative thigh sonograms and pelvic magnetic resonance venograms** are used to screen for deep venous thrombosis (DVT).

a. If a DVT is found, anticoagulation with i.v. heparin is begun (see Chapter 33, Complications of musculoskeletal trauma).

b. An inferior vena cava filter is placed preoperatively on the day of surgery.

5. **Patients are mobilized** on the first day after surgery using a walker. They are restricted to flat-foot weight bearing for 3 months.

6. **Postoperative thigh sonograms** are used to screen for DVT.

7. **All patients who had a Kocher–Langenbeck or extensile approach** undergo a single dose of 600rad (6Gy) of radiation to prevent heterotopic ossification.

8. **Indomethacin is used as prophylaxis** in patients who refuse radiation treatment. At Parkland Memorial Hospital we believe that indomethacin is as effective as radiation in the treatment of heterotopic ossification.

F.   COMPLICATIONS.

1.   **Post-traumatic arthritis** is usually caused by residual articular incongruity, in both surgical and nonsurgical patients.

a.   Femoral head injuries, and posterior wall fractures predispose to post-traumatic arthritis.

b.   This is often due to postoperative collapse of small, marginally impacted fragments of bone and joint surface at the posterior wall.

c.   The best course of action for the surgeon is to strive to achieve a perfect, stable restoration of the joint surface.

2.   **Heterotopic ossification** (HO) can be seen after any acetabular fracture surgery, but is most common after surgery through a posterior or extensile approach.

a.   HO can severely limit hip motion.

b.   Prophylaxis at is accomplished with a single dose of 600rad (6Gy) of radiation.

c.   Alternate treatments include indomethacin orally.

3.   **Sciatic nerve palsy** is most common after posterior approaches. This risk can be limited by flexing the knee and limiting hip flexion during the surgery.

III. PEARLS AND PITFALLS

A.   **Exploratory celiotomy** can be performed with an external fixation frame in place.

B.   **APC-type fractures** are associated with ongoing bleeding, and can be a source of hemodynamic instability.

C.   **APC injuries that are hemodynamically unstable** can, and should, be treated with an anterior pelvic external fixator prior to celiotomy.

D.   **Oral CT contrast** should be avoided in pelvic fracture patients, as it can impede later fluoroscopic imaging of the fractures.

E.   **Prolonged use of MAST** is associated with wound care problems and compartment syndrome of the lower extremities.

IV. REFERENCES

1.   Reinert CM, Bosse MJ, Poka A *et al*. A modified extensile exposure for the treatment of complex or malunited acetabular fractures. *J Bone Joint Surg* 1988, 70A:329–336.

V. FURTHER READING

Dalal SA, Burgess AR, Siegel JH *et al*. Pelvic fracture in multiple trauma: classification by mechanism is key to pattern of organ injury, resuscitative requirements, and outcome. *J Trauma* 1989; 29:981–1002.

Routt MLC, Kregor PJ, Simonian PT *et al*. Early results of percutaneous iliosacral screws placed with the patient in the supine position. *J Orthop Trauma* 1995; 9:207–214.

FRACTURES OF THE PELVIS AND ACETABULUM

FRACTURES AND DISLOCATIONS OF THE LOWER EXTREMITY

I. HIP DISLOCATIONS

A. OCCURRENCE.

1. **Hip dislocations usually occur** after motor vehicle collisions or falls.
2. **They can be missed in multiply injured patients** who have other, more dramatic injuries.
3. **A single anteroposterior (AP) view** of the pelvis is recommended in all trauma patients.

B. EVALUATION.

1. **Sciatic nerve injuries** can occur in 8–19% of posterior dislocations.
   a. The risk is higher with fracture dislocations.
   b. The nerve injury is usually a neuropraxia which will improve with time after the hip is reduced.
2. **Femoral nerve and vessel injuries** have been reported after anterior dislocations, but they are more rare.
3. **Open wounds** should be searched for, and concomitant knee injuries should be ruled out.
4. **Anteroposterior and oblique (Judet) views** of the pelvis should be obtained.
   a. Fractures of the acetabulum and femoral head should be looked for.
   b. These views should be repeated after reduction to assess congruency.
   c. A post-reduction CT scan should be obtained to assure that there are no intra-articular bone fragments. These loose bodies can damage the joint and cause arthritis if left in place.

C. CLASSIFICATION.

1. **Anterior dislocations.**
   a. The femoral head lies anterior to the coronal plane of the acetabulum.
   b. These are classified into two categories:
      1) Type I – 'superior' including pubic or subspinous dislocations.
      2) Type II – 'inferior' including obturator or perineal dislocations.
      3) The injuries are further subclassified as: 'A', no associated fracture; 'B' associated fracture of the femoral head or neck; 'C' associated acetabular fracture.
2. **Posterior dislocations.**
   a. The femoral head lies posterior to the coronal plane of the acetabulum.
   b. These are subclassified into five categories:
      1) Type I – with or without a minor posterior wall acetabular fracture.

2) Type II – with a single-fragment posterior wall fracture.
3) Type III – with comminution of the posterior wall.
4) Type IV – with fracture of the acetabular floor.
5) Type V – with fracture of the femoral head.

c. The type V fractures can be further subclassified according to the location of the femoral head or neck fracture.

D. TREATMENT.

1. **Hip dislocations are an orthopedic emergency.** Results will be worse if reduction is delayed for >12 hours.

2. **Reduction.**

a. Closed reduction is attempted first. Ideally this should be done under a general anesthetic or adequate i.v. sedation.

b. No more than three attempts should be made.

c. Repeated, forceful attempts can damage the articular cartilage, leading to poor results.

d. If closed reduction fails, open methods must be used. In irreducible anterior dislocations, an anterior iliofemoral approach is employed.

e. In irreducible posterior dislocations, a Kocher–Langenbeck approach is used. These approaches are used to try to preserve the remaining blood supply to the femoral head.

3. **Assessment and traction.**

a. Reduction of posterior dislocations is assessed by flexing the hip to 90°. If it redislocates, it is deemed unstable.

b. Instability usually results from an associated posterior wall acetabular fracture.

c. Unstable hip dislocations must be treated with open reduction and internal fixation (ORIF). (Unstable anterior dislocations are rare, so no assessment is done.)

d. After reduction, AP and Judet radiographs of the hip are obtained to assure no intra-articular fragments are present.

e. A pelvic CT scan is also obtained.

f. Any such fragments require surgical removal.

g. If the reduction is stable, the patient is treated with 5–7 days of bed rest and traction. This is followed by limited weight bearing for 6 weeks.

E. COMPLICATIONS.

1. **Recurrent dislocation.**

a. Rare after anterior dislocations.

b. Inadequate length of immobilization is the usual cause.

c. Recurrence is also rare after posterior dislocations (about 1% prevalence), but hip capsule laxity or bony deficiency are usually to blame with these patients.

d. Surgery is often required for recurrent posterior instability.

2. **Avascular necrosis (AVN).**

a. AVN of the femoral head may appear 2–5 years after the dislocation.

b. Delay in reduction and repeated attempts at reduction have been blamed for this complication, although increased severity of the initial injury is the most likely culprit.

c. AVN is rare after anterior dislocations (about 8% prevalence). The rate is higher with posterior dislocations (6–40%).

3. **Post-traumatic arthritis**

a. Usually arises because of associated femoral head or acetabular fractures.

b. It can also result if AVN leads to joint incongruity. As many as one-third of anterior dislocations go on to show arthritic changes.

c. Arthritis has been reported in 17–30% of posterior dislocation patients.

d. The best treatment for this complication is prevention, through congruent, stable reduction of the hip.

II. HIP FRACTURES

1. **Fractures of the femoral neck and intertrochanteric region** are, primarily, injuries of the elderly.

2. **They frequently occur after minor trauma**, and are usually isolated injuries.

3. **While the fractures are often fairly simple**, management of these patients can still be difficult.

4. **Hip fracture patients often suffer from dementia**, and associated medical conditions are usually present.

5. **Mortality rates during hospitalization** for hip fracture treatment can be as high as 10%.

6. **Complications** such as decubitus ulcers, urinary tract infections, and deep vein thromboses are common.

7. **The reported 1-year mortality** ranges from 18 to 30%.

8. **In patients with >3 concurrent medical illnesses**, preoperative medical treatment to optimize the patient's condition has been shown to lessen mortality.

9. **In patients with fewer medical problems**, immediate fracture care seems to improve results.

10. **Improvements in orthopedic implants** have made the orthopedist's job of stabilizing the fracture easier.

III. FEMORAL NECK FRACTURES

A. **EVALUATION.** AP radiographs of the pelvis and lateral view of the hip will generally demonstrate the fracture.

B. **CLASSIFICATION.** Garden classification is most commonly used (Figure 35.1).

1. **Garden I** – valgus impacted neck fracture. May be incomplete, sparing the inferior femoral neck.

2. **Garden II** – complete, nondisplaced fracture.

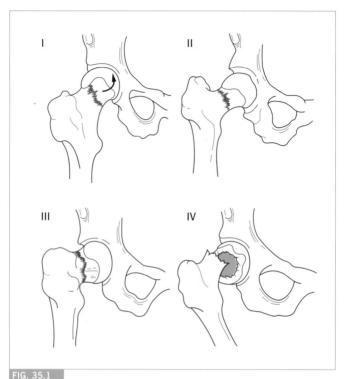

FIG. 35.1
Garden classification of femoral neck fractures. (From Kozin SH, Berlet AC. *Handbook of common orthopedic fractures*. Westchester: Medical Surveillance; 1989.)

3. **Garden III** – complete, partially displaced fracture.
4. **Garden IV** – complete, fully displaced fracture.
C. TREATMENT. The choices for treatment are:
1. **Internal fixation.**
a. Reduction is obtained with the patient on a fracture table.
b. Fluoroscopy is used to judge reduction, and aid guide-wire placement for cannulated screws.
c. Three or four large fragment cannulated screws are placed into the femoral neck and head.
d. Percutaneous technique limits dissection and blood loss.
e. Postoperatively, the patients are made toe-touch weight bearing with crutches or a walker.

2. **Prosthetic replacement**
a. Endoprosthetic use is indicated in patients with:
   1) Severe medical problems.
   2) Physiologic age >75 years (life expectancy <5 years).
   3) Pathologic hip fractures.
   4) Parkinsonism or other neuromuscular disease.
   5) Recently failed internal fixation of a femoral neck fracture.
b. The above criteria are relative indications. Each patient must be considered individually.
3. **Primary total hip arthroplasty** is indicated in patients with a femoral neck fracture in a hip with pre-existing arthritis, such as rheumatoid arthritis.

D. **NONOPERATIVE TREATMENT.**
1. **Traction** has a poor track record for hip fractures.
2. **Only severely ill patients** who are not likely to survive surgery are treated with traction.

E. **COMPLICATIONS.**
1. Lack of blood supply.
a. Fracture and displacement of the femoral neck interrupts all blood flow except that through the ligamentum teres.
b. The intracapsular position of the head means that no callus will form outside the fracture to aid in union.
c. Synovial fluid will lyse any blood clot that forms, which means the femoral neck fracture is dependent on endosteal union alone.
d. After stabilization, revascularization of the avascular head occurs by a process of 'creeping substitution'.
e. As dead segments of bone are reached by the new blood supply, they are resorbed, and replaced with new trabeculae.
f. Understanding this process is the key to understanding the two major complications after femoral neck fracture.
2. **Nonunion.**
a. This occurs in about 20–30% of displaced femoral neck fractures after reduction and stabilization.
b. It is rare after stabilization of nondisplaced fractures.
c. Predisposing factors include:
   1) Increased patient age.
   2) Poor reduction.
   3) Inadequate fixation.
   4) Comminution.
3. **Avascular necrosis.**
a. AVN is death of bone due to ischemia.
b. Prevalence of AVN after a femoral neck fracture varies from 11 to 84%.
c. Prevalence of late segmental collapse ranges from 7 to 35%.

d. Segmental collapse of the infarcted bone results in joint incongruity and post-traumatic arthritis.
e. This segmental collapse can occur as late as 2 years after the fracture.

IV. INTERTROCHANTERIC HIP FRACTURES

A. EVALUATION. AP pelvis and lateral hip radiographs will generally demonstrate the fracture.

B. CLASSIFICATION.

1. **Intertrochanteric fractures** are simply classified as stable or unstable at Parkland Memorial Hospital.

2. **Unstable fractures** involve the posteromedial cortex of the proximal femur, around the lesser trochanter and calcar femoral. They have lost the posteromedial 'buttress'. Stable patterns have not.

3. **Unstable patterns** are more likely to undergo significant bony collapse after stabilization, as the bone settles into a more stable position.

C. TREATMENT.

1. **Surgical stabilization of the fracture** using a dynamic hip screw is the treatment of choice for these injuries.

2. **Nonsurgical treatment** is reserved for severely ill patients.

D. COMPLICATIONS.

1. **Nonunion is rare** after these injuries (1–2%), owing to the rich cancellous blood supply.

2. **AVN** is also rare (<1%).

3. **Nail cutout**. This hardware complication is often due to an unstable reduction, or due to misplacement of the screw inside the femoral head. Recent studies have stressed the importance of central placement of the screw, close to the subchondral bone (about 1 cm from it).

4. **Varus displacement and bony collapse** of the neck is sometimes seen with hardware failure in an unstable fracture pattern.

V. SUBTROCHANTERIC FEMUR FRACTURES

A. OCCURRENCE.

1. **Subtrochanteric femur fractures** can occur after high-energy accidents in young patients, or after minimal trauma in the elderly.

2. **The subtrochanteric region of the femur** is subjected to high compressive and tensile loads. Because of this, implant failure can occur after fixation of these fractures.

B. EVALUATION. AP and lateral radiograph of the entire femur should be obtained.

C. CLASSIFICATION. Seinsheimer classification is most commonly used.

1. **Type I** – nondisplaced.

2. **Type II** – two-part fracture.

3. **Type III** – three-part fracture.
4. **Type IV** – comminuted, with four or more fragments.
5. **Type V** – subtrochanteric fracture with an intertrochanteric extension.

D. TREATMENT.
1. **Nonoperative.**
a. Several authors have reported acceptable results using hip-spica casting with a hinge at the knee. However, the rates of malunion and nonunion are high using conservative methods such as casting.
b. Owing to these problems, casts and traction are not used at Parkland unless the patient is too ill to survive surgery.
c. Subtrochanteric fractures in multiply injured patients should be immediately stabilized to prevent pulmonary complications.

2. **Operative.**
a. Anatomic stabilization of the fracture to allow early mobilization is the goal of treatment. The type of implant used must be determined by the fracture pattern and includes:
   1) Intramedullary (IM) devices (1st- or 2nd-generation nails).
   2) Blade plates.
   3) Dynamic condylar screws.
   4) Dynamic hip screws with long side-plates.
b. Restoration of medial cortical contact is important, since the compressive forces across the medial subtrochanteric region are very high (2–3 times body weight in stance phase of gait).
   1) This force can cause implant failure if the bone has not been aligned to share some of the load.
   2) Some authors have recommended bone grafting the medial cortex at the time of the initial internal fixation.

E. COMPLICATIONS.
1. **Nonunion** (5%).
2. **Comminution of the greater trochanter.**
3. **Fracture of the femoral neck.**
4. **Rotational malalignment** (21%).

VI. FEMORAL SHAFT FRACTURES
A. OCCURRENCE.
1. **Femoral shaft fractures** are high-energy injuries.
2. **These fractures are commonly associated with other injuries,** and can themselves cause life-threatening complications.

B. EVALUATION.
1. **AP and lateral radiographs** of the entire femur.
2. **The hip and knee should be included** in these views.

C. CLASSIFICATION. There is no commonly accepted classification system for femoral shaft fractures.

D. TREATMENT.

1. **A prospective, randomized trial** at Parkland Memorial Hospital showed that, compared with traction, immediate stabilization of femur fractures in multiply injured patients lessens the risk of pneumonia, fat embolism, and ARDS.

2. **Early stabilization** reduces the time spent intubated and in the intensive care unit as well as shortening the hospital stay.

3. **Every effort is made to stabilize femur fractures** within 24 hours of injury.

4. **Indications.**

a. Intramedullary (IM) nailing.

   1) IM nailing has become the treatment of choice for fractures of the femoral shaft. The technique restores anatomy, allows for rapid mobilization, limits the time of bed rest, lessens the pain from fracture instability, and the static locking of the nails lessens the risk of a rotational malunion without adversely affecting union rates.

   2) Methods such as cast bracing and traction for femur fractures have shown consistently poorer results in randomized trials.

   3) Nonoperative treatment methods are reserved for very ill, elderly patients who would not survive a general anesthetic.

b. Retrograde femoral nailing. The relative indications for this technique include:

   1) Need for concurrent celiotomy, or other surgery.

   2) Floating knee (see Part F below, Special situations).

   3) Ipsilateral femoral neck and shaft fractures (see Part F below).

   4) Concomitant femoral vascular injury (Part F below).

   5) Morbidly obese patients with pulmonary or spine injuries.

c. External fixation.

   1) External fixators used for femur fractures are often complicated by pin tract infections, knee stiffness from tethering the quadriceps to the femur, and malunions.

   2) Delayed union is more common with external fixation.

   3) At Parkland, external fixators are primarily reserved for open femur fractures with gross wound contamination, and for fractures which clearly require a flap procedure to cover the fracture site.

   4) External fixators can also be used to stabilize femur fractures in patients who would not survive an IM nailing.

   5) External fixators can be rapidly applied to obtain bony stability in patients with concomitant vascular injuries who present to the hospital late.

E. COMPLICATIONS.

1. **Infections** are rare ($<1\%$).

a. Infections should be treated with irrigation and débridement.

b. The IM nail can usually be left in place until the fracture unites.

2. **Nonunion is rare.**
a. Exchange nailing and placement of a larger nail have proven successful at Parkland.
b. Bone grafting can be used as necessary.
c. Rotational malunions can be treated with nail removal and osteotomy with an IM saw. Derotation and static-locked nailing can then correct the deformity.

F. **SPECIAL SITUATIONS.**

1. **Open fractures.**
a. Rapid stabilization of the femur will prevent pulmonary complications, and limit time spent in the intensive care unit and on the ventilator.
b. Most open femur fractures can be safely treated with immediate IM nailing, after thorough surgical irrigation and débridement.
c. Several series of open femur fractures treated with IM nails have shown functional results comparable to those seen with closed fractures. The infection rates have been reported to be about 2–4%.
d. The presence of gross contaminants in the wound (gravel, dirt, etc.) is an indication for external fixation.
e. Fractures which require flap coverage are usually treated with an external fixator.
f. External fixators on the femur are commonly complicated by pin tract infections.
   1) Malunion and delayed union are also much more frequent than with IM nails.
   2) Placement of the pins through the quadriceps tethers the muscle to the bone and can cause knee stiffness. (More posterior pin placement, nearer to the insertion of the lateral intermuscular septum on the linea aspera, can limit muscle tethering.)
g. Open femur fractures that require flap coverage have a high rate of nonunion and limb loss due to the extensive nature of these injuries.

2. **Ipsilateral femoral shaft and femoral neck fractures.**
a. There are several ways to treat these fractures. The 'recon', or second-generation nail, is one option.
b. The 'miss a nail' method (antegrade femoral nailing followed by placement of percutaneous cannulated screws around the nail) is another option.
c. A third option, now in use at Parkland, is retrograde femoral nailing followed by percutaneous screw fixation of the femoral neck fracture.

3. **Ipsilateral femur and tibia fractures – the 'floating knee'.**
a. This difficult injury pattern is made simpler to treat by approaching both fractures through one incision at the knee.
b. Antegrade tibia nailing in a standard fashion will stabilize the tibia. This is necessary for control of the femur, which can then be stabilized via a retrograde approach. This method saves operating time.

c. The clinician must be aware of the risk of compartment syndrome in floating knee injuries – reported as high as 30% in some series.

4. **Femur fractures with an associated vascular injury.**

a. About 2% of femur fractures have an associated vascular injury.

b. These injuries are managed with immediate fracture stabilization.

c. If the patient arrives at the treating hospital soon enough, standard internal fixation techniques can safely be used.

d. The vascular repair then follows.

e. If the ischemic threshold is approaching (i.e. 3 hours or more since the time of injury), the vascular injury must be addressed first.

   1) This can be done either with direct vascular repair, or with a temporary vascular shunt.

   2) Stabilization of the fracture then follows.

f. Close cooperation among the trauma and orthopedic surgeons is a necessity in the care of these patients.

5. **Gunshot wounds.**

a. IM nailing is a safe, effective form of treatment for femur fractures due to gunshot wounds.

b. The entry wound is debrided, but no attempt is made to remove the bullet unless it is superficial or has entered a joint.

c. Shotgun wounds which produce fractures are close-range, high-energy injuries.

   1) The amount of soft tissue damage is usually extensive.

   2) Fracture comminution and bone loss are often severe.

   3) Wadding from the shell often enters the wound.

   4) This plastic or paper wad (even horsehair in older shells) is not visible radiographically, and can be missed at débridement.

   5) Severe chronic infections can result from these injuries.

   6) Shotgun wounds should be treated as open fractures.

   7) Aggressive, serial irrigation and débridement is necessary.

   8) Antibiotic coverage is mandatory.

VII. SUPRACONDYLAR FEMUR FRACTURES

A. **SUPRACONDYLAR FEMUR FRACTURES,** like subtrochanteric fractures, can either result from high-energy trauma in young patients, or from low-energy trauma in the elderly.

B. **EVALUATION.**

1. **AP and lateral radiographs** of the knee and entire femur.

2. **Oblique views** can occasionally be helpful in delineating the fracture pattern.

C. **CLASSIFICATION.**

1. **The AO classification** is most commonly used:

a. Type A – extra-articular fractures (Figure 35.2).

b. Type B – unicondylar fractures (Figure 35.3).

c. Type C – intercondylar fractures (Figure 35.4).

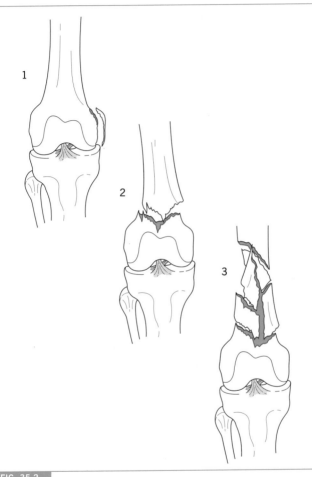

FIG. 35.2

Type A distal femur fracture. (From Kozin SH, Berlet AC. *Handbook of common orthopedic fractures*. Westchester: Medical Surveillance; 1989.)

2. **Each type is subcategorized** as 1, 2, or 3 according to the amount of comminution present.

D. TREATMENT.

1. **Nonoperative.**

a. Nonweight bearing and cast bracing are the forms of nonoperative treatment used at Parkland.

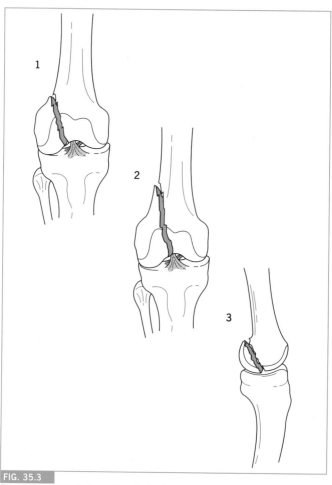

FIG. 35.3

Type B distal femur fracture. (From Kozin SH, Berlet AC. *Handbook of common orthopedic fractures*. Westchester: Medical Surveillance; 1989.)

    b.   Nondisplaced fractures can be safely treated conservatively.

    c.   Very ill, elderly patients who would not tolerate an operation can also be managed conservatively.

2. Operative.

    a.   ORIF.

        1)   Most displaced supracondylar femur fractures will require some form of ORIF.

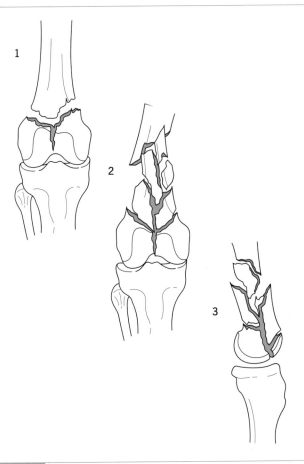

FIG. 35.4
Type C distal femur fracture. (From Kozin SH, Berlet AC. *Handbook of common orthopedic fractures*. Westchester: Medical Surveillance; 1989.)

2) Side-plates, blade plates, dynamic condylar screws, and IM devices have all been used with success.
3) One IM device, the supracondylar nail, has been designed specifically for this fracture type.
4) The implant must be chosen to match the particular 'personality' of the fracture.

     5) The goal is to achieve a stable anatomic reduction, to allow early mobility, and to prevent post-traumatic arthritis.

     6) These fractures are often technically difficult to repair.

     7) Comminution can make exact articular restoration difficult.

     8) Continuous passive motion machines are used.

  b. External fixation.

     1) In patients who are multiply injured, hemodynamically unstable, and near death, there is little time on the day of injury for reconstruction of the distal femoral articular surface.

     2) In patients with large, open wounds with gross contamination, internal fixation is unwise due to the risk of infection.

     3) In these rare types of patients, a knee-bridging external fixator is used at Parkland.

     4) Distraction with this frame will usually give a good reduction of the major fracture fragments.

     5) Fixation can be supplemented by limited internal fixation with percutaneously placed screws.

     6) This type of frame can be easily applied in about 20 minutes.

     7) Minimal blood is lost, and it achieves the goal of stabilizing the fracture.

     8) This makes transport easier, and limits further soft tissue injury.

E. COMPLICATIONS.

1. **Malunion and nonunion.**

2. **Hardware failure** is also fairly common, and can be a sign of nonunion.

3. **Nonunion rates are higher in older patients.**

4. **Some authors have recommended primary bone grafting** to improve union rates.

VIII. PATELLA FRACTURES

A. OCCURRENCE.

1. **Patella fractures** usually result from direct blows to the front of the knee.

2. **Knee ligament injury, femur fracture, and posterior hip dislocation** can be associated with patella fractures.

B. EVALUATION.

1. **AP, lateral, and patellar skyline radiographs.**

2. **The patient's ability to extend the knee** must be evaluated.

C. CLASSIFICATION.

1. **Fractures are usually classified as:**

a. Transverse.

b. Longitudinal.

c. Upper or lower pole fractures.

d. Comminuted.

2. **Comminuted fractures of the lower pole** seem to be the most common.

D. TREATMENT.

1. Nonoperative.

a. This can be used in nondisplaced or minimally displaced (maximum of 2mm step-off) fractures, as long as the patient's extensor mechanism is intact.

b. At Parkland Memorial Hospital these patients are placed in a cylinder cast for 6 weeks, and are kept limited weight bearing.

2. Operative.

a. This is preferable if displacement is present, or if the extensor mechanism is ruptured.

b. Surgery on the patella should be done through a longitudinal midline incision. Transverse incisions can compromise later surgery on the knee.

c. The goal is restoration of articular anatomy with a stable construct which allows early movement.

   1) This can be accomplished with either K-wires or screws.
   2) An anterior tension band wire is passed around the ends of the wires or screws.
   3) Recently, physicians at Parkland have begun passing parts of the tension band through cannulated screws in these fractures.
   4) Cerclage wires are not used as the sole means of stabilization.
   5) The extensor retinaculum is usually torn transversely, and it must be repaired at surgery.
   6) Comminuted inferior pole fractures can be safely excised. The patellar tendon can then be reattached using a nonabsorbable suture woven through the tendon, and passed up through drill holes in the patella.
   7) Postoperatively, most patients are kept in a knee immobilizer for 3–4 weeks, and then are started on active exercises.

E. COMPLICATIONS.

1. **Post-traumatic arthritis** has been reported in as many as 50% of patients in some series.

2. **Nonunion is rare** and has been reported in only 2% of cases.

3. **Painful hardware** is common, owing to the subcutaneous position of the patella. Removal of the hardware when symptomatic usually alleviates this.

IX. TIBIAL PLATEAU FRACTURES

A. EVALUATION.

1. **AP and lateral radiographs** should be obtained.

2. **Oblique views** can sometimes be helpful.

3. **CT scans** are commonly obtained to demonstrate the full extent of depression of the articular surface.

FRACTURES AND DISLOCATIONS OF THE LOWER EXTREMITY

35

4. **Ligamentous stability** must be assessed, either in the operating room under anesthesia, or after injection of an anesthetic in the knee.
B. **CLASSIFICATION.** The Schatzker classification is used at Parkland (Figure 35.5).
1. **Schatzker I** – lateral plateau split.
2. **Schatzker II** – lateral plateau split depression.
3. **Schatzker III** – lateral plateau depression.
4. **Schatzker IV** – medial plateau fracture.
5. **Schatzker V** – bicondylar plateau fracture.
6. **Schatzker VI** – plateau fracture, with associated fracture at metadiaphyseal junction.

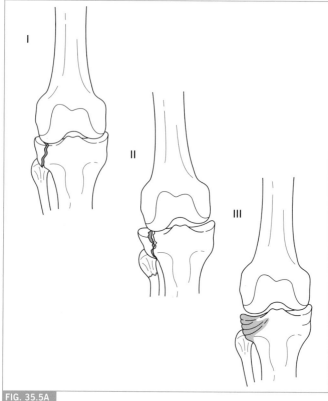

FIG. 35.5A

Schatzker classification of tibial plateau fractures. (From Kozin SH, Berlet AC. *Handbook of common orthopedic fractures.* Westchester: Medical Surveillance; 1989.)

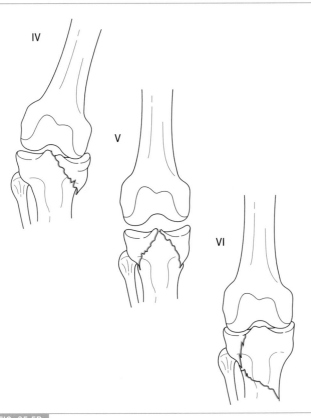

FIG. 35.5B
Schatzker classification of tibial plateau fractures. (From Kozin SH, Berlet AC. *Handbook of common orthopedic fractures.* Westchester: Medical Surveillance; 1989.)

C. TREATMENT.

1. **As with other articular fractures**, stable anatomic reduction and early mobilization are the goals of treatment.
2. **Use of limited exposure and external fixation** as an adjunct is an acceptable form of treatment.
3. **Since 2–3mm of displacement** is commonly accepted as adequate reduction for other articular fractures, it is accepted for tibial plateau fractures as well. Greater displacement is usually an indication for operative reduction.

4. **Varus or valgus instability** of more than 10° is also an indication for surgical stabilization, although this has not been tested in a prospective trial.

5. **Nonoperative.**

a. Nondisplaced or minimally displaced tibial plateau fractures do well when treated with cast bracing.

b. Rapid mobilization prevents stiffness, and nonweight bearing prevents further displacement.

c. In elderly patients greater amounts of displacement can be accepted and nonoperative treatment can be successfully used.

d. In the older population (≥ 60 years) post-traumatic arthritis can be treated with total knee replacement, which has predictably good results.

e. The best predictor of future arthritis is knee instability in the varus or valgus plane. Minor articular irregularities appear to be tolerated well as long as the knee is stable.

6. **Operative.**

a. Internal fixation and buttress plating.

   1) ORIF allows anatomic restoration of articular surfaces.
   2) This prevents future arthritis.
   3) This is normally done through a lateral or medial parapatellar arthrotomy.
   4) The meniscus is lifted off the plateau, and the plateau is reconstructed.
   5) Physicians at Parkland have begun using small fragment plates and 3.5mm screws to limit implant size.
   6) Open fractures or injuries with significant soft tissue contusion or abrasion should probably be treated with other techniques.
   7) Patients with compromised soft tissues are at high risk for infection and wound breakdown.

b. Limited internal fixation.

   1) Depressed plateau fractures can often be elevated using a bone tamp placed through a small anterior cortical window.
   2) Bone graft can be stuffed up into the window to buttress the articular fragment.
   3) Reduction is judged using an image intensifier.
   4) Stabilization is obtained with 2–3 percutaneously placed large fragment cannulated screws.
   5) A screw and a washer placed just below a fracture line can be used as an antiglide plate to hold up metaphyseal fragments.
   6) After surgery, the patients are kept nonweight bearing in a cast brace for 3 months.

c. External fixation.

   1) External fixation can be used to supplement limited internal fixation of plateau fractures.

2) Proximal pins placed into the stable, nonfractured plateau can be used to support the fractured plateau, and hold the tibia out to length.

3) External fixation also obviates the need for cast bracing. This is a very versatile technique that is especially useful in open fractures or fractures with compromised soft tissues. Infection rates are low.

4) As with supracondylar femur fractures, physicians at Parkland use knee-bridging external fixators in patients who have large, contaminated open wounds, or who are hemodynamically unstable. The fixator can be rapidly applied, and a surprisingly good reduction can often be obtained.

d. Hybrid external fixation and ring fixators.

1) Ring fixators (Ilizarov-type fixators) can be used to suspend comminuted articular fragments.

2) The distal rings, anchored in the stable tibial diaphysis, provide the platform for the ring holding up the plateau.

3) As with external fixation, ring fixators limit soft tissue stripping and are less likely to be complicated by wound breakdown and infection. They can also be supplemented with limited internal fixation using cannulated screws.

4) 'Hybrid' fixators use standard external fixator pins in the tibial diaphysis, instead of rings. The pins are connected to the tibial plateau ring using a standard external fixation bar.

D. COMPLICATIONS.

1. **Post-traumatic arthritis** is a common complication of tibial plateau fractures.

a. The major cause of this is instability of the knee in varus or valgus stress.

b. Articular displacement is also a cause of arthritis.

c. Associated ligamentous injuries are repaired using standard techniques after fracture union.

2. **Wound breakdown and infection** are also potential complications, especially with open fractures or those with injured soft tissues.

X. TIBIAL SHAFT FRACTURES

A. OCCURRENCE.

1. **Tibia fracture** is one of the most common long bone injuries seen in trauma centers.

2. **Since much of the tibia is subcutaneous,** open fractures are very common.

3. **Soft tissue damage and bone loss** can be extensive.

4. **The severely mangled leg** remains one of the most difficult injuries to treat.

B. EVALUATION.
1. **AP and lateral radiographs** should be obtained of the entire tibia.
2. **A thorough examination of the soft tissues and neurovascular structures** must be carried out to avoid missing an injury.
C. CLASSIFICATION.
1. **No accepted classification** for tibial fractures exists.
2. **Most surgeons describe fractures according to site** (proximal, middle, or distal third), pattern (transverse, oblique, butterfly, or comminuted), and displacement.
D. TREATMENT.
1. **Nonoperative.**
a. Nonoperative treatment can give good, functional results in many low-energy tibia fractures.
b. Treatment starts with a long-leg, bent-knee cast for about 4 weeks.
c. This is followed by a patellar tendon-bearing cast.
d. Progressive weight bearing is allowed as fracture callus is seen on radiographs.
e. Cast immobilization is continued until the fracture unites. Union commonly takes from 3 to 5 months in tibia fractures (longer in smokers).
f. Maintenance of reduction can be difficult.
g. Close monitoring and frequent radiographs are necessary.
h. Remanipulation or cutting wedges out of the cast to move the fracture are occasionally necessary.
i. The following indications for cast treatment are commonly quoted:
   1) $<5°$ of varus or valgus malalignment.
   2) $<10°$ of anterior or posterior angulation.
   3) <1cm of shortening.
   4) $<5°$ of malrotation.
2. **Operative.**
a. Operative fixation provides excellent stabilization and maintenance of reduction. However, it exposes the patient to all the risks of surgery.
b. The following are commonly quoted as indications for surgical management:
   1) Ipsilateral femur fracture (floating knee).
   2) Segmental tibia fracture.
   3) Concomitant vascular injury requiring repair.
   4) Concomitant compartment syndrome.
   5) Multiply injured patient.
   6) Pathologic fractures.
   7) Inability to maintain reduction with closed methods.
c. Plating, as a means of surgical stabilization, is not used at Parkland.

d. IM nailing is the treatment of choice at Parkland.
   1) Reamed IM nailing gives excellent stabilization of tibial fractures.
   2) Static locking of IM nails prevents rotational deformities, and reaming deposits bone graft at the fracture site.
   3) Reaming allows easy placement of IM nails, and seems to lessen the prevalence of delayed union.
   4) The endosteal blood supply, which reaming destroys, has been shown to return after 6 weeks.
   5) Unreamed-type nails (Delta nails) are still placed, but they are placed after reaming.
   6) The unreamed-type nails are narrower, and can be placed after fewer passes of the reamer.
   7) IM nailing is the surgical treatment of choice for most closed tibia fractures.
e. External fixation.
   1) External fixation is useful in stabilizing open tibia fractures which cannot be managed with an IM nail.
   2) External fixation allows further care of wounds, and does not disturb the fracture site.
   3) In fractures with no soft tissue coverage, external fixation avoids contamination of the medullary canal, which is a possible complication of nailing.
   4) Ring fixators are not used to stabilize acute tibia fractures at Parkland.

E. COMPLICATIONS.

1. **Nonunion or delayed union.**
a. More common after more severe injuries.
b. Prophylactic bone grafting 6–8 weeks after injury is normally done in high-energy fractures, since they will predictably be very slow to unite.
c. The posterolateral approach to the tibia is useful for bone grafting, since it avoids the original injury site.
d. Smoking has been shown to double the time required for healing in practically all types of tibia fractures.
e. Delayed union can be treated with dynamization of the nail, or reamed-exchange nailing.

2. **Malunion.**
a. More common after casting.
b. Correctional osteotomies can be stabilized using plates, IM nails, or Ilizarov-ring fixators.
c. No criteria for defining malunion exist; each case must be individually considered.

3. **Infection and osteomyelitis.**
a. More common after open injuries.

b. Can be prevented with aggressive surgical débridement at the first operation.

c. Established infections should be treated aggressively with removal of all infected tissue, including bone.

4. **Soft tissue loss.**

a. Common after high-energy injuries.

b. Obtaining soft tissue coverage of the wound within 5–6 days of injury has been shown to improve results.

c. Aggressive initial débridement lessens the risk of infection and improves flap success rates.

d. Free flaps or rotational flaps should be used as necessary.

5. **Bone defects.**

a. Common after high-energy injuries.

b. Should be addressed after the soft tissue envelope has healed.

c. Treatment ranges from simple iliac crest-bone grafting to bone transport using Ilizarov-ring fixators.

6. **Compartment syndrome.**

a. Common after tibia fractures, especially open fractures.

b. Up to 10% of open tibia fractures develop compartment syndrome.

c. These must be treated with four-compartment fasciotomy.

XI. SPECIAL SITUATIONS

A. **THE FOLLOWING GUIDELINES FOR OPEN FRACTURES** uses the Gustilo and Andersen classification system. It must be remembered that this classification system has poor interobserver reliability.

B. **EACH OPEN FRACTURE** must be treated according to the fracture's 'personality'.

C. **GRADE I OR II.** These injuries can usually be treated with reamed IM nailing.

D. **GRADE IIIA.** The usual treatment is with an IM nail.

1. **If soft tissue coverage of the bone is available quickly,** IM nailing is usually safe and effective.

2. **If any question about the viability of the soft tissue exists,** external fixation is a safe, reliable alternative.

E. **GRADE IIIB.** This classification is usually best managed with an external fixator.

1. **External fixation** allows good access to the wound, and can easily be modified if needed.

2. **Flap coverage** is not much more difficult with an external fixator in place.

F. **GRADE IIIC.** These injuries should be managed according to the size of the soft tissue defect.

1. **Vascular repair distal to the popliteal fossa** is difficult, and can make later flap coverage harder.

2. **Patients with high-energy injuries** can go through extremely long periods of surgical care and still wind up with an insensate, dysvascular limb.
3. **These are the most difficult patients to manage** and early amputation must be considered as an option.

XII. FURTHER READING

Bone LB, Johnson KD, Weigelt J et al. Early vs delayed stabilization of femoral fractures. A prospective randomized study. *J Bone Joint Surg* 1989; 71A:336–340.

Brumback RJ, Uwagi-Ero S, Lakatos RP et al. Intramedullary nailing of femoral shaft fractures. Part II: fracture healing with static interlocking femoral fixation. *J Bone Joint Surg* 1988; 70A:1453–1462.

Henley MB. Intramedullary devices for tibial fracture stabilization. *Clin Orthop Rel Res* 1989; 240:87–96.

Kenzora JE, McCarthy RE, Lowell JD et al. Hip fracture mortality: relation to age, treatment, pre-operative illness, time of surgery, and complications. *Clin Orthop Rel Res* 1984; 186:45–56.

Starr AJ, Hunt JL, Reinert CM. Treatment of femur fracture with associated vascular injury. *J Trauma* 1996; 40:17–21.

KNEE LIGAMENT INJURIES

I. EVALUATION

A. HISTORY.

1. **Solicit mechanism of injury** (Table 36.1).
2. **Inquire as to** sensations–audible pop, location of pain, feeling of instability, chronology, and quality of effusion.
3. **History of previous injuries or operations on the knee** can be helpful.
4. **History of knee problems since the time of injury** is valuable information in assisting with the diagnosis.

B. PHYSICAL EXAMINATION.

1. **Always examine the good knee** first for comparison.
2. **Inspection** – observe gait, if possible, and look for ecchymosis, edema, effusion, and abrasions.
3. **Palpation** – check for ballottement of the patella as well as tenderness and crepitance along the jointline, epicondyles, apophyses, etc.
4. **Observe the limits** of both active and passive range of motion.
5. **Stability testing** (see Section III).
6. **Be systematic, yet practical**. For example, performing a pivot-shift test prior to other painful stimuli may help gain a diagnosis.

TABLE 36.1

COMMON MECHANISMS OF KNEE INJURY[a]

Mechanism of injury (knee position[b])	Ligament injury
Valgus	
Straight medial opening	Tibial collateral plus capsular ligaments[c]
External rotation	Medial structures, medial meniscus, anterior cruciate – 'terrible triad'
Varus	
Straight lateral opening	Fibular collateral plus capsular ligaments[c]
Internal rotation	Lateral ligaments plus anterior cruciate
External rotation	Lateral ligaments plus posterior cruciate
Hyperextension	Posterior capsule and posterior cruciate[d]
Direct blow driving tibia backward	Posterior cruciate
Direct blow driving tibia forward	Anterior cruciate

[a]Adapted with permission from Hunter-Griffin LY (ed.) *Athletic training and sports medicine*. Rosemount, IL: American Academy of Orthopedic Surgeons; 1991.
[b]Tibia moving with femur fixed.
[c]Severe opening implies injury to either one or both cruciates.
[d]Severe hyperextension may also injure the anterior cruciate ligament.

C. **DIAGNOSTIC TESTS.**
1. **Radiography.**
a. Routine – anteroposterior (AP), lateral, and sunrise patella views.
b. Optional – condylar tunnel and oblique views.
c. Children – comparison and stress views.
2. **Joint aspiration.**
a. Approximately 70% of patients who have acute hemarthroses following an injury have an anterior cruciate ligament injury.
b. Aspiration followed by an injection of lidocaine into the knee joint may relieve the pain and allow a more thorough examination to be obtained.
3. **Magnetic resonance imaging (MRI).**
a. Expensive, very sensitive and specific (>95%).
b. Often unnecessary.
c. This test should not be ordered if an objective finding is not going to be treated surgically.
4. **Arteriograms** are useful in excluding a vascular injury following a knee dislocation.
5. **Arthrometry.** Multiple-instrumented testing devices are available for reliable assessment of AP laxity.

II. CLASSIFICATION OF KNEE LIGAMENT INJURIES
A. **Grade I injury** – usually minor tearing or stretching of the ligament with <5mm of laxity detected.
B. **Grade II injury** – partial tearing of the ligament (50–75%) with 5–10mm of laxity detected.
C. **Grade III injury** – associated with a complete tear, >10mm of laxity, and no endpoint on examination.
D. **Isolated laxities** – involving one plane.
E. **Combined laxities** – involving >1 plane and is usually a rotational instability (i.e. anterolateral rotatory, posterolateral rotatory, anteromedial rotatory, and posteromedial rotatory instabilities).
F. **Knee dislocation** – classification according to the displacement of the tibia in relation to the femur.

III. STABILITY TESTING
A. **ISOLATED LAXITIES.**
1. **Anterior cruciate ligament (ACL) insufficiency.**
a. The Lachman test at 30° of flexion is the most sensitive test (Figure 36.1). The quality of the endpoint (firm or soft) should be noted and compared with the contralateral side.
b. The pivot shift phenomenon describes the anterior subluxation of the tibial plateau in extension pivoting into reduction with knee flexion.
c. The anterior drawer test is less sensitive than the Lachman test (Figure 36.2).

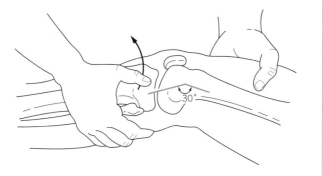

FIG. 36.1
Lachman test for anterior cruciate instability is at 30° of flexion. The extremity does not have to be lifted or the foot stabilized. (Adapted with permission from Hunter-Griffin LY (ed.) *Athletic training and sports medicine*. Rosemount, IL: American Academy of Orthopedic Surgeons; 1991.)

  d. Before determining anterior laxity, assure that the tibia begins in the neutral position for all testing. If the tibia is posteriorly subluxated secondary to a posterior cruciate ligament injury, one may be fooled by anterior–posterior translation.

2. Posterior cruciate ligament (PCL) insufficiency.
  a. Posterior drawer test.
    1) The posterior drawer test is the most accurate method of detecting a PCL injury.
    2) The test is similar to the anterior drawer test except that a posteriorly directed force is applied to the tibia, starting from the neutral position.
    3) The latter point is important because, with a PCL-deficient knee, there is normally a posterior sag of the tibia when flexed to 90°.
  b. Quadriceps active test.
    1) The knee is flexed 90° with the foot stabilized as the patient is asked to contract the quadriceps muscle.
    2) The tibia will translate forward from the posterior subluxed position when a PCL deficiency is present.

3. Medial collateral ligament (MCL) insufficiency with valgus or medial laxity.
  a. Valgus stress test (Figure 36.3).
    1) The primary restraint to valgus stress is the MCL with additional support afforded by the secondary stabilizers (i.e. cruciate ligaments, posterior oblique ligament, and the posteromedial capsule).

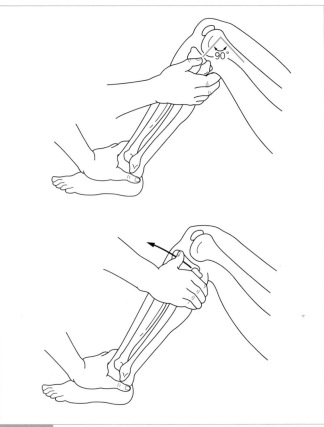

FIG. 36.2
Anterior drawer test determines anterior cruciate instabilitiy. Flex knee to 90° and stabilize foot. Note forward shift of tibia. (Adapted with permission from Hunter-Griffin LY (ed.) *Athletic training and sports medicine*. Rosemount, IL: American Academy of Orthopedic Surgeons; 1991.)

2) The MCL should be stressed at 0° and 30° of flexion.
3) With 30° of flexion, the secondary stabilizers are relaxed, and the superficial and deep MCL fibers are stressed.
4) With full extension, medial laxity implies injury to the MCL and secondary stabilizers, giving anteromedial or posteromedial rotatory instability.

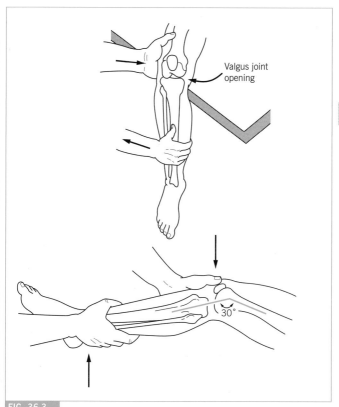

Valgus joint
opening

30°

FIG. 36.3

Valgus test in 30° of flexion. (Adapted with permission from Hunter-Griffin LY (ed.)
Athletic training and sports medicine. Rosemount, IL: American Academy of
Orthopedic Surgeons; 1991.)

4. **Lateral collateral ligament (LCL) insufficiency** with varus or lateral
   laxity.
a. The varus stress test (i.e. varus or adduction stress testing) should be
   performed in the same manner as above in full extension and at 30° of
   flexion.
b. Isolated sectioning of the lateral posterolateral ligaments has
   demonstrated only a small change (1–4°) in varus rotation at all angles
   of flexion with an LCL complete tear.

   c. Further increase in varus laxity or a side-to-side difference in external rotation >10° indicates a posterolateral complex injury usually involving the LCL, popliteus, arcuate ligament complex, lateral head of the gastrocnemius, or posterolateral capsule.

B. COMBINED LAXITIES.

1. Posterolateral complex with ACL deficiency. The external rotation recurvatum test:

   a. Performed with the patient in the supine position.

   b. The big toe is grasped and lifted, lifting the entire leg from the table.

   c. If the tibia externally rotates and the knee falls into varus hyperextension, a combined ACL posterolateral complex injury is present.

   d. Further side-to-side differences in external rotation and Lachman's test at 30° corroborates this diagnosis.

2. Posterolateral complex with PCL deficiency.

   a. Prone (or supine) external rotation test.

      1) Performed at 30° and 90° of flexion[2].

      2) Increases in varus and external rotation at 30° and 90° of knee flexion, compared with the opposite side, indicates an injury to the PCL and posterolateral structures.

   b. Posterolateral drawer test.

      1) A posterior drawer test is applied with the knee flexed 80° and externally rotated 15°.

      2) Laxity indicates a combined injury to the PCL and posterolateral complex.

IV. TREATMENT OF KNEE LIGAMENT INJURIES

A. GENERAL PRINCIPLES.

1. Rest, ice, compression, and elevation (RICE) along with symptomatic treatment is sufficient until the inflammatory phase is completed in several weeks.

2. Gentle, passive-and-active range of motion exercises are performed as tolerated to prevent stiffness and atrophy.

3. Crutches and bracing can be helpful.

B. COLLATERAL LIGAMENT INJURIES.

1. Grades I and IIa.

   a. Treat in a hinged brace with full range of motion until completely nontender and clinically stable.

   b. Rehabilitation should concentrate on quadriceps, hamstrings, and adductor strengthening.

2. Grade III.

   a. Same as above, allowing for more time to heal.

b. MCL tears associated with cruciate ligament injuries may or may not be repaired. This is a controversial subject and should be left to the individual surgeon.

c Posterolateral complex tears should be repaired acutely or reconstructed in chronic situations.

C. ACL INJURY.

1. **Nonoperative treatment.**

a. Treat in a hinged brace and encourage a full range of motion exercises until the acute inflammation has resolved.

b. Rehabilitation concentrating on hamstring and quadriceps strengthening as well as obtaining a full range of motion.

c. Use a functional brace for patients involved in athletics or work requiring pivoting or climbing.

d. Nonoperative treatment may involve arthroscopic surgery for meniscal tears or débridement of the ACL stump to allow a full range of motion.

2. **Operative treatment.**

a. Arthroscopic or open repair should be performed if the ligament has avulsed bone from the tibia or femur (more commonly the former) and is unstable. Primary repairs have a poor success rate and should be considered in only the immature person with open growth plates.

b. Reconstruction of the ACL using patellar bone-tendon-bone, hamstring, or allograft tendon is usually recommended in a young, active patient who wishes to continue an active lifestyle, or has failed nonoperative treatment and has instability with daily activities.

c. This decision should be individualized for each patient with the understanding that the rehabilitation process is lengthy and just as important as the surgery.

D. PCL INJURY.

1. **Isolated PCL injuries are usually treated nonoperatively** with a hinged knee brace, full range of motion, and emphasizing quadriceps straightening. However, in association with disability or combined injuries, surgical reconstruction is advocated.

2. **Arthroscopic or open repair should be performed** if bony avulsion has taken place.

V. KNEE DISLOCATIONS

A. CLASSIFICATION. This is made according to the displacement of the tibia in relation to the femur.

1. **Anterior.**
2. **Posterior.**
3. **Medial.**
4. **Lateral.**
5. **Rotatory.**

36

KNEE LIGAMENT INJURIES

B. OCCURRENCE. Anterior dislocations secondary to a hyperextension force are the most common.

C. VASCULAR INJURY.

1. **Incidence** is about 20–30%. Arteriograms should be performed emergently on all knee dislocations because of the risk.

2. **Absence of pedal pulses, tenderness, swelling, and ecchymosis** in the popliteal fossa, or a cold cyanotic lower extremity, are all danger signals for a vascular injury.

3. **Warm ischemia time** should not exceed 6–8 hours.

a. Vascular surgical repair should precede this time limit.

b. Attempts at arterial repair after 8 hours frequently requires later amputation secondary to nonviable tissues distal to the knee joint.

4. **Compartment syndromes** may accompany these injuries. Treat appropriately with fasciotomies.

D. NERVE INJURY.

1. **The incidence of peroneal nerve injury** varies between 16 and 43%. It is more common following a posterolateral knee dislocation.

2. **Prognosis for return of function** should be guarded.

E. LIGAMENT INJURY.

1. **Usually both cruciates** and one or more collaterals are torn.

2. **Avulsion fractures** at the insertion of the PCL and ACL are common, making repair a possibility.

3. **If the primary repair is tenuous**, then augmentation with the semitendinosus and gracilis, or a reconstruction, should be performed.

F. TREATMENT.

1. **Physical examination** documenting pulses, and a neurologic examination are paramount.

2. **Reduce the dislocation emergently** and splint in slight flexion. Most dislocations can be reduced by closed means.

3. **Re-examine the patient after reduction** for vascular sufficiency and then evaluate the popliteal artery with an arteriogram.

4. **Open dislocations** should undergo:

a. Immediate irrigation and débridement.

b. Vascular exploration and possible repair.

c. Stabilization with either an external fixator, splint, or orthosis.

5. **Ligamentous repair or reconstruction** should be performed within 7–10 days for best results. When this is not possible, nonsurgical management in a hinged brace or cast can yield satisfactory results.

6. **Rehabilitation** should concentrate on range-of-motion therapy and quadriceps and hamstring strengthening.

a. Current data suggest that stiffness and knee pain are much more common than ligamentous insufficiency following knee dislocations.

b. Therefore, rehabilitation is of utmost importance.

7. **Operative results yield better outcomes** than nonoperative results when the literature is fully assessed.

VI FURTHER READING

Fu FH, Harner CD, Vince KG. *Knee surgery*. *Volume I*. Baltimore: Williams and Wilkins; 1994:679–808.

Fu FH, Stone DA. Sports injuries: mechanisms, prevention, treatment. Baltimore: Williams and Wilkins; 1994:949–976.

Gollehon DL, Torzilli PA, Warren RF. The role of the posterolateral and cruciate ligaments in the stability of the human knee. *J Bone Joint Surg* 1987; 69A:233–242.

Insall JN. *Surgery of the knee*. *Volume I*. New York: Churchill Livingstone; 1993:387–560.

Veltri DM, Xiang-Hua D, Torzilli PA et al. The role of the cruciate and posterolateral ligaments in stability of the knee. A biomechanical study. *Am J Sports Med* 1995; 23:436–443.

36

KNEE LIGAMENT INJURIES

FOOT AND ANKLE INJURIES

I. INTRODUCTION

Injuries of the foot and ankle are extremely common. It is essential that the evaluating physician quickly identifies the nature and extent of these injuries through the use of both physical examination and appropriate radiographic studies.

II. INITIAL EVALUATION

1. **Inspection of the skin** is necessary to assess soft tissue injury and determine the presence or absence of an open fracture.
2. **Alignment of the ankle and foot** should be noted. Careful palpation is performed to identify points of tenderness.
3. **Evaluation of the range of motion** of the ankle, subtalar, midtalar, and metatarsophalangeal joints should be performed.
4. **Three standard radiographic views should be obtained** consisting of a mortise view, a standard anteroposterior view, and a lateral view.

III. INITIAL MANAGEMENT PRINCIPLES

1. **All patients with foot and ankle injuries** should be placed on a gurney with their leg or foot elevated above their heart as expeditiously as possible to prevent excessive swelling.
2. **Foot compression devices** are useful in the management of foot and ankle soft tissue swelling.
3. **In general, an attempt at reduction should be made** in any injury in which there is a loss of pulses or severe deformity secondary to fracture or dislocation. This can dramatically improve subsequent care by reducing the risk of skin necrosis and reducing tension on neurovascular structures.
4. **Open fractures or dislocations** should be managed with:
   a. Tetanus prophylaxis.
   b. Immediate i.v. antibiotic therapy.
   c. Emergent surgical irrigation and débridement.

IV. ANKLE SPRAINS AND FRACTURES

1. **Stable ankle sprains** can be managed with:
   a. Compression.
   b. Ice.
   c. Rest.
   d. Nonsteroidal anti-inflammatory drugs.
   e. Early weight bearing.
2. **In the case of severe sprains**, casting or 3D-walker boot immobilization for 2–3 weeks may provide pain relief.

3. **Isolated lateral malleolar fractures** are treated with casting and protected weight bearing.
4. **Bimalleolar fractures and their equivalents** (i.e. Maisonneuve injuries and lateral malleolar fractures with deltoid ligament or syndesmosis ligament disruption), as well as trimalleolar fractures require open reduction and internal fixation.
5. **The decision to treat conservatively vs surgically** is dependent upon the stability of the tibiotalar joint.

V. CLASSIFICATION

There are two major classification schemes that are currently in use of which the Lanuge–Hansen system is the only one that provides information about mechanism and stability.

VI. SPECIFIC PROBLEMS

A. PILON FRACTURES.
1. **This is a subset of ankle fractures** in which the tibial pilon has one or more fractures.
2. **The AO classification groups these injuries** into types I, II, and III with increasing extent and severity of fracture, comminution, and joint incongruity.
3. **Pilon fracture management** can be assisted by CT consisting of both axial and coronal images.
4. **Alignment, joint congruity, and extent of soft tissue injury** dictate the optimal management, which may be cast immobilization or limited open reduction and internal fixation with or without external fixation.
5. **These fractures can be very problematic** to treat and are fraught with potential complications, mostly secondary to the soft tissues.
B. FRACTURES AND FRACTURE DISLOCATIONS OF THE FOOT. These are divided into three areas:
1. **Hindfoot** (talus and calcaneus).
2. **Midfoot.**
3. **Forefoot.**
C. TALUS.
1. **The talus bears more weight** per unit area on the superior surface than any other joint of the body.
2. **This bone is important for motion** between the leg and the foot, as well as the complex motions of the foot through the subtalar joint.
3. **Two-thirds of the talus** is covered with articular cartilage.
4. **There is a distal-to-proximal blood supply** which makes it very difficult for bone to heal once injured and can be the source for prolonged morbidity.
5. **The talus can be divided into three parts:**
a. Dome.
b. Neck.
c. Head.

6. **Defining the anatomy of the injury** is supplemented with a CT scan.
7. **Many of these patients require surgery** consisting of open reduction and internal fixation followed by prolonged cast immobilization and nonweight bearing (up to 3 months).

D. **CALCANEUS.**
1. **Fractures of the calcaneus** are generally caused by a fall from a height or some extreme axial load to the heel.
2. **Fracture of the lumbar spine** is a common associated injury and should be looked for when evaluating a patient with this type of fracture.
3. **These fractures can be divided** into intra- and extra-articular fractures.
4. **Many of these patients have severe soft tissue swelling** and therefore require immediate elevation once identified.
5. **Standard calcaneal views** include a lateral of the foot and a Harris or axial view of the heel.
6. **Most patients will also require a CT scan** to define the anatomy of the injury and to plan operative intervention.
7. **Patients that require surgery** have fewer wound problems if they are nonsmokers and the injury is closed.
8. **Operative management** is almost always open reduction and internal fixation, although there are selected cases in which patients may require a primary fusion.
9. **All patients with calcaneal fractures** need to be made nonweight bearing and immobilized in a short leg cast.

E. **HINDFOOT DISLOCATIONS.**
1. **Dislocations of the hindfoot** include those about the talus ranging from simple talar dislocation from the mortise to total peritalar dislocation.
2. **The most common dislocation** about the talus is a subtalar dislocation, of which medial is most common, but also include lateral, anterior and posterior dislocations.
3. **Reduction of the joint** needs to be performed as expeditiously as possible to prevent embarrassment of the skin or neurovascular structures.
4. **Many of these injuries are accompanied by fractures** and may not be reduced in the emergency or ambulatory setting.
5. **Interposed fracture fragments or interposed soft tissue structures** will require operative intervention.
6. **Once reduction has been performed**, the patient needs to be immobilized in a short leg cast and made nonweight bearing.

F. **FRACTURES NEAR THE MIDTARSAL JOINTS.** These fractures include those of the talonavicular and calcaneocuboid joints.
1. **These are uncommon** and are often accompanied by minor subluxation or fractures of the adjacent joints.
2. **These can often be very difficult to identify** and are often missed.
3. **Radiographic evaluation** is best done with standard foot views.
4. **CT is obtained** to define injury anatomy.

5. **If a fracture is seen in one of these bones**, it must be assumed that there has been at least a sprain with subluxation or dislocation of the adjacent joints, resulting in midtarsal instability.

6. **Some of these injuries** require open reduction and internal fixation, but nearly always will require the patient to be placed in a short leg cast and made nonweight bearing for a prolonged period of time.

G. **TARSOMETATARSAL JOINT.**

1. **The five metatarsals** and their articulations with the cuboid and the three cuneiforms is named the Lis Franc joint.

2. **Injury to this complex of joints is rare**, but not without severe problems.

3. **These injuries are commonly associated with high-energy situations,** such as motorcycle and motor vehicle collisions.

4. **There are many variants of these fractures and dislocations.**

5. **They are best seen with standard views** of the foot and possibly CT.

6. **Nearly all Lis Franc-type injuries** require open reduction and internal fixation followed by prolonged cast immobilization and nonweight bearing.

H. **FOREFOOT FRACTURES.** These fractures involve the metatarsals and phalanges.

1. **These account for the greatest number of fractures in the foot.**

2. **The standard views** of the foot generally identify these injuries.

3. **These fractures are frequently treated nonoperatively.**

4. **Most can be managed with early weight bearing** in a protective device such as a hard-sole shoe or weight-bearing cast.

5. **Phalangeal fractures** may also be 'buddy-taped' to adjacent stable phalanges, not dissimilar from the hand.

6. **Occasionally, there will be significant displacement and malalignment** of a fracture, or significant intra-articular extension and incongruity requiring closed reduction or open reduction with internal fixation.

7. **Simple avulsion fractures** of the base of the 5th metatarsal (i.e. Dancer-type fractures) are best managed with weight bearing in a 3D-walking boot or cast.

8. **Jones' and diaphyseal fractures** of the 5th metatarsal require cast immobilization and nonweight bearing.

9. **Some highly competitive athletes** may recover more quickly with early surgical intervention for these types of injuries.

I. **DISLOCATIONS.**

1. **Dislocations most commonly occur at the metatarsophalangeal joint level**, but can occur at the interphalangeal level.

2. **The majority of these are simple dorsal dislocations** and can be close reduced with longitudinal traction followed by buddy-taping and a hard-sole shoe.

3. **Occasionally a complex dislocation occurs** in which closed reduction cannot be achieved, mandating operative open reduction.

4. **When evaluating dislocations of the forefoot**, it is important to remember that tarsometatarsal or midtarsal injuries may have also occurred.

J. TENDON LACERATIONS.

1. **Simple lacerations of the lesser toe flexors or extensors** without a concomitant traumatic arthrotomy or open fracture can usually be left alone with the only potential long-term problem arising from deformity secondary to muscle imbalance.
2. **Repair of a laceration of the great toe** (flexor hallucis longus) does not change long-term outcome.
3. **Laceration of the extensor hallucis longus** is best treated with primary repair.
4. **Other major tendon lacerations about the ankle** should all be repaired primarily, when possible, to try to maintain proper muscle balance and motion.

K. ACHILLES TENDON RUPTURE.

1. **This is a common entity** seen in athletes and jumpers.
2. **It is usually due to an eccentric loading of the gastrosoleus complex** and is very disabling if not recognized and treated.
3. **A defect can be palpated along the tendon sheath** as well as inability to plantarflex actively.
4. **Lack of plantarflexion** when squeezing the patient's calf just distal to its maximum girth, while the patient is prone, indicates complete Achilles tendon disruption and is a positive Thompson's squeeze test.
5. **Management of these injuries is variable,** but at the minimum requires nonweight bearing cast immobilization in the equinus position.
6. **Surgical repair may decrease the risk of recurrent rupture** and may increase long-term power once healed, but can be fraught with wound problems.

L. COMPARTMENT SYNDROME.

1. **A well-recognized entity** and should be suspected in crush injuries, is Franc's or midtarsal fracture dislocations, or in injury patterns in which there are multiple metatarsal fractures.
2. **Unlike the forearm and leg, there are no consistent signs of foot compartment syndrome** (i.e. pain with passive stretch), and it is therefore incumbent upon the examiner to have a high level of suspicion when the injuries as described above occur.
3. **Invasive catheterization technique** is the 'gold standard' and should be considered positive in those patients with pressures measuring ≥ 30mmHg.
4. **Emergent surgical release** of all compartments involved is necessary.

M. LAWN-MOWER INJURIES.

1. **These injuries often involve** multiple toes or large areas of tissue with multiple fractures or traumatic arthrotomies and amputations.
2. **These patients all require triple-coverage antibiotics** [i.e. cefazolin, gentamicin, and Flagyl (metronidazole) or clindamycin], tetanus prophylaxis, and immediate surgical irrigation and débridement.

FOOT AND ANKLE INJURIES

37

UPPER EXTREMITY FRACTURES AND DISLOCATIONS

I. SCAPULAR FRACTURES AND DISLOCATIONS

A. **THE MOST COMMON FRACTURE PATTERN** is that of the body.

B. **FRACTURES OF THE GLENOID NECK,** scapular spine, acromion, and glenoid also occur, but with less frequency.

C. **ASSOCIATED INJURY.**

1. **The amount of energy** needed to cause such an injury is high.

2. **These patients are generally polytraumatized** and frequently have associated head injuries, clavicle and rib fractures, and injuries of the brachial plexus, C-spine, and lungs.

D. **DIAGNOSIS.**

1. **A routine chest film** may delineate the fracture pattern.

2. **A standard shoulder anteroposterior (AP) radiograph** or a CT scan may help to diagnose glenoid involvement.

E. **TREATMENT.**

1. **Scapular body fractures** can be treated symptomatically.

2. **Union of these fractures is common** because of the great soft tissue coverage.

3. **Glenoid fractures** with >25% of the articular surface involved or shoulder instability need to be addressed surgically.

4. **Fixation** is usually obtained with 3.5mm cortical screws and 3.5mm direct compression or reconstruction plates.

II. SCAPULOTHORACIC DISSOCIATION

1. **This is an uncommon problem** in which the shoulder girdle has been dislocated from the thorax.

2. **It is usually associated with neurovascular compromise**.

3. **Surgical treatment** is usually indicated with revascularization, and open reduction and internal fixation of any associated fractures and dislocations.

4. **Additional treatment** may include amputation, arthrodesis, forearm–hand tendon transfers, and prosthetic fitting.

III. CLAVICLE FRACTURES

A. **THE CLAVICLE** is one of the most common bones fractured. It usually requires minimal treatment and union rates are high.

B. **CLASSIFICATION.** This is based on the fracture location, which may include the middle, distal, or proximal third (Figure 38.1).

1. **Group I** – middle third fractures (80%; most common).

2. **Group II** – distal third fractures (12–18%) (Figure 38.2).

a. Type I – nondisplaced.

b. Type II – coracoclavicular ligament disruption.

c. Type III – intra-articular.

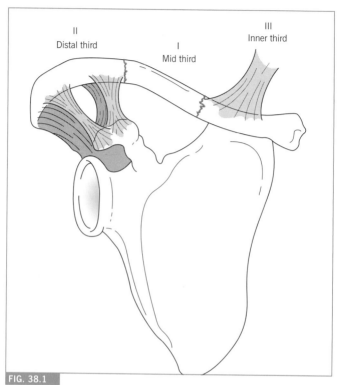

FIG. 38.1

Location of clavicle fracture. (From Kozin SH, Berlet AC. *Handbook of common orthopedic fractures*. Westchester: Medical Surveillance; 1989.)

3. **Group III** – proximal third fractures (5–6%).
a. Type I – minimal displacement.
b. Type II – significant displacement.
c. Type III – intra-articular.
C. **TREATMENT.**
1. **Most fractures heal readily** with a figure-of-eight harness or a sling for 6–8 weeks.
2. Indications for open reduction and internal fixation include:
a. Open fractures.
b. Polytraumatized patients.
c. Neurovascular injury.
d. Scapulothoracic dissociation.
e. Fractures in which the skin is tenting and threatening skin integrity.

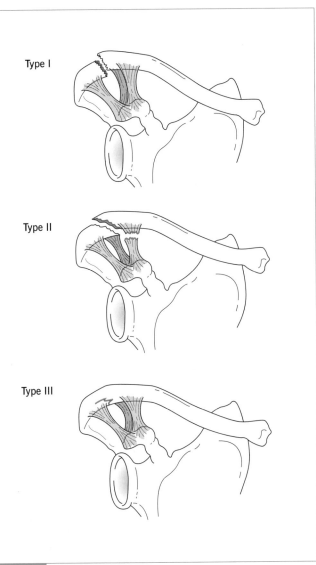

Type I

Type II

Type III

FIG. 38.2

Distal third-types of clavical fractures. (From Kozin SH, Berlet AC. *Handbook of common orthopedic fractures*. Westchester: Medical Surveillance; 1989.)

3. **An incision inferior to the clavicle is preferred**, and fixation is done with a single 3.5mm DC (direct compression) plate.

IV. STERNOCLAVICULAR DISLOCATIONS

A. **THERE ARE TWO TYPES:** anterior and posterior. Both usually result from a direct blow on the clavicle or shoulder.

B. **PHYSICAL EXAMINATION.**

1. **Anterior dislocations** will show a prominent clavicle medially and will be painful.

2. **Posterior dislocations** may give symptoms of dysphagia, dyspnea, or thoracic outlet syndrome because of the mediastinal structures directly underneath the medial part of the clavicle.

3. **A careful neurovascular examination** is required.

C. **RADIOGRAPHIC STUDIES.**

1. **A chest radiograph and apical lordotic views** may be all that is needed.

2. **Since the medial part of the clavicle does not ossify** until age 25 years, CT may aid in the diagnosis of a dislocation with an associated growth plate-type injury (i.e. Salter type I or II). It may also help to determine the mediastinal structures being compromised.

D. **TREATMENT.**

1. **Anterior dislocations.**

a. Conservative treatment is recommended unless symptoms or cosmesis are unacceptable.

b. Closed reduction is performed with a towel placed between the scapulae and with gentle abduction of the affected shoulder.

2. **Posterior dislocations.**

a. Closed reduction is similar to that of anterior dislocations.

b. Open reduction is done only when mediastinal structures are compromised or there is intractable pain.

c. Surgery in this area needs to be performed in conjunction with a cardiothoracic surgeon.

V. ACROMIOCLAVICULAR INJURIES

A. **A DIRECT BLOW TO THE SUPERIOR ASPECT OF THE SHOULDER** will commonly injure the acromioclavicular (AC) and the coracoclavicular (CC) ligaments.

B. **CLASSIFICATION.** There are six grades of AC joint separation (Figure 38.3):

1. **Type I** – sprain of the ligaments.

2. **Type II** – AC joint disrupted and partial disruption of the CC ligament.

3. **Type III** – AC and CC ligament disruption.

4. **Type IV** – type III plus posterior distal clavicle dislocation.

5. **Type V** – type III plus the deltoid and trapezius are detached from the distal third of the clavicle.

6. **Type VI** – type III plus inferior dislocation of the clavicle.

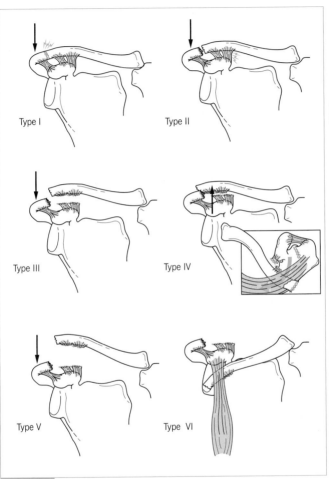

FIG. 38.3

Classification of acromicroclavicular joint injuries. (From Rockwood, Williams, Young. Injuries to the acromicroclavicular joint. In: Rockwood CA Jr, Green DP, Bucholz RW et al. (eds.) *Fractures in adults. Volume 2.* 4th edn. Philadelphia: Lippincott-Raven; 1996:1354.)

C. TREATMENT.
1. **Types I–III** – conservative treatment with sling and early motion.
2. **Types IV–VI** – surgical reconstruction of the CC ligament, with the coraco-acromial ligament and suture augmentation.

VI. SHOULDER DISLOCATION

A. ANTERIOR DISLOCATION (84%) is the most common, but posterior and inferior dislocation also occur.

B. A GOOD HISTORY will determine the most efficacious treatment. Important factors are:

1. Timing since injury.
2. Frequency of dislocations.
3. Location of the upper extremity when the shoulder dislocates.
4. Traumatic vs atraumatic.
5. Current psychiatric illness.
6. Connective tissue disorder.
7. Voluntary vs involuntary dislocation.
8. Unilateral vs bilateral.
9. Neuromuscular causes (i.e. seizures, encephalitis).
10. Direction of dislocation.

C. PHYSICAL EXAMINATION.

1. Asymmetry of the shoulders can often be seen.
2. Palpable humeral head (anterior dislocations).
3. External rotation and slight adduction (anterior dislocations).
4. Adduction and internal rotation (posterior dislocations).
5. Limited range of motion.
6. A detailed neurologic examination is mandatory before and after an attempt at a reduction.

D. RADIOGRAPHIC STUDIES.

1. Two radiographs at 90° orientation to each other are needed.
2. An AP and an axillary lateral are the two most commonly requested.
3. A posterior dislocation will sometimes look normal on the AP film, which is why two views at 90° orientation to each other are essential.

E. ASSOCIATED INJURIES.

1. Axillary (most common, 2–30%) and musculocutaneous nerve injuries are almost all neuropraxic in nature.
2. Vascular compromise (not common) is seen most frequently in the elderly who have stiff and fragile vessels. Injury may occur at the time of either injury or reduction.
3. Rotator cuff tears are also seen with increased incidence in patients over 35 years of age.

F. TREATMENT.

1. Acute dislocations need to be reduced as soon as possible.
2. Intravenous analgesics and muscle relaxants may aid in the reduction.
3. A chronic dislocation (several days) may require general anesthesia with or without open reduction.
4. There are several reduction techniques but generally it should be remembered that allowing the muscles to relax with gentle traction is more effective than forceful, shorter attempts.

a. Technique I.
   1) Traction on the affected arm with a sheet around the flexed forearm and physician's waist, and countertraction with a sheet passed under the patient's arm, around the chest and around the assistant's waist.
   2) This technique appears to be the easiest.
b. Technique II.
   1) With the patient supine, the physician's foot is used as countertraction in the patient's axilla.
   2) Traction is made longitudinally in a slow and gentle manner.
   3) Unreduced chronic dislocations (>3 weeks) or irreducible acute dislocations may necessitate open reduction in the operating room.
5. **Postreduction management.**
a. Radiographs are obtained to assess reduction adequacy and to detect possible fractures.
b. Repeat neurovascular examination is performed.
c. Immobilization is usually accomplished with a sling or shoulder immobilizer.

VII. PROXIMAL HUMERUS FRACTURES

A. THERE IS A GREATER INCIDENCE of these fractures in the osteoporotic population.

B. THE FRACTURES ARE CLASSIFIED as a two-, three-, or four-part fracture pattern according to displacement (>1cm) or angulation (>45°) of each part.

C. REGARDLESS OF THE NUMBER OF FRACTURE LINES, unless displaced or angulated as stated above, the fracture is considered a one-part fracture.

1. **Two-part fractures** are usually seen in dislocations of the humeral head with the greater or lesser tuberosity fractured off (Figure 38.4).

2. **Three-part fractures** are usually a shaft fracture associated with a tuberosity fracture (Figure 38.5).

3. **Four-part fractures** involve both tuberosities and the humeral neck (Figure 38.5).

D. TREATMENT.

1. **It is important to assess the fracture classification**, as well as the bone quality, age, patient expectations, functional demands, and the patient's overall health.

2. **Nondisplaced fractures** may be treated with a sling and early range of motion.

3. **Two-part fractures are first treated with a closed reduction**. If reduction is not satisfactory then either open reduction and internal fixation or closed reduction and percutaneous pin fixation is performed.

4. **Three-part fractures are seldom amenable to closed reduction,** and operative treatment with tension-band wiring or a blade plate is commonly performed.

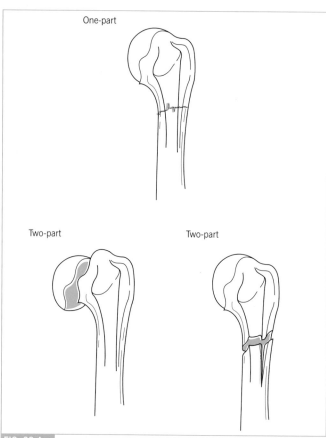

One-part

Two-part   Two-part

FIG. 38.4

Two-part fractures of the proximal humerus. (From Kozin SH, Berlet AC. *Handbook of common orthopedic fractures*. Westchester: Medical Surveillance; 1989.)

5. **Four-part fractures are associated with loss of vascularity** to many of the fractured fragments. Prosthetic replacement should be performed in the elderly patient.

VIII. HUMERAL SHAFT FRACTURES

A. **THE LOCATION OF THE FRACTURE** is important for developing a treatment plan since attachment of the pectoralis major and the deltoid muscles will cause different deforming forces according to the fracture pattern.

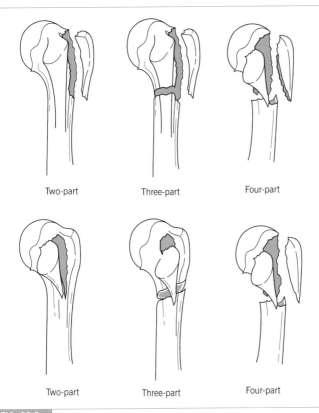

FIG. 38.5

Three-part and four-part fractures of the proximal humerus. (From Kozin SH, Berlet AC. *Handbook of common orthopedic fractures*. Westchester: Medical Surveillance; 1989.)

B. CLASSIFICATION. The AO classification is the most widely used and it is divided into three main types:
1. **Simple** (type A).
2. **Wedge** (type B).
3. **Complex** (type C).
C. RADIOGRAPHIC STUDIES.
1. **AP and lateral views of the entire humerus** are usually all that is necessary.
2. **If pathologic changes are apparent**, then further studies need to be obtained for staging and for planning treatment.

38

D. TREATMENT.

1. **Owing to the close proximity of the radial nerve** in relation to the humeral shaft, a pre- and postreduction neurovascular examination should be performed.

2. **Nonsurgical treatment** is with closed reduction and immobilization in a plaster U-splint or in a humeral cuff orthosis, which yield good results in most patients.

3. Surgical.

a. Indications for surgical intervention include:
   1) Open fractures.
   2) Polytraumatized patients.
   3) Neurovascular injury.
   4) Failed closed treatment.
   5) Pathologic fractures.
   6) Bilateral fractures.
   7) Segmental fractures
   8) Floating elbow.

b. Open reduction and internal fixation through an anterolateral approach (fixation with a 4.5mm or 3.5mm dynamic compression plate) or locked intramedullary fixation are commonly used for shaft fractures.

c. External fixation may be used when there is extensive soft tissue damage or bone loss.

d. Radial nerve palsy.
   1) Associated radial nerve palsy is reported from 1–24%.
   2) Spontaneous recovery occurs in about 75% of the patients.
   3) Exploration of the nerve is indicated when the nerve was intact prior to reduction or open reduction and internal fixation (ORIF) and demonstrates impaired function after reduction or ORIF.

IX. DISTAL HUMERUS FRACTURE

A. Restoration of the anatomy should be the primary goal.

1. **The osseous anatomy** has a medial and lateral osseous column that supports the articular surface.

2. **Because early range of motion and restoration of anatomy are important,** nonsurgical treatment is rarely capable of meeting these goals.

B. CLASSIFICATION.

1. Extra-articular.

a. Transcondylar and supracondylar fractures are more common in children than adults.

b. Supracondylar fractures in children may be classified as:
   1) Nondisplaced (type I).
   2) Minimally displaced, but stable once reduced (type II).
   3) Displaced and unstable (type III).

2. Intra-articular.
a. These may be subdivided into unicondylar (medial or lateral) or bicondylar.
b. These may also be accompanied by extra-articular extension or comminution.

C. NONOPERATIVE.
1. **Supracondylar type I and most type II fractures** can be treated with conservative measures in children.
2. **Small, avulsion-type fractures** that are extra-articular or nondisplaced may also be treated with splints, casts, or functional braces.

D. OPERATIVE.
1. **Supracondylar type III fractures** are commonly treated with closed reduction and are percutaneously pinned in children.
2. **Intra-articular fractures** in adults are treated by internal fixation.
3. **External fixation** may be used for fractures in which the soft tissues have been severely damaged.
4. **Ulnar nerve transposition** is routinely performed to minimize the incidence of neuropathy, which is the most common complication following treatment of distal humerus fractures.

X. ELBOW DISLOCATIONS

A. **ELBOW STABILITY** is determined by the articular congruity between the proximal ulna and radius with the distal humerus, as well as the capsular ligament complexes

B. **STABILITY TO VALGUS STRESS** is most dependent on the medial collateral ligament (especially the anterior bundle of the ligament).

C. **CLASSIFICATION.** These dislocations are classified according to the position of the radius and ulna segments.
1. **Posterior dislocations** are the most common.
2. **Other dislocations** include lateral, medial, anterior, and divergent.

D. **ASSOCIATED INJURIES.**
1. **Radial head and neck fractures** are seen in about 50% of patients.
2. **Humeral epicondyle fractures, coronoid fractures, and neurovascular injury** occur, but are less common.

E. **DIAGNOSIS.**
1. There is usually **gross deformation and swelling** about the elbow.
2. **The range of motion** will be limited.
3. **Radiographic studies** include an AP and a lateral of the affected elbow.

F. **TREATMENT.**
1. **Dislocations need to be reduced** as soon as possible.
2. **Many methods of closed reduction have been described** and involve traction and translation of the ulna relative to the humerus.
3. **A detailed neurovascular examination** is mandatory prior to and after an attempt at a reduction.

4. **Postreduction radiographs** need to be obtained to assess adequacy of the reduction.
5. **If the elbow is stable postreduction**, it is kept in a sling at 90° of flexion for 2–3 weeks.
6. **Range-of-motion exercises** are begun 2–3 weeks after reduction.
7. **Unstable elbow dislocations** may need ORIF.
8. **Dislocations with concomitant humerus, radius, or ulna fractures** are best served with ORIF of the fracture and reduction of the dislocation.

XI. CORONOID FRACTURES

A. **THESE ARE UNCOMMON INJURIES** of the proximal ulna.
B. **CLASSIFICATION.**
1. **Type I** – avulsion of the tip.
2. **Type II** – fragment involves <50%.
3. **Type III** – fragment involves >50%.
C. **TREATMENT.**
1. **Types I and II** may be treated with closed reduction and early mobilization.
2. **Type III** is best treated with ORIF.

XII. OLECRANON FRACTURES

A. The olecranon is the triceps tendon attachment to the ulna.
B. The examination should include checking for active extension of the forearm.
C. **TREATMENT.**
1. **Nondisplaced fractures are treated** with a long arm splint or cast.
2. **Displaced fractures** may be comminuted, transverse, or oblique.
3. **Displaced fractures are treated** with ORIF through a posterior approach.
4. **Fixation may be obtained** with circlage wires and Steinman pins or a 3.5 DC plate.
5. **Early range of motion** is encouraged.

XIII. RADIAL HEAD FRACTURES

A. These are common injuries whenever elbow trauma occurs.
B. **CLASSIFICATION** (Figure 38.6).
1. **Type I** – nondisplaced.
2. **Type II** – displaced.
3. **Type III** – comminuted.
4. **Type IV** – radial head fracture and elbow dislocation.
5. **Essex–Lopresti fractures** – radial and ulnar interosseous membrane and distal radio-ulnar joint disruption may occur with complex radial head fractures.

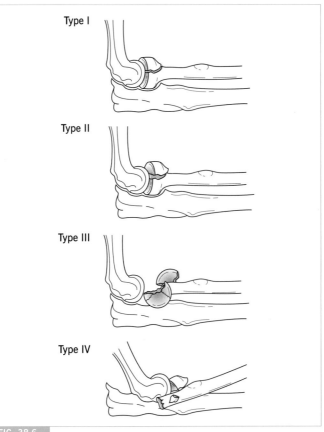

FIG. 38.6

Classification of radial head fractures. (From From Kozin SH, Berlet AC. *Handbook of common orthopedic fractures*. Westchester: Medical Surveillance; 1989.)

C. TREATMENT.

1. **Check for a mechanical block** during pronation and supination.
2. **Presence of such a block** often precludes surgical intervention.
3. **Type I fractures** require a sling and early range of motion.
4. Type II and III fractures indicate either ORIF or radial head excision including angulation of >30°, depression of more than one-third of the joint surface, or a mechanical block.

XIV. RADIAL AND ULNAR SHAFT FRACTURES

A. RADIAL AND ULNAR shaft fractures are described by their location, the amount of comminution present, and the degree of displacement.

B. RADIOGRAPHIC STUDIES. Radiographs should include the whole forearm, wrist, and elbow to identify any associated injury.

C. TREATMENT.

1. Nondisplaced.

a. Isolated fractures are treated with splint-and-cast immobilization.

b. Polytraumatized patients may need ORIF.

2. Displaced fractures are best treated with ORIF.

3. Gustillo type III open fractures can be externally fixated.

4. Intramedullary rodding may also be done for both ulna and radius diaphyseal fractures.

5. Galeazzi fractures are those in which there is a mid or distal third radius fracture and an associated subluxation of the distal radio-ulnar joint. Treatment is with ORIF.

6. Monteggia fractures involve a fracture of the proximal ulna with an associated dislocated radial head. Treatment is with ORIF (Figure 38.7).

D. TYPES OF DISLOCATIONS.

1. Anterior (type I).

2. Posterior (type II).

3. Lateral or anterolateral (type III).

4. Anterior dislocation with fracture of the radius and ulna (type IV).

a. Treatment is with ORIF of the shaft fracture and closed (open if unsuccessful) reduction of the radial head.

b. Immobilization for types I and III is then done at 110° and for type II in 70° of flexion.

XV. DISTAL RADIAL FRACTURES

A. These fractures are more common in elderly osteoporotic bone.

B. The distal radial fragment may be dorsal (Colles' fracture) or volar (Smith's fracture).

C. The position of the extremity at the time of the injury may help in the understanding of the mechanism of injury.

D. PHYSICAL EXAMINATION.

1. Soft tissue integrity and a neurovascular examination should be assessed.

2. Range of motion of both the affected and unaffected upper extremities should be evaluated.

E. RADIOGRAPHIC STUDIES.

1. AP, lateral, and oblique films of the wrist should be obtained.

2. A high clinical suspicion for hand, elbow, or forearm injuries should be maintained and the associated radiographs should be obtained.

3. The degree and location of the comminuted bone in the distal radius will determine the stability of the fracture pattern.

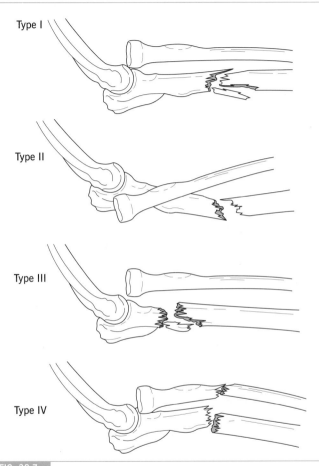

Type I

Type II

Type III

Type IV

FIG. 38.7

Types of Monteggia's fracture of the proximal third of the ulna with dislocation of the radial head. (From Kozin SH, Berlet AC. *Handbook of common orthopedic fractures*. Westchester: Medical Surveillance; 1989.)

F. CLASSIFICATION.
1. **Frykman's classification** is the most widely accepted (Table 38.1 and Figure 38.8).
2. **It divides the fractures** based on involvement of the radiocarpal or the distal radio-ulnar joints.

TABLE 38.1

FRYKMAN CLASSIFICATION OF FRACTURES TO DISTAL RADIUS

Fracture	Distal ulna fracture	
	Absent	Present
Extra-articular	I	II
Intra-articular involving radiocarpal joint	III	IV
Intra-articular involving radio-ulnar joint	V	VI
Intra-articular involving both radiocarpal and radio-ulnar joints	VII	VIII

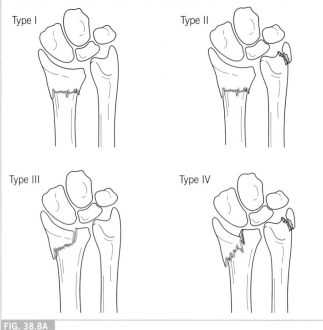

FIG. 38.8A

Distal radius fractures types I–IV. (From Kozin SH, Berlet AC. *Handbook of common orthopedic fractures*. Westchester: Medical Surveillance; 1989.)

G. TREATMENT.

1. **Restoration of the radial height** (normal 11–12mm), volar tilt (normal 11°), radial inclination (normal 22–23°), and the joint congruity should be maximized.

2. **Nondisplaced fractures** can be managed with a sugar-tong splint or a long arm cast. Frequent radiographs are mandatory to assess loss of reduction.

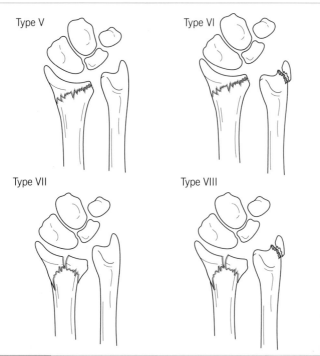

Type V   Type VI

Type VII   Type VIII

FIG. 38.8B
Distal radius fractures types V–VIII. (From Kozin SH, Berlet AC. *Handbook of common orthopedic fractures.* Westchester: Medical Surveillance; 1989.)

3. **Displaced fractures** may be treated closed, with open reduction and internal fixation, with percutaneous pinning, or with external fixation.
4. **The stability of the fracture** will be dependent on the amount and the pattern of the comminution.
5. **Fracture reducibility does not equal fracture stability**, which needs to be assessed on the prereduction and not the postreduction radiographs.

XVI. FURTHER READING

Ebraheim NA, An S, Jackson WT et al. Scapulothoracic dissociation. *J Bone Joint Surg* 1988; 70A: 428–432.

Frykman G. Fracture of the distal radius? *Acta Orthop Scand* 1967; 108(Suppl.):1–153.

Grant JCB. *Method of anatomy,* 7th edn. Baltimore: Williams and Wilkins; 1965.

Green DP. *Operative hand surgery,* 2nd edn. New York: Churchill Livingstone; 1988.

Kazar B, Polvozsky E. Prognosis of primary dislocation of the shoulder. *Acta Orthop Scand* 1969; 40:216–224.

Lindblom A, Leven H. Prognosis in fractures of the body and neck of the scapula. *Acta Chir Scand* 1974; 140:33–47.

Neer CS. Displaced proximal humeral fractures: I classification and evaluation. *J Bone Joint Surg* 1970; 52A:1077–1089.

Reckling FW. Unstable fracture-dislocations of the forearm (Monteggia and Galeazzi lesions). *J Bone Joint Surg* 1982; 64A:857–863.

Rockwood CA Jr, Green DP, Bucholz RW et al. *Fractures in adults,* 4th edn. Lippencott-Raven;1996.

Rockwood CA Jr, Matsen FA III (eds.) *The shoulder*. Philadelphia: WB Saunders; 1990.

Rockwood CA Jr, Wilkins KE, Beaty JH. *Fractures in children,* 4th edn. Lippincott-Raven; 1996.

HAND INJURIES AND INFECTIONS

I. HISTORY AND MECHANISM OF INJURY

1. Timing – age of injury.
2. Position of hand when injured.
3. Extent of contamination.
4. Prior hand injury.
5. Dominant hand.
6. Occupation.
7. Medical history (e.g. diabetes, hypertension, etc.).
8. Demands patient places on hands (i.e. activities of daily living).
9. Age of patient.

II. PHYSICAL EXAMINATION

A. **OBSERVE RESTING POSITION** of hand and fingers (tendon lacerations can cause asymmetry of position).
B. **INSPECT SOFT TISSUE** (discoloration, abrasions, lacerations, puncture wounds, erythema, swelling, drainage, crepitus).
C. **VASCULAR.** Pulses (radial and ulnar), Doppler flow in palmar arch, and capillary refill in digits (normal <2 seconds).
D. **SENSATION.** Two-point discrimination (normal 5mm) can use ends of opened paper clip placed 5mm apart on fingers.
E. **MOVEMENT.** Passive and active motion – specify which muscles tested (Figures 39.1 and 39.2).

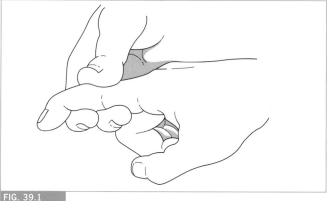

FIG. 39.1

If the distal interphalangeal joint can be actively flexed while the proximal interphalangeal joint is stabilized, the profundus tendon has not been severed. (Redrawn from Canale T. In: *Campbell's Operative Orthopedics,* 9th edn. St. Louis: Mosby; 1998.)

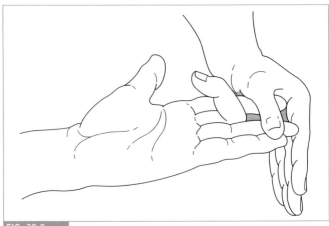

FIG. 39.2
If the proximal interphalangeal joint can be actively flexed while adjacent fingers are held completely extended, the sublimis tendon has not been severed. (Redrawn from Canale T. In: *Campbell's Operative Orthopedics,* 9th edn. St. Louis: Mosby; 1998.)

F. SWEATING. Normally hand and fingers should have fine film of moisture on palmar surface – smooth and dry skin may indicate nerve damage.
G. STRESS EXAMINATION. Laxity at joints may indicate ligament instability. This test should be performed under local anesthetic.

III. ANESTHETIC TECHNIQUES USED IN THE HAND

A. LIDOCAINE 1% OR 2% may be used, but never use lidocaine with epinephrine in the hand.
B. WRIST BLOCK. Can do all or one of these depending on the area to be examined (use about 5–7mL at each location):
1. Median nerve.
a. A 25-gauge needle is inserted on the ulnar side of the palmaris longus at the level of the proximal crease of wrist at an angle of 45° to the wrist.
b. If paresthesia is encountered, pull the needle back and be careful not to inject into the substance of the nerve (Figure 39.3).
2. Ulnar nerve – a 25-gauge needle is inserted just medial to the flexor carpi ulnaris tendon at the level of the proximal wrist crease (Figure 39.3).
3. Radial sensory nerve – raise a subcutaneous weal over radial styloid and to dorsum of midline wrist.

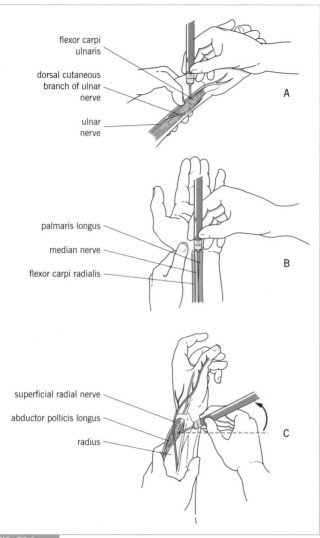

flexor carpi
ulnaris

dorsal cutaneous
branch of ulnar
nerve

ulnar
nerve

A

palmaris longus

median nerve

flexor carpi radialis

B

superficial radial nerve

abductor pollicis longus

radius

C

FIG. 39.3

Technique for peripheral nerve blocks. (A) Ulnar nerve, superficial branch. (B)
Median nerve. (C) Superficial radial nerve. (Redrawn from Abadir AR. In: Omer GE
Jr, Spinner M, Van Beek A. *Management of peripheral nerve problems*. Philadelphia:
WB Saunders; 1988.)

C. **DIGITAL BLOCK** (Figure 39.4).

1. Inject into the web space at the base of the finger on both sides.
2. Use about 3–5mL.

D. **CIRCUMFERENTIAL BLOCK.** This is not recommended because it can cause necrosis.

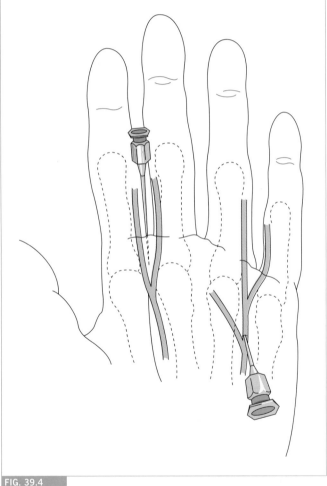

FIG. 39.4

Digital nerve blocks. (Redrawn from Canale T. In: *Campbell's Operative Orthopedics, 9th* edn. St. Louis: Mosby; 1998.)

IV. RADIOLOGIC EXAMINATION

A. **RULE OF THUMB** – order radiograph of exact part under suspicion (i.e. 'finger' not 'hand' for a look at the finger, etc.).

B. **STANDARD VIEWS** – anteroposterior (AP), lateral, and oblique.

C. **STRESS VIEWS** – best test for instability if ligament damage is suspected.
1. Best results if examiner performs stress test.
2. Requires local anesthetic.

D. **COMPARISON VIEWS** of opposite normal side are essential for children (especially elbow) and may be helpful in adults if the anatomy is confusing, particularly the wrist.

V. OTHER DIAGNOSTIC TESTS

A. **ALLEN'S TEST.**
1. Evaluates the patency of the radial and ulnar arteries at the wrist level.
2. Procedure.
   a. Digitally occlude both radial and ulnar arteries at the wrist.
   b. Patient pumps fist 2–3 times to exsanguinate the hand (can be done in the unconscious patient by exsanguinating the extremity with an Esmarch bandage or gravity and using a blood pressure cuff).
   c. Patient opens hand about 90%.
   d. Examiner releases one artery and observes time and area of filling.
   e. Repeat with other artery.
3. A positive Allen's test is when there is no arterial flush in the hand within 10–15 seconds (normal 3–5 seconds).
4. Interpretation – that particular artery is not patent and the hand is dependent upon another arterial supply, which must be preserved.

B. **ARTERIOGRAM.**
1. Evaluates continuity and patency of the vascular supply of the upper extremity.
2. Risks – allergic reaction, bleeding, arterial injury, and renal failure.

C. **ELECTRODIAGNOSTIC STUDIES.**
1. Identify neuropathy by demonstrating a nerve conduction deficit along the course of a nerve.
2. In the acute setting these studies are not useful.
3. Often not helpful until more than 3 weeks after the injury to the nerve.

D. **INTRACOMPARTMENTAL PRESSURES.**
1. Fasciotomy is recommended when the intracompartmental pressure is >30mmHg.
   a. The diagnosis of compartment syndrome is clinical.
   b. Pressure readings serve only as a guideline.
2. CT scan – useful for bone and joint evaluation.
3. MRI – useful for soft tissue evaluation.
   a. May need small coils for hand evaluation to get useful images.
   b. Not all centers have this equipment.

39

HAND INJURIES AND INFECTIONS

A. TENDONS.

1. **Anatomy.**

a. Flexor tendons (Figure 39.5).

   1) Two flexors to each digit – flexor digitorum superficialis and profundus.

   2) Pulley system anchors tendons, prevents bowstringing of tendons, and improves mechanical power.

   3) A2 and A4 pulleys are the most important.

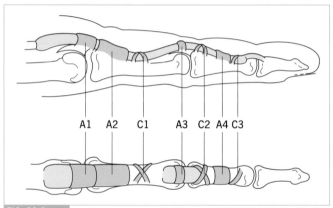

FIG. 39.5

This anatomical diagram of various parts of the flexor sheath is helpful in understanding gliding of tendon. Maintenance of the second annulus (A2) and fourth annulus (A4) is essential to retain appropriate angle of approach and prevent 'bowstringing' of flexor tendons or tendon graft. (Redrawn from Doyle JR, Blythe W. The finger flexor tendon sheath and pulleys: anatomy and reconstruction. *In: American Academy of Orthopaedic Surgeons: Symposium on tendon surgery in the hand*. St. Louis: Mosby; 1975.)

b. Extensor tendons are interconnected by the juncturae tendinum which helps extend the digit even if the tendon to that digit is lacerated.

2. **Type of injury** – classified by zone of injury:

a. Five flexor zones (Figure 39.6).

b. Nine extensor zones (Figure 39.7).

3. **Flexor tendon.**

a. Closed injury.

   1) Commonly an avulsion injury from the insertion of tendon on to the bone.

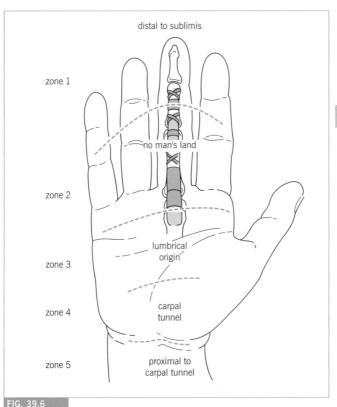

FIG. 39.6
Flexor zones of the hand. Designated zones on the flexor surface of the hand are helpful, since treatment of tendon injuries may vary according to the level of severance. (Redrawn from Canale T. In: *Campbell's Operative Orthopedics,* 9th edn. St. Louis: Mosby; 1998.)

    2) Midsubstance rupture in a closed injury is not as common.
    3) Treatment – open repair in operating room.
b. Open injury.
    1) Zone II injuries are notorious for poor gliding of tendons through the scar.
    2) Level of tendon injury may be at a different site than that of the skin laceration secondary to the position of the hand and fingers at the time of injury (i.e. if the fist was clenched the tendon laceration will be distal to the skin laceration).

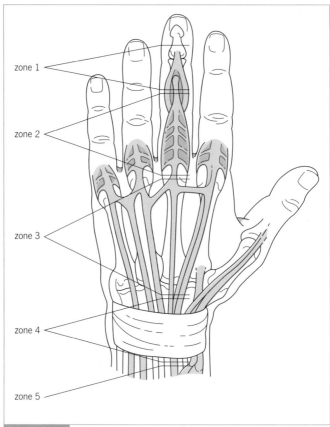

FIG. 39.7
Indications for surgery of extensor tendon lacerations vary according to the level of pathological condition; therefore, various zones have been designated. (Redrawn from Canale T. In: *Campbell's Operative Orthopedics,* 9th edn. St. Louis: Mosby; 1998.)

3) Requires open repair in operating room.
4) Rehabilitation is as important as the actual repair.
5) If the repair is to be delayed, clean and close lacerations, and splint the hand with the digits and wrist in slight flexion.

4. Extensor tendon.

a. Closed injury.

1) Extensor tendon avulsion from dorsum of distal phalanx as a result of hyperflexion, often with a small chip of bone, can lead to mallet deformity of distal phalanx.
2) Treatment – closed reduction with a premade splint or aluminum foam splint placed on either volar or dorsal surfaces, though volar application is preferred leaving the proximal interphalangeal (PIP) joint free, for 6–8 weeks (Figure 39.8).

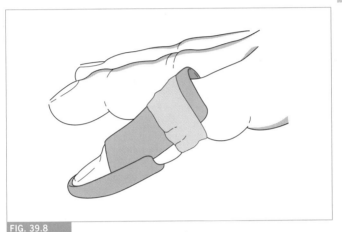

FIG. 39.8

Stack splint. (Redrawn from Canale T. In: *Campbell's Operative Orthopedics,* 9th edn. St. Louis: Mosby; 1998.)

b. Open injury.
1) If laceration – best repaired in operating room.
2) If the repair is to be delayed, close the wound, and splint the wrist with 45° extension with the metacarpophalangeal (MP) joints flexed to 30–40°.

5. **Boutonnilidocainere deformity.**
a. Disruption of the extensor tendon central slip at the PIP joint with volar migration of the lateral bands leading to flexion of the PIP joint and hyperextension of the distal interphalangeal (DIP) joint.
b. Treatment.
1) If open: incision and debridement; and repair tendon.
2) If closed: either splint PIP joint in full extension or pin PIP joint with K-wire, leave DIP joint free for active flexion, and splint for 6 weeks.

39

HAND INJURIES AND INFECTIONS

B. **NERVES.**

1. **Digital nerves.**

a. Examination – light touch sensibility, two-point discrimination, and sweat pattern.

b. Treatment – repair the following nerves to preserve pinch and protective sensation:
   1) Index radial digital branch.
   2) Thumb ulnar digital branch.
   3) Small finger ulnar digital branch.
   4) Other digital branches may be indicated depending on situation.
   5) Best done in operating room by experienced microsurgeon.

2. **Peripheral nerves.**

a. Median, radial, ulnar nerves.

b. Examine for sensation and motor function.

c. Repair is mandatory and best performed by an experienced microsurgeon.

d. If repair is to be delayed:
   1) Clean and close wound.
   2) Splint hand or arm in neutral position depending on level of injury.

C. **OFTEN ASSOCIATED WITH TENDON INJURY.**

1. **If isolated nerve injury is suspected** it is prudent to re-examine in a few days to see if sensation has returned as neuropraxia is not uncommon.

2. **If repair is to be delayed**, clean and close wound, and splint hand in neutral position.

D. **BLOOD VESSELS.**

1. **Examine** for color, pulses, Doppler flow, and capillary refill.

2. **If complete flow is disrupted** to one or more fingers, microvascular repair in the operating room is necessary.

3. **In the presence of an isolated digital artery injury** where the involved finger is pink with good capillary refill, repair is not indicated.

4. **Do not clamp blindly in the hand** as a nerve runs along almost every artery in the hand and could be crushed and damaged.

E. **NAIL BED INJURIES.**

1. **Administer adequate regional anesthesia** (a digital block is commonly used).

2. **Remove nail** by spreading small hemostat or Freer elevator gently under nail and explore the nail bed.

3. **Repair** with small chromic (7-0) or plain gut (6-0) suture with meticulous débridement and approximation of laceration.

4. **Replace nail under nail fold** and secure with a suture at the distal fingertip to act as a splint to help keep the eponychial fold open, thereby preventing nail deformation.

5. **Drill hole in nail** prior to replacing in nail fold to help allow drainage from subungual area.
6. **If nail is not available,** place contoured xeroform gauze beneath eponychial fold.
7. **Warn patient** about possible problems with nail regrowth or deformity.
8. **Complete new nail growth** can take between 70 and 160 days.

F. FINGER TIP INJURIES.
1. **Most common** type of finger amputation injury in the upper extremity.
2. **Usual mechanism** is finger slammed in door.
3. **Under digital block,** clean and debride.
4. **If a large enough part is amputated,** it may be amenable to replantation (consult microvascular surgeon).
5. **If replantation is not feasible** and injury is distal to DIP joint, irrigation, débridement, and primary closure is performed.
6. **In the setting of exposed bone,** the preferred method is irrigation, débridement, and bone resection to allow primary closure.
7. **May allow closure by secondary intention,** but primary closure gives best results.

G. INJURY THROUGH DIP JOINT OR PIP JOINT.
1. **Shorten phalanx and close primarily.**
2. **Do not suture flexor and extensor tendons together.**

H. INJURY THROUGH MIDDLE PHALANX.
1. **Distal to flexor digitorum superficialis tendon** – shorten bone and close primarily
2. **Proximal to flexor digitorum superficialis tendon** – may want to preserve PIP joint for cosmetic reasons or shorten and close as the patient wishes.

I. INJURY PROXIMAL TO PIP JOINT.
1. **Treatment** depends on the length of the injury.
2. **Will still have gripping motion** with intrinsic muscles and common extensors.
3. **If injury is close to MP joint,** stump may be more of a hindrance than a help and the patient may want to consider ray resection, especially of the long and ring fingers.

J. THUMB.
1. **May be quite functional** if amputation is distal to the interphalangeal joint.
2. **Treatment.**
a. Shortening of bone and primary closure.
b. Replant.
c. Reconstruct if possible or if proximal to IP joint.

K. LIGAMENT INJURIES AND DISLOCATIONS.
1. **Basic treatment regimen** – attempt closed reduction under digital block and stress joint to test stability after reduction.
a. Joint stable – immobilize.

    b. Joint unstable or unable to reduce – consider operative intervention.

    c. Open injuries require irrigation and débridement in operating room.

2. DIP joint and thumb IP joint.

    a. Usually dorsally or laterally dislocated.

    b. Closed reduction and immobilize with slight flexion for 3 weeks.

3. PIP joint.

    a. Most common ligament injury in the hand.

    b. May be dorsal, lateral, or volar dislocation (refers to position of midphalanx).

    c. Most can be closed reduced and treated in a splint with 20–30° flexion for 2 weeks followed by buddy taping and range of motion.

    d. An unstable joint may indicate a fracture dislocation.

    e. If >40% of articular surface is involved, proceed to open reduction and pinning to restore articular surface.

4. MP joint.

    a. Usually dorsally dislocated.

    b. Index finger is most common.

    c. Must distinguish between simple (subluxation) and complex (complete) dislocation.

    d. Simple.

        1) Be careful not to convert to complex dislocation.

        2) Reduce with flexion of wrist and pressure distally and volarly over dorsum of proximal phalanx.

    e. Complex.

        1) Irreducible – metacarpal head buttonholes through volar structures and prevents reduction.

        2) Reducible – joint is markedly hyperextended (60–80°) with dislocated phalanx directly on top of the metacarpal head. The joint is commonly held in extension and may be slightly angulated and the volar skin may be puckered. Closed reduction, splint, and start early range of motion with dorsal extension block splint in neutral. Open reduction and immobilization in 30° flexion for 2 weeks followed by dorsal block splint to 0° flexion for an additional 2 weeks.

5. Carpometacarpal joint.

    a. Majority are dorsal.

    b. Fifth carpometacarpal joint is most common.

    c. Attempt closed reduction under wrist block.

        1) Usually successful if performed within 12 hours of injury.

        2) Reduction maneuver: flex wrist; traction on metacarpal with dorsal pressure on displaced metacarpal base followed by extension of metacarpal head; hold with K-wire if unstable; and cast for 4 weeks.

    d. May require open reduction.

6. **Thumb MP joint.**
a. Dorsal.
   1) Under adequate anesthesia apply dorsal pressure to base of proximal phalanx with wrist and metacarpal flexed and adducted.
   2) Immobilize in 25° flexion for 4 weeks.
b. Lateral.
   1) Associated with ulnar collateral ligament injuries (gamekeeper's or skier's thumb).
   2) Stress joint under block: if degree of laxity is <30°, suspect partial rupture; if >30°, suspect complete ligament rupture.
   3) Treatment is a thumb spica cast for 4 weeks for partial rupture and surgical repair for complete rupture.
   4) Radial collateral ligament – less commonly injured – similar treatment as for ulnar collateral ligament.
7. **Thumb carpometacarpal joint.**
a. Quite rare.
b. Usually an injury of the volar ligament which is thought to be main capsular reinforcement.
c. May be difficult to diagnose.
d. Stress radiography may be helpful.
e. Immobilize – 4 weeks in thumb spica cast.
f. If grossly unstable pin with K-wire.

L. **FRACTURES.**
1. **Metacarpal head.**
a. Metacarpal head (intra-articular).
b. Simple two-part fracture (open reduction and internal fixation with screws).
c. Comminuted fracture treatment
   1) Closed injury – immobilize for 2 weeks followed by aggressive range of motion exercises.
   2) Open injury – incise and drain initially followed by external fixation, with arthrodesis of joint as salvage procedure.
2. **Metacarpal neck (boxer's fracture).**
a. Acceptable angulation of neck fractures:
   1) Index finger 15°.
   2) Long finger 15°.
   3) Ring finger 30–40°.
   4) Small finger 50–60°.
b. Angulation greater than above or shortened >3mm is an indication for reduction.
c. Most commonly treated closed in ulnar gutter splint including adjacent intact finger.
d. Recommended duration of immobilization is 2–3 weeks and then range of motion started, but the splint is often left on longer (4–6 weeks) depending upon patient reliability.

e. If unable to hold reduction use crossed percutaneous K-wires, but may also use plate and screw fixation.

3. **Metacarpal shaft.**

a. Types.
    1) Transverse.
    2) Oblique.
    3) Spiral.
    4) Comminuted.

b. Most can be treated by closed reduction and splinting.

c. If reduction is unstable, percutaneous pinning vs open reduction with internal fixation should be performed (Figure 39.9).

d. Indications for open reduction:
    1) Open fractures.
    2) Multiple fractures.
    3) Unstable fractures.
    4) Rotational or angulatory malalignment.

e. Fixation options include:
    1) K-wires – most commonly used.
    2) Plates and screws.
    3) Intramedullary pins.
    4) Wiring.
    5) External fixation.

f. If there is a large amount of metacarpal bone loss consider external fixation.

4. **Distal phalanx.**

a. Most common fracture in the hand.

b. Reduction usually not necessary.

c. Splint for protection and pain control with aluminum finger splint for 3–4 weeks.

d. Often associated with nail bed injuries which may require nail removal and suture repair.

e. Associated subungual hematoma may be decompressed using a sterile 18-gauge needle with a twisting motion on top of nail.

5. **Proximal and middle phalanx shaft.**

a. Stable, nondisplaced fractures
    1) Treat with splint in safe position at 70° MP joint flexion and IP joint extended.
    2) Splint one joint proximal and one joint distal to fracture for 3–4 weeks.
    3) Buddy tape to adjacent finger and start gradual range of motion over 4–6 weeks.

b. Displaced fractures are closed reduced under digital block and splinted as above.

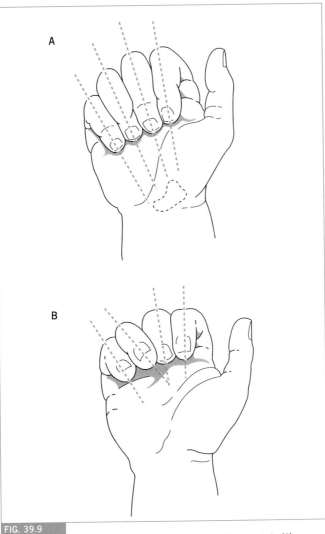

FIG. 39.9
Any malrotation of metacarpal or phalangeal fractures must be corrected. **(A)**
Normally all fingers point toward the region of scaphoid when a fist is made. (B)
Malrotation at fracture causes affected finger to deviate. (Redrawn from Canale T. In:
Campbell's Operative Orthopedics, 9th edn. St. Louis: Mosby; 1998.)

   c.   Unstable fractures are treated by open vs closed reduction in the operating room followed by percutaneous pinning with K-wires, miniplate, and screws, or external fixation.

6. Condylar.

   a.   Best treated by open reduction to reduce the joint surface and fixation with parallel K-wires or mini screws unless severely comminuted, in which case immobilization and early protected range of motion is desirable.

   b.   Head fractures, if badly comminuted – immobilize for 2 weeks and begin early protected range of motion.

7. Thumb.

   a.   Phalanx shaft.

      1)   Repair nail bed if necessary.

      2)   Splint and immobilize for 4 weeks.

      3)   Decompress subungual hematoma if necessary.

      4)   Percutaneous pinning of shaft if displaced.

      5)   If comminuted, immobilize for 2 weeks and begin early protected range of motion.

   b.   Phalanx head.

      1)   Goal is to reduce articular surface as anatomically as possible by open reduction and internal fixation.

      2)   If severely comminuted, immobilize for 2 weeks and begin early range of motion.

   c.   Thumb metacarpal shaft.

      1)   Angulation <20–30° is well tolerated.

      2)   If angulation is greater, reduce closed and percutaneously pin.

8. Thumb metacarpal base (intra-articular).

   a.   Bennett's fracture.

      1)   If fragment is <20% of articular surface reduce closed and pin.

      2)   If fragment >20% of articular surface reduce open with internal fixation using K-wires or screws.

   b.   Rolando's fracture – all comminuted intra-articular fractures require open reduction with internal fixation if fragments are large enough to hold fixation.

VII. WRIST INJURIES

A. SPRAIN.

1. In the presence of normal radiographs and no tenderness in anatomic snuffbox, treat with normal range of motion and anti-inflammatory drugs as needed.

2. If tenderness is present in the anatomic snuffbox, but radiographs are normal, splint in a thumb spica splint and repeat radiographs in 7–10 days to rule out an occult scaphoid fracture.

3. Consider bone scan if symptoms continue.

B. **DISLOCATIONS.**

1. **Radiocarpal.**

a. Pure dislocation without associated fracture of distal radius is extremely rare and can be treated by closed reduction.

b. Check neurovascular status closely.

2. **Radiocarpal and intracarpal** – this combination generally requires open reduction with internal fixation.

3. **Intracarpal dislocations** are frequently associated with a high-energy injury and marked soft tissue damage.

a. Careful assessment of neurovascular status is important, especially median nerve which may often be injured.

b. Incorrect treatment may lead to chronic instability and degeneration of the wrist.

4. **A spectrum of injury patterns** is often seen – the two most common are:

a. Perilunate (dorsal or volar).

   1) Look for 'spilled teacup' sign on lateral radiograph (Figure 39.10).

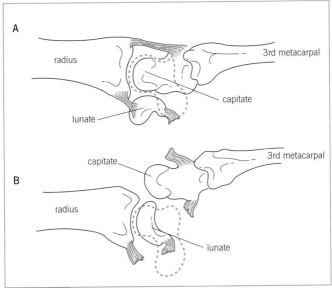

FIG. 39.10

(A) Anterior dislocation of the lunate. (B) Dorsal perilunar dislocation of the carpus. (Redrawn from Hill NA. Fractures and dislocations of the carpus. *Orthop Clin North Am* 1970; 1:275.)

      2) Can often be reduced by closed methods: longitudinal traction with fingertraps for 5–10 minutes prior to attempted reduction; extend the wrist and pull longitudinal traction with one hand while stabilizing the lunate with the thumb of the other hand; slowly flex the wrist allowing the capitate to slip on to the lunate concavity. May require pinning to hold the reduction.

      3) If unable to obtain a closed reduction or stability, open reduction in the operating room is indicated.

      4) Splint in 30° flexion with a dorsal thumb spica splint.

   b. Trans-scaphoid perilunate.

      1) Same means of closed reduction as for perilunate.

      2) Associated with incidence of avascular necrosis of proximal pole of scaphoid ranging from 50 to 100%.

      3) May require open reduction with internal fixation of scaphoid fracture.

C. CARPAL FRACTURES.

1. Scaphoid.

a. Usually caused by a fall on dorsiflexed wrist and may be dismissed as only a sprain.

b. Examine patient for pain and swelling in anatomic snuffbox.

c. Confirm radiographically, including AP, lateral, and oblique.

d. If clinically tender, but radiographs negative, presume fracture and immobilize in a thumb spica splint and repeat radiograph in 10–14 days.

      1) If fracture present and there is no displacement or angulation, apply a thumb spica cast for 8–12 weeks.

      2) In the presence of flexion, angulation, or >1mm displacement perform open reduction with internal fixation using K-wires or screws.

      3) High risk of avascular necrosis or nonunion secondary to tenuous blood supply to the proximal pole which may be injured during the fracture.

2. Lunate.

a. Very rare.

b. Fracture of volar pole is most common.

c. May require open reduction with internal fixation to help avoid disruption of the blood supply.

d. Most may be treated by conservative splinting.

3. Triquetrum.

a. Often associated with other carpal injuries.

b. Impaction is the most common mechanism.

c. Usually treated with cast immobilization for 6 weeks.

4. Pisiform.

a. Uncommon.

b. Direct blow is the most common mechanism.

c. Often missed secondary to difficulty seeing on standard X-rays.
d. Often need supination oblique or carpal tunnel view to make the diagnosis.
e. Cast for 4–6 weeks.

5. **Trapezium.**
a. Infrequent.
b. Often seen in cyclists.
c. If nondisplaced, treat with thumb spica splint for 4–6 weeks.
d. If displaced or intra-articular, treat with open reduction with internal fixation using screws or K-wires.

6. **Trapezoid and capitate.**
a. Very rare as an isolated injury.
b. Often seen with other carpal injuries.
c. Splint if nondisplaced.
d. Open reduction with internal fixation if displaced.

7. **Hamate.**
a. Fracture of hook is most common, particularly in golfers.
b. Carpal tunnel view is helpful in diagnosis.
c. Cast if acute.
d. Chronic fracture may require excision of the fragment.

VIII. AMPUTATIONS
A. INDICATIONS FOR REPLANTATION.
1. **Thumb.**
2. **Amputation in a child.**
3. **Multiple digits.**
4. **Amputation proximal to the digits.**
B. CONTRAINDICATIONS.
1. **Crushed or mangled part.**
2. **Other life-threatening injuries.**
3. **Amputation proximal to the flexor digitorum superficialis tendon insertion** on the digit (zone II).
4. **Prolonged ischemia time** of >6 hours of warm or 12 hours of cold ischemia.
C. TRANSPORTATION OF AMPUTATED PARTS. Wrap the part in gauze moistened with Ringer's lactate solution and then place in a bag on ice.

IX. INFECTIONS
A. HUMAN BITES.
1. **High index of suspicion** – obtain a good history.
2. **Must be treated aggressively** with irrigation and débridement in the operating room.
3. **Leave wound open.**
4. **Extended-spectrum penicillins,** ampicillin, sulbactam, or ticarcillin

HAND INJURIES AND INFECTIONS

clavulanate are the i.v. antibiotics of choice.

5. **Oral agent of choice** is amoxicillin clavulanate.
6. **Tooth may penetrate** into the metacarpophalangeal or the interphalangeal joint during the clenched fist blow to the mouth.
7. **The most common organism** is *Eikanella corrodans*.

B. ANIMAL BITES.

1. **Most common organism** in cat and dog bites is *Pasteurella multocida*.
2. **Antibiotic of choice** is amoxicillin clavulanate.

C. HERPETIC WHITLOW.

1. **Seen in medical and dental personnel** who care for orotracheal area.
2. **Respiratory therapists** are often affected.
3. **Herpes simplex infection** – patches of fluid-filled vesicles often with a rim of erythema.
4. **Do not incise and drain.**
5. **Treatment** includes splinting and elevation.
6. **Antiviral medication,** such as acyclovir, may be considered.

X. HIGH-PRESSURE INJECTION INJURIES

1. **Pinpoint wound appears deceptively benign** and often is more painful than its appearance would suggest.
2. **A history of cleaning a pressure gun** is often given.
3. **Must be treated aggressively** with surgical irrigation and débridement as the injected material often enters the tendon sheath and travels proximally into the hand or forearm.
4. **Oil-based injection material** (i.e. paint) may be especially difficult to remove completely and is an ominous condition for good long-term outcome.
5. **This is a very serious injury** with an amputation rate of 60–70%.

XI. BURNS

A. THERMAL.

1. **First degree** – treat symptomatically as one would a sunburn with topical lotion or anesthetic.
2. **Second degree** – partial-thickness injury requires treatment with daily dressing changes and topical antibiotic, such as silver sulfadiazine.
3. **Third degree** – full-thickness injury requires excision and skin grafting.
4. **Fourth degree** – deep injury to bone may require amputation.

B. ELECTRICAL.

1. **Extent of injury** is proportional to the amount, pathway, and type of current.
2. **Alternating current is particularly dangerous** as it causes muscle tetany and the patient is unable to withdraw from the current source.
3. **Must undertake complete physical examination** looking for entrance and exit sites which commonly are distant from each other.

4. **Should consider cardiovascular evaluation** and monitoring in these patients.
5. **Be alert for the development of a compartment syndrome** which may require fasciotomy.
6. **May require surgical débridement** of nonviable tissue and skin grafting or flap coverage as indicated.

C. **CHEMICAL.**
1. **Copious water irrigation** is the mainstay of treatment.
2. **Extent of injury** depends on duration of contact, amount, and concentration of the chemical.
3. **Hydrofluoric acid burns** should be treated with subcutaneous 10% calcium gluconate or topical calcium gluconate gel.
4. **White phosphorus burns** should be treated with 1% copper sulfate.

D. **FREEZING INJURIES.**
1. **Tissue damaged from cellular injury** via formation of ice crystals and vascular damage via endothelial injury.
2. **Treatment is by rapid rewarming of frozen extremity** in 38°C water for 15–30 minutes, followed by daily dressings and débridement.
3. **May require amputation.**

XII. COMPARTMENT SYNDROME

A. **DIAGNOSIS.** See Chapter 33.
1. **Remember, this is a clinical diagnosis.**
2. **Accentuation of pain by passive muscle stretching** is the most reliable clinical test.
3. **Diminished sensation.**
4. **Weakness and decreased muscle function.**
5. **Palpation in hand and forearm** reveals tenseness and tenderness.
6. **Must have high index of suspicion.**
7. **Do not elevate extremity** because it can increase the ischemia.
8. **Look for this in massive crush injuries, burns, and infections** in which the fascia is intact.
9. **Measure compartment pressure** – rule of thumb for abnormal pressure is >30mmHg.

B. **TREATMENT.**
1. **Surgical release** (Figure 39.11).
a. Extend incision distally through the carpal tunnel.
b. Tendons and nerves should be covered loosely.
c. Leave rest of wound open.
2. **Digital fasciotomy.**
a. Decision to do fasciotomy is made clinically based on the degree of swelling.
b. Most common error is failure to perform this after doing the proximal fasciotomy.

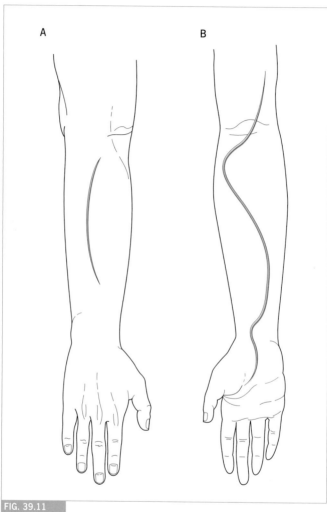

FIG. 39.11
Incisions used in the forearm in severe Volkmann contracture. (A) Extensive opening of fascia of the dorsum of forearm in dorsal compartment syndromes. (B) Incision used for anterior forearm compartment syndromes in which skin and underlying fascia are released completely throughout. (Redrawn from Gelberman RH, Zakib GS, Mubarak SJ, et al. Decompression of forearm compartment syndromes. *Clin Orthop* 1978; 134:225.)

c. Incisions should be made on the ulnar sides of the index, long, and ring finger and on the radial sides of the small finger and the thumb through a midaxial lateral incision.

XIII. FURTHER READING

Dray GJ, Eaton RG. Dislocations and ligament injuries in the digits. In: Green DP (ed.) *Operative hand surgery*, 3rd edn. New York: Churchill Livingstone; 1993:767–798.

Kiefhaber TR. Intra-articular fractures in joint injuries. In: Manske PR (ed.) *AAOS: hand surgery update*. American Association of Orthopedic Surgery; 1996:17–28.

Leddy JP. Flexor tendons – acute injuries. In: Green DP (ed.) *Operative hand surgery*, 3rd edn. New York: Churchill Livingstone; 1993: 1823–1852.

Neviaser RJ. Infections. In: Green DP, ed. *Operative hand surgery*, 3rd edn. New York: Churchill Livingstone; 1993:1021–1038.

Ramamurthy S, Hickey R. Anesthesia of hand. In: Green DP (ed.) *Operative hand surgery*, 3rd edn. New York: Churchill Livingstone; 1993:25–52.

Schneider LH. Flexor tendon injuries. In: Manske PR (ed.) *AAOS: hand surgery update*. American Association of Orthopedic Surgery; 1996:141–148.

Seyfer AE. Injection and extravasation injuries. In: Manske PR (ed.) *AAOS: hand surgery update*. American Association of Orthapedic Surgery; 1996:405–412.

Stern PJ. Fractures of the metacarpals and phalanges. In: Green DP (ed.) *Operative hand surgery*, 3rd edn. New York: Churchill Livingstone.

39

HAND INJURIES AND INFECTIONS

FRACTURES IN CHILDREN

I. ETIOLOGY
1. Etiologies are strongly age dependent.
2. 37% of all childhood fractures occur in the home environment.

II. PATHOPHYSIOLOGY
1. **The immature skeleton of children** is a more dynamic system than that of adults.
2. **Pediatric bone is more narrow and flexible**.
3. **A large potential for remodeling exists** in the bones of children.
4. **Pediatric bones may contain cartilaginous components** of varying size that are radiolucent and which may cause difficulty in diagnosing fractures.
5. **Immature bones contain a physis** or 'growth plate'.
6. **The periosteum is a much more significant structure** when compared with adult bone.

III. FRACTURE PATTERNS
A. **INCOMPLETE PATTERNS.** These include:
1. **Torus (buckle fracture).**
a. An impaction fracture of childhood primarily involving the metaphysis.
b. This is a stable injury which presents as pain without deformity.
2. **Greenstick.**
a. Commonly seen in the ulna and fibula, in which the cortex is incompletely fractured with plastic deformation of the remaining intact cortex and periosteum.
b. This often results in angular deformity which may necessitate conversion to a complete fracture to correct the deformity.
3. **Longitudinal** fractures occur along the axis of the bone and they may be associated with other fracture patterns.
B. **COMPLETE FRACTURE PATTERNS.**
1. Transverse.
2. Oblique.
3. Spiral.
4. Comminuted.
C. **EPIPHYSEAL AND APOPHYSEAL INJURIES.**
1. **Avulsion fractures** (e.g., tibial spine, ulnar styloid, etc.):
a. Stronger soft tissues (e.g., ligament).
b. Avulse a portion of the bone.

   2. **Osteochondral fractures** (e.g., capitellum, femur):
   a. Intra-articular bone and cartilage fragments.
   b. May result in loose bodies within the joint.
   D. **PHYSEAL INJURIES.** These are most commonly categorized by the
       Salter–Harris scheme. The more recent classification by Peterson[1] is
       based on the first population-based epidemiological study and is
       presented below (Figure 40.1).

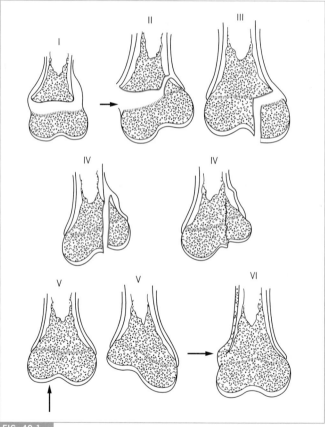

FIG. 40.1

Rang's version of the Salter–Harris classification of epiphyseal fractures adds type VI.
This classification has been the basis for communication and discussion of fracture
types since shortly after its publication in 1963. (From Rang M. *The growth plate and
its disorders.* Baltimore: Williams and Wilkins; 1969.)

1. **Type I.**
a. Transverse fracture of the metaphysis with one or more fracture lines extending to the physis.
b. No fracture along the physis and no displacement of the epiphysis.
c. No Salter–Harris equivalent.
2. **Type II.**
a. Separation of part of the physis with a portion of the metaphysis attached to the epiphysis.
b. Salter–Harris II.
3. **Type III.**
a. Separation of the epiphysis from the diaphysis through any of the layers of the physis, disrupting the complete physis.
b. Salter–Harris I.
4. **Type IV.**
a. Fracture of the epiphysis extending to and along the physis.
b. More common in older children in whom part of the physis has begun to close.
c. Salter–Harris III.
5. **Type V.**
a. Fracture traversing the metaphysis, physis, and epiphysis.
b. Salter–Harris IV.
6. **Type VI.**
a. Fracture with missing physis.
b. No Salter–Harris equivalent.
7. **Type II injury is most common** (54%) and the need for both immediate and late surgery increases with increasing type number.

IV. PRINCIPLES OF PEDIATRIC FRACTURE MANAGEMENT

1. **Ligament injuries are rare in children**, while physeal fractures are common.
2. **Stress radiographs** or other imaging modalities may clearly delineate a suspected fracture through the physis.
3. **Vascular injuries.**
a. Occur in association with fractures in children, but are rare.
b. Prompt recognition and treatment are essential.
c. Most commonly seen with supracondylar fractures of the humerus.
4. **Compartment syndrome does occur** in the pediatric population, especially with fractures of the distal humerus and tibia.

V. CHILD ABUSE

1. **Approximately 2.4 million reports of child abuse** are filed annually in the United States.
2. **The incidence of physical abuse** is roughly 4.9 children per 1000.
3. **The orthopedist will see about 30–50% of abused children.**

40

FRACTURES IN CHILDREN

4. **The risk of abuse** is greatest for the child under 3 years of age, firstborn children, premature infants, stepchildren, and handicapped children[2].
5. **Radiographic evidence for child abuse** includes:
a. Multiple fractures in various stages of healing.
b. This finding indicates child abuse and should be considered as such until proven otherwise.
6. **Fractures of the extremities** (usually humerus, femur, or tibia), skull, and ribs are most frequently seen.
7. **Suspicious patterns** include:
a. Fractures in children under the age of 3 years without reasonable explanation.
b. Metaphyseal and epiphyseal fractures of the long bones.
c. Buckle fractures of the metaphyses are commonly associated with child abuse.
d. Spiral long bone fractures.
e. Periosteal hematomas from direct trauma will be evident on radiographs at 10–14 days.
f. Bucket-handle fractures of the metaphyses are thought to be pathognomonic of abuse. Radiographs reveal a 'chip' at the edge of the metaphysis with no gross displacement of the epiphysis.
8. **Any child suspected of being abused** should be undressed completely and examined for other signs of abuse such as bruises or burns.
9. **Several states have laws requiring physicians to report any case of suspected abuse** and physicians should be aware of such laws in their areas of practice.

VI. OPEN FRACTURES IN CHILDREN

A. **THE MAJORITY OF OPEN FRACTURES** are the result of high-energy trauma.
B. **10% OF THOSE FRACTURES** seen in multiply injured children are open.
C. **ONE-HALF** will have additional injuries.
D. **CLASSIFICATION** is principally based on the Gustilo–Anderson system (see Chapter 32).
E. **TREATMENT**
1. **Initial resuscitation (ABCs) and a detailed musculoskeletal examination**, to include neurologic and` vascular examination of the extremities.
2. **Tetanus prophylaxis.**
3. **Removal of gross contamination** and sterile coverage of wound.
4. **Application of a splint** with realignment of the limb to prevent further soft tissue injury.
5. **Intravenous antibiotics are initiated** in the emergency room.
a. Type I fractures require a first-generation cephalosporin for 48–72 hours.

b. Type II and III fractures require a cephalosporin and aminoglycoside for 48–72 hours.
c. Injuries sustained on a farm benefit from the addition of penicillin to the above regimen.
d. Regimen may be repeated at the time of delayed closure or bony reconstruction.
e. Emergency room cultures are of questionable benefit.
F. SURGICAL DÉBRIDEMENT.
1. **All open fractures should be treated in the operating room**.
2. **Wound edges should be excised** and the open wound extended to explore the depths of the wound and to debride all necrotic tissues and contamination.
3. **Fasciotomies should be performed** as indicated.
4. **Débridement should be aggressive** since multiple modalities now exist for soft tissue and bony reconstruction.
a. Return to the operating room as many times as needed to gain control of the wound.
b. Decisions on definitive fracture treatment can be made at this time depending on fracture type, location, and condition of the soft tissues.
c. Options include:
    1) Splint or cast with or without percutaneous pins (e.g., radius).
    2) External fixation (commonly employed for the tibia and femur).
    3) Internal fixation.
    4) Intramedullary fixation (e.g., type I open femur fracture in a 12-year-old female).

VII. AMPUTATION
1. **Every attempt should be made to salvage amputated limbs in children**.
2. **Even type III-C injuries**, which may suggest amputation in the adult, should be salvaged, if possible, in the child.
3. **Length should be preserved,** given the potential for growth in children.
4. **As in adult trauma patients, multiply injured children benefit from early fracture stabilization** and definitive treatment of all fractures as soon as they are stable.

VIII. FRACTURES AND DISLOCATIONS OF THE UPPER EXTREMITY
A. HAND.
1. Basic principles.
a. The number of hand fractures peaks around age 13 years.
b. Almost all children's hand fractures can be treated by closed reduction and splinting for 3–4 weeks.
c. Repeated attempts at reduction of physeal fractures are not advised.

    d. Repeat radiographs should be obtained at 5–7 days to confirm maintenance of reduction.

    e. 'Buddy-taping' and short arm immobilization are acceptable for fractures of the phalanges and metacarpals, but more proximal fractures should be addressed with long arm immobilization.

    f. The most common hand fracture is either the distal phalanx injury or Peterson type II (Salter II) of the proximal phalanx.

    g. Open reduction is generally reserved for:

        1) Displaced intra-articular fractures.

        2) Displaced Peterson type IV or V fractures (Salter–Harris type III and IV).

        3) Unstable fractures.

2. Distal phalanx.

    a. Extraphyseal injury.

    b. Nail removal with careful débridement, irrigation, and nail-bed repair may be in order.

    c. If there is insufficient stability, the fracture may be pinned.

    d. Most can be treated simply by splinting the tip of the distal interphalangeal joint leaving the proximal interphalangeal joint free.

3. Mallet finger (distal phalanx physeal injury).

    a. There are five types, as follows:

        1) Peterson type III or II (Salter–Harris I or II).

        2) Peterson type IV or V (Salter–Harris III or IV).

        3) Peterson type III or II with joint dislocation.

        4) Avulsion of extensor with Salter–Harris fracture.

        5) Reverse Mallet with flexor avulsion with bone.

    b. Treatment depends on the type of fracture:

        1) Closed, nonoperative treatment; open injuries may require nail-bed repair, etc.

        2) Nonoperative treatment is favored except in the presence of inadequate reduction or joint subluxation, both of which require operative treatment.

        3) Open reduction to restore joint and extensor mechanism.

        4) Treat as Patterson type III or type II with joint dislocation.

        5) Repair under minimal tension within 1 week through volar approach.

4. Proximal phalanx

    a. Fracture classification:

        1) Physeal fractures.

        2) Shaft fractures.

        3) Condylar and phalangeal neck fractures.

    b. Treatment for type A fractures includes closed reduction and immobilization for 3 weeks.

c. Indications for operative reduction include:
    1) Irreducibility.
    2) Unstable reductions.
    3) >25% articular surface involvement.
    4) Displacement of >1.5mm.

B. FRACTURES OF THE RADIUS AND ULNA.

1. Distal radius fractures are the most common of childhood fractures.

2. Classification.

a. Type A – dorsally displaced.

b. Type B – volarly displaced.

3. Treatment is nonoperative.

a. Timely and gentle closed reduction is ideal.

b. For type A fractures a good three-point mold of the splint or cast with the wrist in neutral is essential.

c. For type B fractures a three-point mold with the wrist dorsiflexed 30° and the forearm in full supination is desirable.

d. Acceptable results for a child with 1 year of growth remaining are at least 50% apposition (which should remodel to almost normal) and <25° of angulation.

e. Immobilize for 4–6 weeks in a short or long arm cast with follow-up radiographs at 4–6 months to ensure the resumption of normal growth.

4. Operative treatment may be required in patients with:

a. Severe local soft tissue or ipsilateral proximal fractures.

b. Open fractures.

c. Median nerve compression or compartment syndrome.

d. Comminuted epiphyseal fractures.

e. Failure to obtain an adequate closed reduction.

C. FRACTURES OF THE SHAFT OF THE RADIUS AND ULNA.

1. Basic principles.

a. Rotation and angular deformities must be corrected.

b. <10° of deformity in all planes is desirable.

c. Children <10 years old have more potential for remodeling.

d. Bayonet apposition does not limit rotation.

e. Avoid narrowing of the interosseous membrane and use the bicipital tuberosity to aid in rotational alignment.

2. Greenstick fractures.

a. Necessity of 'completing' the fracture is controversial.

b. Angular components must be corrected as follows:
    1) For apex–volar angulation, a pronation force must be applied during reduction.
    2) For apex–dorsal angulation, a supination force must be used during the reduction maneuver.

40

FRACTURES IN CHILDREN

     3) Immobilize in a well-molded, sugar-tong splint or long arm cast.
     4) Slight overcorrection may be preferable to prevent recurrence of deformity.
     5) Repeat radiographs within the first few days, then every week for 2–3 weeks to ensure maintenance of reduction.
     6) Remanipulate fracture if reduction is lost after 2–5 days.

3. Complete fractures of the radius and ulna.
a. Closed reduction.
     1) Confirm correct rotational and angular alignment by radiographic examination.
     2) Bayonet apposition is acceptable if the interosseous distance, and angular and rotational alignment are acceptable.
     3) Apply a well-molded, sugar-tong splint and change to a long arm cast as swelling permits.
     4) In older children, difficulty in obtaining or maintaining the reduction may require open reduction and plate fixation.
     5) Close radiographic follow-up is required to confirm maintenance of alignment.

4. Monteggia fractures (fractures of the ulnar shaft associated with radial head dislocation).
a. Treatment varies with the direction of the dislocation.
b. Anterior or lateral dislocation requires closed reduction and immobilization of the arm in a long arm splint or cast for 6–8 weeks.
c. Flexion and supination are the appropriate positions for these variants.
d. Posterior dislocation may require immobilization in extension to maintain stability of the reduction.
e. Check for alignment of the proximal radius with the capitellum on the anteroposterior (AP) and lateral radiograph.

5. Galeazzi fractures (fracture of the radial shaft with distal radio-ulnar joint dislocation).
a. Unlike adults, results are good with closed reduction in children.
b. Closed reduction of the radius and long arm immobilization in supination or pronation (depending on the deforming forces) is recommended.
c. Operative reduction is reserved for unstable closed reduction.

D. FRACTURES OF THE ELBOW.
1. Radiographic evaluation should include AP, lateral, and oblique views.
2. Comparison views may be helpful.
3. Stress radiographs may be helpful if ligamentous or physeal injury is suspected.
4. Documentation of neurologic and vascular examination is critical.
5. If there is a suspected fracture but negative radiographs, splint the extremity and re-evaluate at 10–14 days.

E. SUPRACONDYLAR HUMERUS FRACTURES.

1. **Initial treatment** includes:
    a. Complete neurologic and vascular examination.
    b. Reduction of gross displacement.
    c. Splint application.
    d. Radiographic evaluation.
2. **These fractures are one of the most common causes of compartment syndrome** in children and require a high index of suspicion, with careful examination and frequent monitoring.
3. **Inpatient observation** is recommended for at least 24 hours for the majority of supracondylar humerus fractures.
4. **Classification.**
    a. Type I – nondisplaced or minimally displaced.
    b. Type II – displaced with an intact posterior cortex.
    c. Type III – a completely displaced fracture or one lacking intrinsic stability with the elbow flexed.
5. **Treatment.**
    a. Type I fractures are treated with splinting in 90° of flexion, with conversion to a long arm cast (when swelling permits) for 3–4 weeks.
    b. Type II and III fractures are treated with closed reduction and, after assessment for stability, treated by either splint, cast, or percutaneous pin fixation if unstable.
    c. At Parkland, the majority of type III and many type II fractures are stabilized with K-wires: crossed medial and lateral pins are used.
    d. Anatomic reduction is critical.
    e. The reduction maneuver involves longitudinal traction to obtain length and the correction of angulation (restoring a normal carrying angle), followed by hyperflexion and then pronation.
    f. Open reduction may sometimes be necessary.
    g. Anteromedial or anterolateral exposure may be used as appropriate.
    h. Frequent, early radiographic follow-up is mandatory to ensure maintenance of reduction.
6. **Associated injuries and vascular compromise.**
    a. The incidence of associated nerve injury, previously estimated at 7%, is now felt to be somewhat higher with the anterior interosseous nerve most commonly affected.
    b. Vascular compromise is not uncommon, especially with type III fractures (Figure 40.2).
        1) Fractures that present with diminished or absent pulses are best treated by immediate reduction followed by percutaneous pin fixation if pulses return after reduction.
        2) There is very little role for angiography in the treatment of these patients because it may result in a significant delay in appropriate treatment.

40

FRACTURES IN CHILDREN

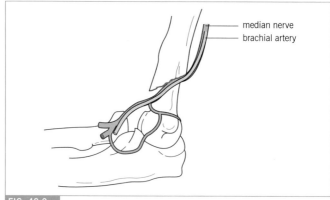

FIG. 40.2

The brachial artery, along with the median nerve, can be compressed between the fracture fragments. (From Rockwood CA, Wilkins KE, King RE. *Fractures in children,* 3rd edn. Philadelphia: JB Lippincott; 1991.)

    3) Persistent vascular compromise after reduction mandates open vascular exploration.

7. **Loss of reduction after closed treatment** is an indication for percutaneous pin fixation.

F. MEDIAL EPICONDYLE FRACTURES.

1. **The injury mechanism** is an extension force at the wrist and valgus force at the elbow.

2. **Comparison radiographs are frequently helpful for diagnosis,** although children <5 years old will not have an ossified epicondyle.

3. **Treatment.**

a. Nondisplaced fractures are treated in a long arm cast for 3–4 weeks.

b. Fractures with >5mm displacement, instability of the elbow joint, or a fragment incarcerated in the joint require open reduction and internal fixation.

c. Carefully document ulnar nerve status prior to instituting therapy.

4. **Lateral epicondyle fractures** are very rare and are treated the same as the medial epicondyle.

G. LATERAL CONDYLE FRACTURES.

1. **Peterson type V** (Salter–Harris type IV) pattern.

2. **The injury mechanism** is commonly elbow extension with a valgus force.

3. **Nondisplaced fractures** are treated with a long arm cast for 3–4 weeks with radiographic follow-up at 3–4 days to assure maintenance of reduction.

4. **Anatomic reduction** is mandatory for displaced fractures.
a. Closed reduction with percutaneous pins is acceptable if reduction is anatomic.
b. Most of these fractures require open reduction and pin fixation.
H. MEDIAL CONDYLE FRACTURES.
1. **These fractures are a relatively uncommon injury** in children.
2. **Classification.**
a. Milch type I is a Peterson type V (Salter–Harris type IV) pattern.
b. Milch type II is a Peterson type II (Salter–Harris type II).
c. Also classified in terms of displacement, which may assist in determination of appropriate treatment.
   1) Type I – fracture line from the medial condylar metaphysis extending to the physis. Generally nondisplaced.
   2) Type II – fracture line from the medial condylar metaphysis extending into the medial condylar physis.
   3) Type III – the fragment is displaced and rotated.
3. **Treatment.**
a. Type I is best treated with a long arm splint or cast for 3–4 weeks, with range-of-motion exercises begun at the appearance of abundant callous.
b. Types II and III are treated at Parkland by open reduction and pin fixation.
I. RADIAL HEAD AND NECK FRACTURES.
1. **These are often associated with other fractures or dislocations**.
2. **Angulation of >30° requires an attempt at closed reduction.**
3. **Poorer results** are associated with initial angulation of >30° or translocation >3–4mm.
4. **Treatment.**
a. For fractures with <30° angulation and no translation, long arm immobilization for 7–10 days followed by early motion is usually adequate.
b. Angulation >30° requires closed manipulation followed by long arm immobilization for 1–2 weeks.
c. Angulation >45° requires closed manipulation or percutaneous pin reduction followed by long arm immobilization for 1–2 weeks.
d. Open reduction, with or without fixation, is required for fractures with residual angulation fixed at >40° with translation >3mm, and <60° of supination or pronation, or complete displacement of the radial head.
e. Acceptable results are <45° of angulation, no translation, and supination or pronation arc of 50–60°.
J. OLECRANON FRACTURES.
1. **Very uncommon** and highly associated with other injuries.

2. **Most minimally displaced fractures and nondisplaced fractures** can be treated by simple immobilization in 75–80° of flexion.
3. **Displaced fractures** require open reduction and internal fixation.

K. **ELBOW DISLOCATION.**
1. **Commonly associated** with other fractures and injuries.
2. **Closed reduction** is generally the successful treatment for these injuries.
3. **Confirm joint congruity on postreduction radiographs**, and examine the joint for stability.
4. **Beware of entrapment of the median nerve** or a nonossified medial condyle which may prevent reduction.
5. **Treatment** is long arm immobilization for 5–7 days, followed by active range of motion.

L. **SUBLUXATION OF THE RADIAL HEAD (NURSEMAID'S ELBOW).**
1. **Commonly the result of pulling the outstretched arm**, although about one-third of presentations may be atypical.
2. **The child will usually present with the elbow flexed and pronated,** and will refuse to use the arm.
3. **Radiographs may be negative**.
4. **The reduction maneuver** involves supination and gentle traction in extension, followed by hyperflexion.
5. **The child will usually begin to use the arm immediately** and without pain with a successful reduction.
6. **Parents should be warned against causing recurrence** by pulling on the child's arm.

M. **FRACTURES OF THE HUMERUS.**
1. **Humeral shaft fractures.**
   a. Frequently transverse or spiral fracture patterns which can be treated in a coaptation splint, humeral cuff orthosis, or collar and cuff for 3–4 weeks.
   b. Be wary of child abuse when spiral fractures are seen.
   c. Overgrowth of the humerus by 1cm can be expected.
   d. Neuropraxic injury to the radial nerve can be apparent on presentation and is managed as follows:
      1) Observation only is recommended if nerve palsy is present at initial patient presentation.
      2) If neuropraxic injury occurs after manipulation, surgical exploration is warranted.
   e. Rarely, soft tissue interposition may block an adequate reduction and require surgical intervention.
2. **Metaphyseal fractures.**
   a. These are usually greenstick injuries and can be treated in a sling for 3–4 weeks.

b.   Displaced fractures require closed reduction and immobilization.
c.   The fracture may buttonhole through the deltoid and require surgical extraction to achieve reduction.

N.   INJURIES AROUND THE SHOULDER GIRDLE.

1.   Proximal humerus fractures.
a.   AP and axillary lateral radiographs are ncessary for adequate evaluation.
b.   These injuries are usually Peterson type II (Salter–Harris II) patterns caused by a variety of mechanisms.
c.   The vast majority of these fractures can be treated by nonoperative means.
d.   No hard and fast rules exist for operative treatment, but possible indications are:
   1)   Marked displacement with little growth remaining.
   2)   Multiple trauma.
   3)   Open fracture with significant periosteal disruption.

2.   Traumatic shoulder dislocations.
a.   AP and axillary lateral or trans-scapular views are necessary to evaluate.
b.   Occurrence is more frequent in the adolescent with closed physes.
c.   Treatment is by closed reduction, sling immobilization, and early motion.
d.   Anterior dislocations far exceed posterior dislocations in frequency.
e.   The axillary nerve is the most frequently injured neurovascular structure with anterior dislocations.
f.   Open reduction may rarely be required if closed reduction is unsuccessful.

3.   Clavicle fractures.
a.   Shaft fracture.
   1)   Very common in the pediatric population and usually midshaft.
   2)   Treated in a figure-of-eight splint for 3–6 weeks.
   3)   Most heal in malunited position, but remodel within 1 year.
   4)   Occasionally may be implicated in brachial plexus or vascular injury.
   5)   Greenstick fractures with posterior bowing may also result in neurovascular compromise.
b.   Proximal clavicle fracture.
   1)   Usually represents an epiphyseal separation which can occur up to age 25 years.
   2)   Anterior displacement is manifested by prominence of the clavicle and may be treated conservatively.
   3)   Posterior displacement may compromise the trachea or vascular structures.
   4)   Reduction to anatomic position by closed or open means.

5) Unstable reductions may require internal fixation.
6) Rockwood 45° upshot view provides the best radiographic visualization.

c. Distal clavicle fracture.
1) Usually epiphyseal separation.
2) Treated in a sling for 2–3 weeks.

4. Scapular fractures.

a. Usually associated with severe trauma.

b. Majority may be treated with a sling, analgesia, and early motion.

c. Avulsion of the coracoid with complete acromioclavicular separation may require open reduction and internal fixation.

d. Some glenoid fractures with joint incongruity or instability may require open reduction and internal fixation.

IX. FRACTURES OF THE PELVIS AND ACETABULUM

A. APOPHYSEAL FRACTURES are usually the result of a sudden, violent muscle contraction.

B. ANTERIOR SUPERIOR ILIAC SPINE AND ISCHIAL AVULSIONS are the most commonly seen.

C. SYMPTOMATIC TREATMENT is sufficient unless there is marked displacement.

D. 'ISOLATED' FRACTURES OF THE PUBIC RAMUS, ISCHIUM, OR ILIUM.

1. Pubic ramus fractures are common pelvic injuries in children.

2. They are associated with high-energy trauma.

3. The superior ramus fracture is most commonly seen.

4. Treatment is symptomatic, but these patients have a high incidence of associated injuries.

5. Ischial fractures are rare and treatment is generally symptomatic.

6. Iliac wing fractures result from high-energy trauma and are highly associated with other injuries.

7. The majority are nondisplaced or minimally displaced.

8. Treatment is conservative with protected weight bearing on the affected side for 4–6 weeks.

E. FRACTURES OF THE SACRUM AND COCCYX.

1. These fractures may be associated with neurologic injury.

2. Most are treated conservatively.

F. PELVIC RING DISRUPTIONS.

1. Classification is the same as in adults.

2. Most are treated conservatively with protected weight bearing.

3. Pelvic ring disruptions can be associated with other significant injuries.

G. ACETABULAR FRACTURES.

1. These fractures are uncommon in the pediatric population.

2. Classification is similar to adults.

3. **Most are treated conservatively** with protected weight bearing, traction, or spica cast.
4. **The goal is to maintain a congruent joint** until healing has occurred.
5. **Injuries to the triradiate cartilage** may lead to growth arrest and acetabular insufficiency

X. FRACTURES AND DISLOCATIONS OF THE LOWER EXTREMITY

A. FRACTURES AND DISLOCATIONS OF THE HIP.

1. **Hip fractures are rare injuries** in the pediatric population.
a. Transepiphyseal fracture, with or without hip dislocation.
  1) Expect poor results.
  2) Treatment is closed or open reduction with secure pin fixation.
  3) In very young children, closed reduction and traction can be used.
b. Transcervical fracture.
  1) These account for the majority of pediatric hip fractures.
  2) There is a 15–40% incidence of associated avascular necrosis.
  3) Anatomic reduction with internal fixation is standard treatment.
c. Cervicotrochanteric fracture.
  1) A nondisplaced fracture is treated in an abduction hip spica cast, and followed by frequent radiographs to confirm maintenance of reduction.
  2) A displaced fracture is treated with closed or open reduction with internal fixation.
d. An intertrochanteric fracture is generally treated with skin or skeletal traction followed by spica cast or internal fixation in the older child.

2. **Hip dislocations.**
a. Careful neurovascular examination is important.
b. Obtain prereduction radiographs to identify associated fractures.
c. Treatment is urgent, gentle reduction, usually under a mask anesthesia.
d. If closed reduction fails or the joint is incongruent, open reduction is indicated.
e. Beware of occult physeal injuries which may displace during reduction.
f. Document joint congruency with good postreduction radiographs or CT scan if necessary.
g. After reduction, traction followed by protected weight bearing.

B. FRACTURES OF THE SHAFT OF THE FEMUR.

1. **Infants 0–2 years of age.**
a. Consider the possibility of child abuse.
b. Almost all can be treated by immediate hip spica application for 4–6 weeks.
c. Acceptable reduction is <1.5cm of shortening and 30° of angulation.

2. **Children 2–6 years of age.**
a. Most can be treated by closed reduction and immediate hip spica application.

b. Shortening >2–3cm or multiple injuries contraindicate immediate spica cast application.

c. Treat with skeletal or split Russell's traction for 2–3 weeks until fracture is stable.

d. Spica cast for 4–6 weeks.

e. Acceptable reduction is up to 2cm of shortening, and angulation 20–30° in the sagittal plane and 15–20° in the coronal plane.

3. Children 6–16 years of age.

a. Treatment goal currently revolves around healing the fracture without deformity, low cost of care delivery, and rapid return to function.

b. Treatment modalities are currently evolving with several options.

c. Immediate spica cast:
  1) This is still the best and arguably the least expensive form of treatment.
  2) Tends to apply to the younger children in this age group.

d. Traction followed by spica cast: low major complication rate and a cost comparable to surgical treatment.

e. External fixation:
  1) May be useful for open injuries or comminuted fractures, but is associated with a high major and minor complication rate (and complications are expensive, making this procedure less cost-effective.)
  2) Performs poorly on purely transverse fractures.
  3) Average time to device removal in the above series was 18 weeks, and to full weight bearing 22 weeks.

f. Flexible intramedullary nails:
  1) Excellent choice for transverse fractures with early healing and a low complication rate.
  2) Also useful for other fracture patterns, but use is technique dependent with a learning curve.
  3) Average time to device removal is 44 weeks, and to full weight bearing 8 weeks.
  4) This modality is currently used at Parkland for patients up to age 14 years.

g. Plate fixation: this technique is useful in special situations.

h. Reamed intramedullary nails:
  1) This may have a use in older children, but sporadic cases of avascular necrosis of the femoral head are being reported.
  2) For this reason, this method is not currently used at Parkland.

4. Acceptable reduction is no more than 1.5mm shortening, 5–10° of varus or valgus, and 10–15° of AP angulation, with more exacting standards applied with increasing age of the child.

5. **Hardware removal.**
a. Timing of hardware removal is controversial.
b. At Parkland, hardware is generally removed in children under age 10–11 years or if parents are insistent.

C. **SUPRACONDYLAR FEMUR FRACTURES.**
1. **These are often occult fractures.**
2. **They are often misdiagnosed** as a 'knee sprain' or ligament injury.
3. **Comparison views of the unaffected leg are often helpful**, as are stress views of the injured extremity.
4. **These injuries are usually Peterson type II or III injuries**, but often result in growth arrest or deformity because of the undulating nature of the femoral physis.
5. **Supracondylar metaphyseal fractures in young children** may be the result of child abuse.
6. **Long term follow-up is necessary** to assess growth.
7. **Treatment of nondisplaced fractures** should be immobilization in a cast.
8. **Displaced fractures need closed reduction** followed by cast application for 4–6 weeks.
9. **Unstable fractures** may require smooth pin fixation or internal fixation.
10. **Document neurovascular status** pre- and postreduction.

D. **KNEE INJURIES.**
1. **Knee dislocation is uncommon** in the pediatric population.
a. Physeal injury is much more common.
b. There is a high incidence of vascular injury with knee dislocation.
c. Treatment is by closed reduction and casting; in some instances ligament repair may be appropriate.
d. External fixation is required for:
    1) Open joint injuries.
    2) Vascular injury.
    3) Gross instability.
2. **Knee ligament injuries.**
a. Variable prognosis.
b. Be alert for epiphyseal fractures presenting as a 'ligament sprain'.
3. **Patellar dislocations.**
a. These are common pediatric injuries.
b. Diagnosis is arrived at by history and physical examination.
c. Dislocations commonly reduce spontaneously with knee extension, and frank dislocation may not be present by the time the patient seeks out the physician.
d. Treatment is with a long leg cast for 3–6 weeks.
e. If a dislocation is present on presentation, closed reduction by knee extension, then cast application is required.

f.   In the presence of an associated chondral or osteochondral fracture, this may be addressed by closed reduction and fixation or excision of the fragment.

4.   **Patella fractures.**

a.   AP, lateral, and sunrise patella views should be obtained.

b.   A nondisplaced fracture with preserved active extension is treated in a cylinder cast for 6 weeks

c.   Greater than 2mm displacement or loss of active knee extension needs open reduction and internal fixation.

E.   **TIBIAL SPINE FRACTURES.**

1.   **These injuries are usually caused by a direct blow** or fall on the knee.

2.   **Classification and treatment.**

a.   Type I (nondisplaced) – require casting for 6 weeks.

b.   Type II (hinged fracture of the spine) – require closed reduction and casting in 0–10° for 6 weeks.

c.   Type III (displaced tibial spine fracture) – may be treated by closed reduction with casting for 6–8 weeks, otherwise failed closed reduction requires open reduction and internal fixation.

F.   **PROXIMAL TIBIAL EPIPHYSEAL FRACTURE.**

1.   **Assess for vascular injury.**

2.   **Stress radiographs and comparison views** may aid diagnosis.

3.   **Treatment for nondisplaced fractures** is a long leg cast for 6 weeks.

4.   **Displaced fractures** require anatomic closed reduction and cast or pin fixation, or open reduction and internal fixation.

G.   **TIBIAL TUBERCLE FRACTURES.**

1.   **Similar to avulsion of the patellar ligament.**

2.   **Classification.**

a.   Type I – fracture at the secondary ossified center.

b.   Type II – fracture at the primary and secondary ossification centers.

c.   Type III – fracture extending across the tibial epiphysis into the knee joint.

3.   **Treatment** is with closed reduction and immobilization if anatomic reduction is obtained and the patient is able to extend the knee.

4.   **Open reduction and internal fixation** is necessary for any displacement in this epiphyseal fracture.

H.   **PROXIMAL TIBIAL METAPHYSEAL FRACTURES.**

1.   **Assess for vascular injury.**

2.   **All valgus greenstick fractures** should be reduced anatomically or over-reduced into varus.

3.   **Overgrowth into valgus is common.**

4.   **Warn parents of possible valgus deformity.**

5.   **Most valgus deformities** correct spontaneously over time.

I. TIBIAL SHAFT FRACTURES.

1. Greenstick fractures.
a. Greenstick deformity of the fibula may prevent reduction of the tibia.
b. Anatomic reduction should be attempted.
c. Treatment is with a long leg cast for 6 weeks.

2. Nondisplaced fractures.
a. These injuries can be treated in a long leg cast for 6–8 weeks.
b. Some may need hospital admission for observation.

3. Displaced fractures.
a. Treatment is closed reduction and a long leg cast for 6–8 weeks.
b. Most warrant overnight observation to rule out compartment syndrome.

4. Unstable fractures.
a. Treatment is closed reduction and pin fixation with cast immobilization.
b. Internal or external fixation may be used if above treatment is unsuccessful.

J. INTRA-ARTICULAR FRACTURES OF THE DISTAL TIBIA.

1. **Best results** are obtained with anatomic reduction.
2. **A CT scan may be necessary** to evaluate fracture or reduction.
3. **Closed reduction is successful** if anatomic reduction is achieved, and is followed by immobilization in a long leg cast for 4–6 weeks.
4. **If unable to achieve anatomic reduction**, perform open reduction, internal fixation.

K. FRACTURES OF THE DISTAL TIBIAL PHYSIS.

1. **AP, lateral, and mortise radiographs** are helpful.
2. **Most of these are Peterson type II or III.**
3. **Beware of 'triplane' fractures in older children** in whom the physis has begun to close.
4. **Treatment** is closed reduction by reversing mechanism of injury, followed by a long leg cast for 6 weeks.
5. **Intra-articular fractures require anatomic reduction.**

XI. REFERENCES

1. Peterson HA. Physeal fractures: part 3 classification. *J Pediatr Orthop* 1994; 14(4):439–448.
2. Dormans JP. Acute neurovascular complications with supracondylar humerus fractures in children. *J Hand Surg (Am)* 1995; 20:1–4.

XII. FURTHER READING

Rang M. *The growth plate and its disorders*. Baltimore: Williams and
Cheng JC, Shen WY. Limb fracture pattern in different age groups: a study of 3350 children. *J Orthop Trauma* 1993; 7:15.
Gustilo RB, Anderson JT. Prevention of infection in the treatment of 1025

open fractures of long bones, retrospective and prospective Analysis. *J Bone Joint Surg* 1976; 58A:453–458.

Kreder HJ, Armstrong P. The significance of peri-operative cultures in open pediatric lower extremity fractures. *Clin Orthop* 1994; 302:206–212.

BITES AND STINGS

I. INTRODUCTION

1. Each year, approximately 2 million Americans are victims of animal and human bites.
2. The majority of bite wounds are minor and resolve without complications in lieu of medical attention.
3. Wound infection is the most common bite-related complication.

II. DOG BITES

1. Canines account for 80–90% of animal bites, affecting the upper, then lower, extremities most often (Figure 41.1).
2. Dog bites to the head and neck region are often seen in young children.
3. Large dogs may generate jaw pressures >450psi (3105 kPa), which result in significant avulsion or crush injury.
4. Bite wounds to the hand are at increased risk for tenosynovitis, septic arthritis, and abscess formation.
5. The incidence of infection ranges from 2 to 20%. Infecting agents include:
   a. α-Hemolytic streptococci – most frequent.
   b. Methicillin-susceptible *Staphylococcus aureus* – 20–30%.
   c. *Pasteurella multocida* – 20–30%. Clinical infection with *P. multocida* is characterized by development of intense inflammation with localized pain and swelling within 24–48 hours.
   d. *Capnocytophaga canimorsus* is a fastidious Gram-negative rod isolated in the normal flora of 16% of dogs and 18% of cats that can cause severe sepsis, disseminated intravascular coagulation, and renal failure in immunocompromised hosts.

III. CAT BITES

1. Cat bites are the second most common type of mammalian bites in the United States.
2. 60–70% of bite injuries occur in the upper extremity with an associated infection rate of 30–50%.
3. Septic arthritis or osteomyelitis may result from penetrating bone injuries.
4. Cat scratches inoculate the same microorganisms as bites and should be treated as such.
5. *P. multocida* is isolated more often from infected cat bites than dog bites.
6. Inoculation with *Afipia felis*, via a scratch or bite, may result in cat-scratch disease, which is characterized by fever and lymphadenitis.
7. Cat-scratch disease is usually a self-limited disease with complete resolution of symptoms within 2 months.

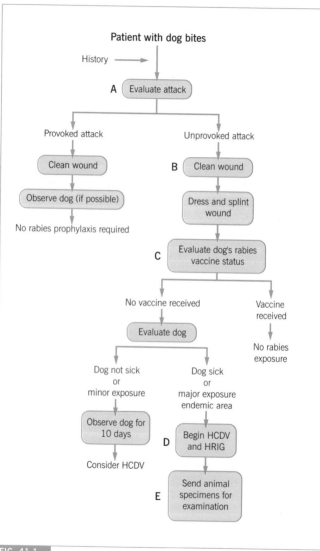

FIG. 41.1

Treatment of patient with dog bite. HCDV = human cell diploid vaccine; HRIG = human rabies immunoglobulin.

IV. HUMAN BITES

A. **HUMAN BITES** are less common than dog or cat bites, but cause more serious infection owing to the mechanism of injury and oral flora.

B. **CLENCHED-FIST INJURIES** are the most serious of human bite wounds and usually occur at the third metacarpophalangeal (MCP) joint of the dominant hand.

1. The MCP joints are in flexion at the time of injury, facilitating tooth penetration into the joint space.

2. Tendon or nerve laceration, or phalangeal or metacarpal fracture, may occur occasionally.

3. Clenched-fist injuries should be evaluated by a hand surgeon for possible joint injury or tendon involvement, or need for exploration.

C. **OCCLUSIONAL BITES TO THE HAND,** not involving a clenched fist, have a higher risk of infection and complication than simple occlusional bites to other areas.

D. **PARONYCHIA IN CHILDREN** who suck their fingers should be managed as bite wounds, though their rate of infection is less than that in adults.

V. INITIAL MANAGEMENT

1. **In patients sustaining animal bites,** determine the type of animal involved and whether the attack was provoked or unprovoked. This information is useful in establishing the need for rabies prophylaxis.

2. **Elicit a history of allergies** to local anesthetics or other medications, as well as tetanus and rabies immune status.

3. **Record important medical data** including history of splenectomy, liver disease, malignancy, or immunosuppressive therapy.

4. **Perform a thorough neurovascular examination** with emphasis on wound type and depth, as well as tendon, ligament, bone, or joint involvement.

5. **Document initial and subsequent range of motion and level of discomfort**.

6. **Obtain a radiograph** to exclude bone or joint involvement, as well as to determine if a foreign body (e.g., tooth) is present.

7. **Gram stain and culture all infected wounds before treatment**, as 90% of infected dog-bite wounds yield pathogenic bacteria.

8. **Irrigate** under 15lb (6.75kg) of pressure using an 18–20 gauge angiocath, a 60mL syringe, and a minimum of 150mL of normal saline or Ringer's lactate. Pressure irrigation significantly decreases the bacterial inoculum and may reduce the rate of infection by up to 20-fold.

9. **Immobilize and elevate** the wounded extremity.

10. **Do not close human or cat-bite wounds** as secondary infection is common.

41

BITES AND STINGS

11. **Dog bites without signs of infection or hand involvement** may be sutured if <8 hours old.
12. **Bite wounds older than 24 hours** should be left open, even if infection is not obvious.
13. **Bites to the head and face** may be closed at the discretion of a plastic surgeon.

VI. ANTIBIOTIC TREATMENT

A. **PROPHYLACTIC ANTIBIOTIC THERAPY** is recommended in:
1. Late presentations (>8 hours).
2. Moderate to severe or deep puncture wounds.
3. Cat bites.
4. Facial or hand involvement.
5. Diabetic, asplenic, or immunocompromised patients.
B. **A 3–5 DAY COURSE OF PROPHYLACTIC ORAL ANTIBIOTICS** is recommended.
1. **Amoxicillin–clavulanic acid 500mg p.o. three times a day** is the treatment of choice as it adequately covers *P. multocida*, *Eikenella corrodens*, *C. canimorsus*, *S. aureus*, and anaerobes.
2. **Alternately, cefuroxime 500mg p.o. twice daily** or ceftriaxone 1g i.m. daily may be given.
3. **For penicillin-allergic patients, doxycycline 100mg p.o. twice daily,** ciprofloxacin 500mg p.o. every 12 hours, and ofloxacin 400mg p.o. every 12 hours are adequate substitutes.
4. **Erythromycin, clindamycin, and first-generation cephalosporins are not recommended,** owing to their poor activity against *P. multocida*.

VII. INDICATIONS FOR HOSPITAL ADMISSION

1. Systemic signs of infection (e.g., fever, chills).
2. Head injury.
3. Severe cellulitis.
4. Peripheral vascular disease.
5. Poorly controlled diabetes mellitus.
6. Penetration of a joint, nerve, bone, tendon, or central nervous system.
7. Failed outpatient therapy, or likelihood of noncompliance with outpatient treatment.

VII. TETANUS IMMUNIZATION

1. Patients with no history of tetanus vaccination or uncertain immunization history should receive tetanus IG 250–500 units intramuscularly plus the first of three doses of tetanus toxoid, given 1 month apart.
2. Tetanus toxoid 0.5mL s.c. or i.m. is recommended for patients who have not received a booster in the last 10 years.

IX. RABIES

1. **The risk of contracting rabies** from a rabid animal bite ranges from 5 to 80%.
2. **Nonbite exposures** include scratches, abrasions, and contamination of an open wound by potentially infectious material including saliva, cerebrospinal fluid, and brain tissue.
3. **Cats, followed by cattle and dogs**, are responsible for the majority of domestic animal rabies cases.
4. **The principal wildlife vectors** in the United States are raccoons, foxes, skunks, and bats.
5. **All unprovoked animal attacks are considered high risk** and the highest risk of infection occurs with bites to the face and hands.
6. **A healthy domestic dog or cat**, with current vaccination status, should be confined and observed for 10 days. Postexposure prophylaxis may be postponed for 48 hours under these circumstances.
7. **Direct fluorescent antibody microscope identification** of egri bodies in brain stem, hippocampus, or frontal cortex is the only reliable method of rabies diagnosis.
8. **If the animal is not immediately available for quarantine or testing,** the patient should undergo local wound care followed by passive immunization with rabies immunoglobulin 20 units/kg (half the dose infiltrated around the wound and the remainder given i.m. in the gluteal area).
9. **Human diploid cell vaccine** (HDCV) or rabies vaccine adsorbed (RVA), 1mL i.m. to the deltoid area, is given on days 0, 3, 7, 14, and 28.
10. **Previously vaccinated patients** do not need rabies immunoglobulin but should receive rabies vaccine on days 0 and 3.

X. SNAKE BITES

A. **TWO FAMILIES OF POISONOUS SNAKES** exist in the United States (Figure 41.2).

1. **Crotalidae** which includes copperheads, cottonmouths, and rattlesnakes.

a. Members of the Crotalidae family are also known as pit vipers because a heat-sensitive pit is located between the eye and the nostril.

b. Pit vipers can be distinguished from nonvenomous snakes by their elliptical pupils, curved fangs, subcaudal scale pattern, and rattles (only in rattlesnakes).

c. Pit viper venom contains 15–20 proteolytic enzymes.

  1) These enzymes alter cell membrane permeability, disrupt hemostasis, and catalyze disseminated intravascular coagulation (DIC).

  2) In addition to proteases, Mojave rattlesnake venom contains neurotoxins, as does the venom of coral snakes.

41

BITES AND STINGS

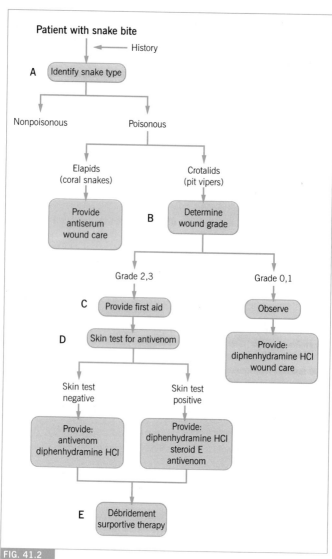

FIG. 41.2
Treatment of patient with snake bite.

d. Signs of pit viper envenomation are more caustic.
   1) Initial symptoms include severe pain and burning, followed by edema, ecchymosis, vesicle and bleb formation, nausea, vomiting, hypotension, hemolysis, and DIC.
   2) Patients also report perioral numbness, a metallic taste in the mouth, lethargy, muscle weakness, ptosis, tremors, or seizure activity.

2. Elapidae, which includes the coral snakes.
a. Coral snakes are small with black snouts and alternating bands of yellow, red, and black.
b. The immediate symptoms following a coral snake bite are mild, but may progress to nausea, vomiting, weakness, diplopia, photophobia, bulbar paralysis, and death.

B. **THE MAJORITY OF SNAKE BITES** occur in July and August with up to 30% of recognized snake bites resulting in no signs or symptoms of envenomation.

C. **TREATMENT.**

1. Immediate transport to the nearest emergency department is key.
a. Field therapy includes immobilization and alignment of the affected extremity below heart level.
b. Constriction bands should be placed 5–10cm proximal to the bite with periodic readjustment to compensate for edema.
c. Distal pulses should be evaluated every 5 minutes.
d. The goal is to minimize absorption in the lymphatics without restricting deep venous and arterial blood flow.
e. Incision and suction is discouraged and cryotherapy is contraindicated.

2. On arrival at the hospital the patient should undergo routine assessment for ABCs and placement of two large-bore i.v. lines, followed by evaluation for degree of envenomation and need for antivenin.
a. Grade 0 – no envenomation.
b. Grade 1 – envenomations are mild and may be treated symptomatically without antivenin.
c. Grade 2 – envenomations are moderate to severe and should be treated with 10–15 vials of anitvenin.
d. Grade 3 – envenomations manifest with severe systemic signs that require an initial dose of 15–20 vials of antivenin.

3. Antivenin is effective only when given intravenously.
a. The initial dose of antivenin should be diluted in 25–50mL of normal saline per vial and given at a rate of 1 drop per 5 seconds.
b. If no adverse effects occur within 30 minutes, the remaining solution may be administered over 2 hours.

    c.   Skin testing is required prior to administration of antivenin in order to prevent anaphylaxis.
       1)   Subcutaneous injection of 0.02–0.03mL of a 1:10 dilution of antivenin is applied to the forearm with a normal saline control.
       2)   If the patient has a positive skin test, but requires antivenin for severe envenomation, i.v. diphenhydramine and hydrocortisone should be given 20 minutes before antivenin infusion. Furthermore, the antivenin should be diluted 1:10 and infused slowly.
    d.   Patients that receive antivenin should be monitored for development of serum sickness which may develop within 3 weeks of administration

4. **If the patient is stable**, the bite wound may be cleansed and debrided.
5. **Tetanus prophylaxis** should be given and broad-spectrum antibiotics initiated, providing coverage against normal skin flora and anaerobic organisms.
6. **Recommended initial lab tests** include CBC, PT, PTT, FSP, fibrinogen, bleeding time, electrolytes, CPK, urinalysis, and arterial blood gases.
7. **Lab work should be repeated every 6 hours** until abnormal parameters stabilize.
8. **Fasciotomy is indicated** only with multiple intracompartment pressure readings >30mmHg.
9. **Pit viper bite victims** that present without signs or symptoms of envenomation and remain asymptomatic in the emergency department for 6 hours may be discharged.

XI. ARTHROPOD AND INSECT BITES

A.   **BLACK WIDOW SPIDER (*LATRODECTUS MACTANS*).**
1. **Venom is neurotoxic to humans** (Figure 41.3).
2. **Bite victims** may present with chest pain following upper extremity bites or abdominal pain after lower extremity bites.
3. **The abdominal pain** is crampy in character and accompanied by abdominal rigidity, mimicking pancreatitis, peptic ulcer, or appendicitis.
4. **Other symptoms** include nausea, vomiting, diaphoresis, vertigo, ptosis, dyspnea, myalgias, and weakness.
5. **Treatment includes:**
    a.   Direct application of an ice pack to the bite area.
    b.   Acute hypertension may be treated with nitroprusside if diastolic blood pressure is >130mmHg.
    c.   Muscle cramps may be relieved with diazepam, methocarbamol, or dantrolene.
    d.   Patients >65 years and <16 years old should receive latrodectus antivenin.

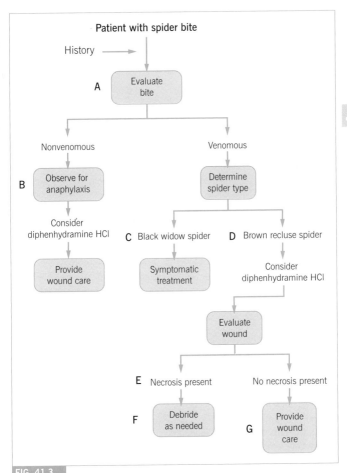

FIG. 41.3
Treatment of patient with spider bite.

B. **BROWN RECLUSE SPIDER** (*LOXOSCELES RECLUSA*).
1. Bites are known to cause local tissue destruction and necrosis.
2. Local effects are due to a levarterenol-like substance that induces severe vasoconstriction and hemolytic enzymes, like sphingomyelinase D.
3. Systemic envenomation may manifest with:
a. Fever.
b. Chills.

c. Rash.

d. Petechiae.

e. Nausea, vomiting, and weakness.

4. **Severe cases of envenomation may lead to:**

a. Intravascular hemolysis.

b. Thrombocytopenia.

c. Renal failure.

d. Pulmonary edema.

e. Death.

5. **Treatment.**

a. Placement of an i.v. line and routine labs (CBC, electrolytes, PT, PTT, urinalysis) should precede local wound care.

b. Excision of the target-like lesion will not prevent local necrosis and may result in more disfigurement.

c. Methylprednisolone 100mg i.v. followed by a prednisone 5-day tapered dose is recommended if the patient presents within 24 hours of the spider bite.

d. Dapsone, 50–200mg p.o. daily, is useful in treating local symptoms.

e. Analgesics and antibiotics should be prescribed if indicated.

C. **POISONOUS SCORPIONS** (*CENTRUROIDES SCULPTURATUS* AND *C. GERTSHI*).

1. **Scorpion venom** exerts its neurotoxic effect by activating sodium channels, thereby inducing repetitive neuronal axon firing.

2. **Initial symptoms** include severe pain at the sting site accompanied by local edema, erythema, hyperesthesia or paresthesia, and weakness.

3. **Later, the patient may develop** blurred vision, muscle spasms, diaphoresis, pseudoseizures, syncope, hemiplegia, cardiac arrhythmias, or respiratory arrest.

4. **Treatment**

a. Apply an ice pack to the sting site.

b. Diazepam may be given for muscle spasms and convulsions.

c. Antivenin is required for severe envenomation.

d. Narcotic analgesics and barbiturates increase venom toxicity and should not be used.

D. **OTHER ARTHROPODS AND INSECTS.** This group includes wasps, yellowjackets, hornets, bumblebees, honeybees, and fireants (Hymenoptera).

1. **Most common reaction** to an insect sting is pain, erythema, and edema.

2. **Treatment includes analgesia** and the application of ice to the affected area.

3. **IgE-mediated hypersensitivity reactions** may manifest within 2–7 days of the incident, and may be difficult to differentiate from cellulitis.

4. **Diphenhydramine**, 50mg p.o. every 6 hours, is recommended along with a prednisone tapered dose.

5. **Anaphylactic reactions** tend to occur within 30 minutes of an insect sting.

a. This may be reversed with epinephrine (1:1000) 0.3mL given subcutaneously or intramuscularly.

b. If the systolic blood pressure is <60mmHg, cutaneous blood flow is insufficient for local absorption. In this case, i.v. epinephrine (1:10,000) should be used and titrated to effect.

c. Diphenhydramine, 50mg i.v., will help reverse bronchoconstriction, coronary artery vasoconstriction, intestinal cramping, and laryngeal edema.

d. Numerous studies have demonstrated a synergistic effect with concomitant use of i.v. H_1 and H_2 antagonists in the treatment of anaphylaxis.

e. Biphasic reactions, characterized by the reappearance of symptoms 6–10 hours after initial treatment and resolution of anaphylaxis, require 80–120mg of i.v. methylprednisolone.

f. Patients with stridor, airway compromise, hypotension, or biphasic response require hospital admission.

XII. FURTHER READING

Dire DJ. Emergency management of dog and cat-bite wounds. *Emerg Med Clin North Am* 1992; 10:719–736.

Fishbein DB, Robinson LE. Rabies. *N Engl J Med* 1993; 329(22):1632–1638.

Forks TP. Evaluation and treatment of snakebites. *Am Fam Physician* 1994; 50(1):123–130.

Griego RD, Rosen T, Orengo IF et al. Dog, cat, and human bites: a review. *J Am Acad Dermatol* 1995; 33(6):1019–1029.

Jerrard DA. Emergency department management of insect stings. *Am J Emerg Med* 1996; 14(4):429–433.

Kelleher AT, Gordon SM. Management of bite wounds and infection in primary care. *Cleve Clin J Med* 1997; 64(3):137–141.

Lewis KT, Stiles, M. Management of cat and dog bites. *Am Fam Physician* 1995; 52(2):479–485.

41

BITES AND STINGS

TRAUMA IN THE PREGNANT PATIENT

I. INTRODUCTION

A. **TRAUMA** is the most frequent cause of death in women younger than 35 years of age and is a leading cause of nonobstetric maternal death.

B. **PROMPT AND PROPER CARE** for the injured obstetric patient requires knowledge of the specific anatomic and physiologic changes that occur in pregnancy.

C. **COOPERATION OF A TRAUMA TEAM** that includes the trauma surgeon, the obstetrician, the emergency department physician, and at times the pediatrician, is essential.

II. ANATOMIC AND PHYSIOLOGIC CHANGES OF PREGNANCY

A. **CARDIOVASCULAR.**

1. **Maternal blood volume.**
   a. Begins to increase in the 1st trimester and near term averages 40–50% above nonpregnant values.
   b. Because more plasma than red blood cells is added to the maternal circulation, an 'anemia' results.
   c. Normal hematocrit levels in the pregnant woman during the 2nd and 3rd trimesters should be between 30 and 36%.
   d. A low hematocrit may be due to an iron deficiency state (common in pregnancy), or, in the trauma patient, to acute blood loss.

2. **Cardiac output.**
   a. Increases by 30–50% by 28–32 weeks over pregravid levels (6.2 ± 1.0L per minute).
   b. Resting heart rate increases by 10–20 beats per minute (83 ± 10 beats per minute).
   c. Blood pressure (BP) decreases in the 1st trimester with a nadir in the 2nd trimester, then begins to return to the prepregnant baseline in the latter part of the 3rd trimester:
      1) 1st trimester mean BP 105/60.
      2) 2nd trimester mean BP 100/54.
      3) 3rd trimester mean BP 110/70.

B. **PULMONARY.**

1. **Minute ventilation** increases by 50%, tidal volume increases by 40%, and minute oxygen consumption increases.

2. **There is a decrease in functional residual capacity and and residual volume** as a result of the elevated diaphragm.

3. **Hormonal changes in pregnancy** cause hyperventilation and a sensation of dyspnea, although the respiratory rate does not change in pregnancy.

4. **Hyperventilation** produces an increase in the partial pressure of oxygen (Po$_2$ 100–105mmHg), as well as a respiratory alkalosis (Pco$_2$ 30mmHg) which is compensated for by a reduction in plasma bicarbonate level.

5. **Pregnant women are in a state of compensated respiratory alkalosis** with an essentially normal blood gas pH measurement.

C. **HEMATOPOIETIC.**

1. **Several coagulation factors** (fibrinogen, VII, VIII, IX, X) as well as the white blood cell count are increased in normal pregnancy.

2. **Fibrinogen levels** average 450mg/dL (4.5g/L) in late pregnancy.

3. **If a trauma patient presents in the latter half of pregnancy** with a normal or low fibrinogen level as well as with elevated fibrin degradation products, consider a consumptive coagulopathy, as with placental abruption.

D. **GASTROINTESTINAL.**

1. **Owing to hormonal factors**, there is decreased lower esophageal sphincter pressure, as well as delayed gastric emptying and intestinal transit time, which increases the risk of gastroesophageal reflux and aspiration.

2. **There is displacement of abdominal viscera cephalad** in the latter part of pregnancy which increases the risk of complex bowel injuries with penetrating trauma to the upper abdomen.

3. **Abdominal tenderness and peritoneal signs** are less obvious in later pregnancy owing to stretching of abdominal musculature and peritoneum.

E. **GENITOURINARY.**

1. **The glomerular filtration rate and renal plasma flow** increase about 50% in pregnancy.

2. **Glucosuria may be present** and is not necessarily abnormal.

3. **Proteinuria and hematuria** are not normal.

4. **There is a mild to moderate amount of hydro-ureter and hydronephrosis** (right > left) in the 2nd and 3rd trimesters due to compression of the ureters by the gravid uterus.

III. INITIAL EVALUATION AND PRIMARY SURVEY

A. **TREATMENT PRIORITIES** are directed toward the injured pregnant woman as they would be to the nonpregnant person.

B. **THE FETUS.** If attention is drawn to the fetus before the patient has been adequately resuscitated and stabilized, life-threatening maternal injuries may be overlooked.

C. **NO RESTRICTION** should be placed on using the usual diagnostic, pharmacologic, or resuscitative procedures or maneuvers.

D. **BASIC RULES OF RESUSCITATION.**

1. **Airway and breathing.**

a. Maintaining a patent airway is of primary importance.

b. Supplemental oxygen should be given because a small increase in maternal oxygen concentration will improve the blood oxygen concentration and reserve for the fetus.

c. Maternal Sao_2 should be maintained >90%.

2. **Circulation**

a. Owing to the hypervolemia of pregnancy, the patient's blood loss may be substantial before she manifests signs of shock.

b. Minor volume depletion may shunt blood from the placenta and comprise the fetal blood supply.

c. Two large-bore peripheral i.v. lines should be placed and crystalloid infused generously.

d. It may be necessary to administer large quantities of fluid and blood to resuscitate the pregnant patient adequately because of her expanded blood volume.

3. **If the patient is >20 weeks pregnant** and her spine has been stabilized, she should be placed in the lateral decubitus position to avoid the supine hypotension syndrome.

4. **In late pregnancy**, in the supine position, the gravid uterus will impede blood return to the heart and therefore decrease cardiac output.

a. This so-called supine hypotension syndrome is characterized by hypotension, dizziness, pallor, tachycardia, sweating, and nausea.

b. The uterus may also compress the aorta, thereby reducing blood flow to the fetus.

c. If the patient is strapped to a backboard, a wedge can be placed beneath her laterally to deflect the uterus.

d. A Foley catheter should be inserted to decompress the bladder, to monitor urine output, and to detect hematuria or hemoglobinuria.

IV. THE SECONDARY SURVEY

1. **Once resuscitation is complete**, a complete history and physical examination are performed.

2. **Obstetricians should be called immediately** to help with determination of fetal gestational age (Figure 42.1) as well as fetal condition, management of the fetus, and any obstetric emergencies.

3. **Fetal heart rate auscultation**, fundal height measurement, cervical examination, assessment of the presence and frequency of contractions using electronic monitoring, and sonographic evaluation of the placenta and fetus are all important in determining fetal age and status and the need for obstetric intervention.

4. **It may be necessary to evaluate the pregnant patient further** using diagnostic peritoneal lavage or radiographic studies.

5. **Irradiation studies**, including CT and angiography, should be performed when indicated, regardless of fetal age, but with the uterus shielded when possible.

42

TRAUMA IN THE PREGNANT PATIENT

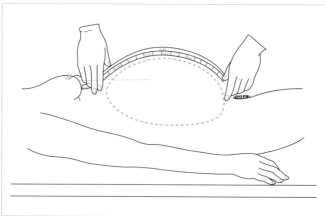

FIG. 42.1
Measuring fundal height in centimeters from the pubic symphysis to the dome of the uterus. (From Alger L, Crenshaw M Jr. Management of the obstetric patient after trauma. In: Siegel JH, ed. *Trauma: emergency surgery and critical care.* New York: Churchill Livingstone; 1978.)

6. **Unnecessary and duplicate films** should be avoided to minimize fetal doses of radiation.
7. **Special consideration should be given to the possibility of splenic injury and retroperitoneal hemorrhage** following blunt trauma, as these are thought to occur more frequently in the pregnant patient, than in the nonpregnant female.
8. **Pelvic fractures are not unique to pregnant patients**; however, there is increased blood flow through the pelvis, which can lead to greater bleeding than in the nonpregnant patient.

V. OPERATIVE PRINCIPLES AND MANAGEMENT

1. **Indications for exploratory celiotomy** are unchanged by pregnancy.
2. **All patients with gunshot wounds should be explored,** as well as patients with stab wounds or blunt trauma who have a positive physical examination or lavage.
3. **If the patient has been adequately resuscitated,** the fetus will usually tolerate the stress of surgery and anesthesia.
4. **Prior to celiotomy,** if possible, the fetus should be examined for gestational age and condition using sonography, cardiotocographic monitoring, and possibly amniocentesis.
5. **During the exploration, the uterus may be retracted** out of the operative field provided that blood flow to the uterus is not compromised.

6. **The uterus must be carefully examined** for evidence of penetrating injury, at the time of exploratory celiotomy.
7. **If the uterus has been injured** and there is evidence for fetal jeopardy in a viable fetus (i.e. >25 weeks estimated gestational age), cesarean delivery should be considered.
8. **If the fetus appears to be in good condition or is previable,** repair of the uterus and expectant management may be indicated.
9. **If the fetus is dead,** either cesarean delivery or induction of labor with vaginal delivery may be indicated, depending on the location and extent of the uterine injury.
10. **Celiotomy itself is not an indication for cesarean section:** consideration is given to fetal age and condition, extent of uterine injury, and whether treatment or evaluation of the mother's injuries at the time of operation is hindered by the gravid uterus.
11. **Cesarean section prolongs the operative procedure** and increases blood loss by approximately 100mL, so therefore should be performed only as indicated.

VI. OBSTETRIC EMERGENCIES IN THE TRAUMA PATIENT

A. TRAUMATIC PLACENTAL ABRUPTION.

1. **Abruptio placentae, or premature separation of the normally implanted placenta,** complicates 1–6% of minor injuries and up to 50% of major injuries.
2. **This should be high on the list of differential diagnoses** when the injured gravid patient presents with shock, disseminated intravascular coagulation, uterine tenderness, vaginal bleeding, ruptured fetal membranes, fetal jeopardy, or fetal death.
3. **In some cases of placental abruption,** there may be no vaginal bleeding or other physical findings and the abruption may be confused with labor.
4. **Cardiotocographic monitoring** is the most sensitive method for detecting abruption and subtle signs of fetal jeopardy.
5. **Monitoring should begin as soon as possible** after maternal stabilization in women of 20–22 weeks estimated gestational age (EGA).
6. **Women are typically monitored** in the labor and delivery suite for a minimum of 4–6 hours.
7. **If contractions or an unreassuring fetal heart rate tracing is noted,** monitoring is usually extended for at least 24 hours.
8. **The following blood tests should be performed:** CBC, PT, PTT, d-dimers, Kleihauer–Betke stain, fibrinogen, group, screen and hold (GSH), and a red-top tube (thrombin clot).
9. **Placental abruption is one of the most common causes of consumptive coagulopathy** in obstetrics, and in abruption severe enough to kill a fetus.
10. **Blood loss accompanied by hypofibrinogenemia may be substantial.**

11. **In a patient with placental abruption and a live fetus of viable gestational age**, the decision to deliver the fetus and the mode of delivery must be made by experienced obstetricians after stabilization of the mother.

12. **In Rh negative women** with evidence of fetomaternal hemorrhage, Rhogam must be given to prevent Rh iso-immunization.

B. UTERINE RUPTURE.

1. **This an uncommon event** occurring in <1% of blunt trauma, but it must be considered especially if the patient has suffered direct and intense force to the uterus.

2. **Rupture of the uterus** results in rapid deterioration of the mother and the fetus.

3. **The diagnosis** of uterine rupture may be suspected by history, physical examination, or radiologic studies, but often the diagnosis is not confirmed until celiotomy.

4. **Repair of the uterus is possible**, but emergency hysterectomy is often required.

C. FETAL INJURY AND FETAL JEOPARDY.

1. **The risk of fetal injury is high** when factors such as hypoxia, head injury, pelvic fracture, placental injury, and shock are present in the mother.

2. **Direct fetal injury** occurs two-thirds of the time when the uterus sustains penetrating trauma.

3. **Fetal skull and brain injury** are especially common with pelvic fractures in gravid women in which the fetal head is presenting and engaged in the pelvis.

4. **Fetal jeopardy in a viable fetus** can be diagnosed with electronic monitoring and an experienced obstetrician.

5. **If the mother has been adequately stabilized**, emergency cesarean section may be considered.

D. UMBILICAL CORD PROLAPSE.

1. **Spontaneous rupture of fetal membranes** has been seen either with or without contractions following blunt trauma.

2. **If the presenting fetal part is not well engaged in the maternal pelvis**, the fetal umbilical cord may prolapse into the vagina.

3. **This condition requires emergency cesarean delivery** in a viable fetus, as fetal hypoxia and death will quickly ensue.

E. IMPENDING MATERNAL DEATH

1. **In the case of a dead or moribund pregnant patient**, the decision to perform emergency cesarean delivery must be made quickly, as fetal survival is unlikely if >20 minutes have elapsed since the death of the mother.

2. **Consideration is given to fetal age** (>25 weeks EGA is considered viable), and fetal condition (presence and rate of fetal heart tones).

3. **The senior pediatrician,** the pediatric resuscitation team, and, if possible, the neonatologist should be present at delivery.

VII. FURTHER READING

Alger L, Crenshaw M Jr. Management of the obstetric patient after trauma. In: Siegel JH, ed. *Trauma: emergency surgery and critical care.* New York: Churchill Livingstone; 1978:1075–1098.

American College of Obstetricians and Gynecologists. *Trauma during pregnancy.* Technical Bulletin No 161. ACOG Nov 1991.

Crosby WM. Trauma during pregnancy; maternal and fetal injuries. *Obstet Gynecol Surg* 1974; 29:683.

Cunningham FG, Clark SL et al. Trauma. In: *Operative obstetrics,* 1st edn. Norwalk: Appleton and Lange; 1995.

Cunningham FG, MacDonald PC, Gant NF et al. Critical care and trauma. In: *Williams obstetrics,* 20th edn. Norwalk: Appleton and Lange; 1997.

Esposito TJ, Gens DR, Smith LG et al. Trauma during pregnancy: a review of 79 cases. *Arch Surg* 1991; *126*:1073.

Kissinger DP, Rozycki GS, Morris JA Jr et al. Trauma in pregnancy: predicting pregnancy outcome. *Arch Surg* 1991; 126:1079.

PEDIATRIC TRAUMA

I. INTRODUCTION
1. **Priorities, evaluation, and management** same as for the adult.
2. **Remember the ABCs.**

II. ANATOMIC DIFFERENCES AND THEIR SEQUELAE
1. **Relatively larger head** – increased frequency of head injury.
2. **Larger tongue and anterior larynx** – different intubation technique.
3. **Increased body surface area** – increased heat loss.
4. **Compliant chest and abdomen** – internal injury without evidence of external trauma.

III. PHYSIOLOGIC DIFFERENCES
1. **Stroke volume relatively fixed;** thus increased heart rate required for increased cardiac output.
2. **Hypotension** is a late manifestation of blood loss.
3. **Hypothermia** is common, especially with increased body surface area.

IV. OCCULT INJURIES
1. **Spine dislocation from torn ligaments** in the absence of a fracture.
2. **Myocardial and pulmonary contusion** without rib or sternal fracture.
3. **Vascular injury** – intimal disruption with delayed occlusion.
4. **Nondisplaced fractures** in the unconscious child.
5. **Intestinal injuries.**

V. RESUSCITATION
A. AIRWAY.
1. **Similar to the adult using an oral or nasopharyngeal airway** preceded by a chin lift or jaw thrust.
2. **Indications for intubation** include:
   a. Apnea.
   b. Severe head injury – Glasgow Coma Score (GCS) <9.
   c. Facial injury.
   d. Severe hypotension.
3. **Infants and young children have an anterior airway** and a relatively larger tongue.
4. **Intubation is accomplished without neck extension** using a noncuffed endotracheal tube.
   a. Tube size should approximate the patient's fifth finger size.
   b. Tube size can also be calculated by taking the patient's age plus 16 and dividing by 4.

5. **A surgical airway** is rarely required.
6. **A tracheostomy** should be performed in children under the age of 7 years.
7. **Children over the age of 7 years** may have a cricothyroidotomy performed.
8. **The cricoid cartilage is the only complete ring in the upper airway** and damage to this cartilage, in young children, may necessitate tracheal reconstruction.

B. BREATHING.
1. **Oxygen is indicated** whether or not the patient is intubated.
2. **Tidal volumes** of 10–15mL/kg with respiratory rate varying by age (Table 43.1).

C. CIRCULATION.
1. **Frequent assessment of volume status** is needed.
a. A normal heart rate and good capillary refill are signs of adequate volume status.
b. Do not rely on blood pressure alone.
2. **Preferred vascular access:**
a. Two upper extremity i.v. lines.
b. Saphenous vein cutdown or interosseous lines are indicated if unable to achieve i.v. access.
3. **Fluid administration** is 20mL/kg of Ringer's lactate as a bolus.
a. Bolus may be repeated 1–2 times.
b. If the patient remains unstable, then transfuse with 10mL/kg of packed red blood cells.
4. **Cardiopulmonary resuscitation** in accordance with the Pediatric Advanced Cardiac Life Support guidelines is indicated for the patient in cardiac arrest (Table 43.2).

VI. PHYSICAL EXAMINATION

1. **The physical findings and injury pattern** in children vary from those in the adult.

TABLE 43.1

NORMAL PEDIATRIC VITAL SIGNS

Age	Blood pressure (mmHg)	Pulse (beats per minute)	Respiration rate (breaths per minute)
Neonate	70/40	120–160	30–60
3–12 months	90/50	90–140	30–60
1–6 years	95/60	80–110	20–35
6–12 years	100/70	70–100	16–25
>12 years	120/70	60–90	8–16

TABLE 43.2

PEDIATRIC PATIENT IN CARDIAC ARREST

Medication	Dosage (mg/kg)
Atropine	0.02
Calcium chloride	20
Dextrose	0.5
Epinephrine	0.1
Lidocaine	1
Sodium bicarbonate	1
Succinylcholine	1

43

PEDIATRIC TRAUMA

2. **Knowledge of these differences** will allow accurate assessment and prompt treatment as the physician completes the primary and secondary surveys.

VII. SPECIFIC INJURIES

A. BRAIN INJURIES.

1. **Brain injury is the primary cause of death** and disability in children.
2. **Most injuries are traumatic brain injuries** without subdural or epidural hematomas.
3. **Prevention of secondary injury** is aided by maintaining adequate oxygenation and cerebral perfusion as well as preventing brain swelling.
4. **The GCS** has been adapted for children (Table 43.3). Rapid assessment of neurologic status with a thorough examination and liberal use of CT scan in those patients with a suspicion of injury is indicated.
5. **Indications for a CT scan** include:
a. Loss of consciousness.
b. Neurologic deficit.
c. GCS <15.

TABLE 43.3

GLASGOW COMA SCORE ADAPTED FOR CHILDREN

Verbalization:	
Appropriate for age, fixes and follows, social smile	5
Cries but consolable	4
Persistently irritable	3
Restless, lethargic	2
None	1
Motor:	
Spontaneous movement	6

All other motor and all eye-opening scores are the same as for an adult.

6. **Epidural hematomas** are the most common surgical mass lesion seen in children as opposed to subdural hematomas in adults.
7. **Patients with increased intracranial pressure** (ICP) should have their ICP monitored with the goal of maintaining cerebral perfusion pressure (CPP) of 50mmHg.
a. CPP = mean arterial pressure − ICP.
b. Maintaining CPP can be done by:
    1) Hyperventilation to Pco_2 of 30–35mmHg (not generally recommended).
    2) Mannitol.
    3) Judicious fluid management.
    4) Adequate sedation.
    5) Occasionally pentobarbital coma.
8. **Bulging fontanelles** can be an indication of intracranial swelling or bleeding in the very young child.
9. **Traumatic brain injury** is a significant problem in the pediatric population and is implicated in as many as 75% of the deaths in children resulting from blunt trauma.
B. **SPINE INJURIES.**
1. **Dislocation of the spine** can occur without fracture.
2. **Ligamentous injuries to the cervical spine** will result in an unstable spine with possible cord injury.
3. **Children with altered consciousness**, or those under the age of 8 years, should be maintained with the neck in neutral position until cervical spine films are obtained regardless of the presence or absence of tenderness.
4. **The neutral position of the spine in children** under age 5 years is accomplished by having the shoulders elevated 2.0–2.5cm on a foam pad or blanket.
5. **Elevation of the shoulders** in this fashion will eliminate the pseudosubluxation that is seen on the lateral cervical spine films of these patients.
6. **Evaluation of the ligaments**, in patients without a reliable examination, can be done with sagittal magnetic resonance imaging (MRI) of the cervical spine.
7. **Knowledge of the mechanism of the injury** will help determine which patients will benefit from MRI studies.
8. **Children over the age of 8 years** may be evaluated for cervical injury in a similar fashion to adults.
9. **Lumbar spine injury** (Chance fracture) must be ruled out in children with lap belt injuries.
C. **CHEST.**
1. **Pulmonary contusion, pneumothorax, and hemothorax** may be present in the absence of rib fractures.

2. **Significant force is required** to break the pliable ribs.
3. **A high index of suspicion should be present** for underlying injuries, including cardiac contusion, pulmonary contusion, aortic injuries, and liver and splenic injuries in patients with rib fractures.

D. **ABDOMEN.**

1. **A CT of the abdomen** remains the standard for evaluation of children with blunt abdominal trauma.
2. **Diagnostic peritoneal lavage** (DPL) is occasionally performed in patients with lap-belt imprints and suspected bowel injury.
3. **The majority of solid organ injuries** are managed nonoperatively with careful assessment of the hemodynamic status as well as hematocrit.
4. **A blush of contrast seen in the liver or spleen** on a CT scan is an indication of active bleeding and is likely to increase the need for surgery.
5. **Most deaths from abdominal trauma** result from injuries to the liver, which involve either the portal or hepatic veins.
6. **Successful management** depends on:
   a. Early recognition of the need for surgery.
   b. Adequate pre operative and intraoperative blood volume replacement.
   c. Control of bleeding by clamping of the porta hepatis.
   d. Exposure and suture of the bleeding veins before blood loss exceeds one blood volume.
   e. Avoiding hypothermia and coagulopathies.
7. **Pancreatic injury** seen on CT warrants early exploration.
8. **Distal pancreatectomy with splenic salvage** is indicated when the patient has a transection to the left of the superior mesenteric vessels.
9. **Renal injuries** are most often managed by observation.
   a. Nonfunction of a kidney on CT should be evaluated with angiography.
   b. Operative repair should be completed within 4–6 hours of injury if renal function is to be salvaged.
10. **Hyperflexion mechanisms,** secondary to lap belts plus deceleration, are associated with injuries to the:
    a. Small bowel.
    b. Duodenum.
    c. Pancreas.
    d. Lumbar spine.
    e. Liver and spleen, to a lesser extent.
11. **Unrestrained children in motor vehicle collisions** have a higher incidence of head and solid organ injuries.
12. **Motor–pedestrian collisions** have a higher incidence of head injury as well as solid organ injuries and long bone fractures.
13. **DPL is used in the evaluation** of the hemodynamically unstable patient or in the patient who needs to go immediately to the operating room.

43

PEDIATRIC TRAUMA

14. **Warmed Ringer's lactate should be infused** into the peritoneal cavity as follows:
a.   1000mL in adult patients.
b.   500mL in a child.
c.   250mL in an infant.
15. **DPL is considered positive if:**
a.   Blood is aspirated prior to instillation of the lavage fluid.
b.   The red cell count is >200,000/mm^3 in a child.
c.   The red cell count is >400,000/mm^3 in an infant.
d.   The white blood cell count is >500/mm^3.
e.   There is bile, amylase, or particulate matter in the lavage fluid.

E.   MUSCULOSKELETAL TRAUMA.
1.   **Radiologic examination** of the contralateral extremity is helpful in making an accurate diagnosis.
2.   **Supracondylar fractures of the humerus** and fracture dislocations of the knee and ankle have a high likelihood of vascular injury.
3.   **Concern for child abuse should be raised** any time there is variation in the history or the history is not consistent with the injuries present.
4.   **Abuse should be suspected** if a young child has had multiple previous injuries or old fractures are seen radiographically.
5.   **When abuse is suspected** the appropriate authorities must be notified.

VIII. FURTHER READING

Committee on Trauma. *Advanced trauma life support program instructor manual*. Chicago: American College of Surgeons; 1997.
Oneal JA (ed.) *Pediatric Surgery*, 5th edn. St Louis: Mosby; 1998:235–365.

GERIATRIC TRAUMA

44

I. DEMOGRAPHICS

A. **THE ELDERLY** is the fastest-growing sector of the United States population and it is estimated that by the year 2050, 40% of all trauma patients will be ≥ 65 years of age.

B. **THE MORTALITY RATE FOR ELDERLY TRAUMA PATIENTS** is six times higher than younger trauma patients, even after controlling for injury severity.

C. **PATIENTS >65 YEARS OF AGE** consume nearly one-third of the health care resources expended for trauma care in the United States.

II. PHYSIOLOGIC CHANGES

A. **CARDIOVASCULAR.**

1. **Decrease in cardiac output and stroke volume** secondary to decreased compliance.

2. **Decrease in the number of β-adrenergic receptors,** resulting in decreased responsiveness to catecholamines.

B. **RENAL.** There is a decrease in the glomerular filtration rate and in concentrating ability.

C. **THESE CHANGES** can make measurements such as heart rate, blood pressure, and urine output difficult to use as end points of resuscitation in the elderly trauma patient.

III. TREATMENT

A. **INITIAL TREATMENT.** Although initial resuscitation of an elderly patient is no different than for other patients (airway, breathing, and circulation), these patients require very close monitoring and consideration of their physiologic reserve. The key to their care is recognizing subtle signs of decompensation and avoiding iatrogenic complications.

B. **MONITORING.** Early invasive monitoring in the ICU with pulmonary artery catheterization may improve survival in geriatric blunt trauma patients.

1. **Patients who appear hemodynamically stable** by standard monitoring may have dangerously low cardiac outputs after placement of pulmonary artery catheters.

2. **By identifying these patients,** fluid, blood, or inotropes can be used to improve hypoperfusion.

C. **INTENSIVE CARE.** At Parkland Memorial Hospital elderly trauma patients are admitted to the ICU within 2 hours of arrival at the emergency room.

1. **Evaluation is completed in the ICU** while these patients undergo aggressive resuscitation with pulmonary artery catheter, arterial lines, serum lactate levels, and gastric tonometry.
2. **Monitoring** of all but the most mildly injured geriatric trauma patients is routine in the ICU using pulmonary artery catheters and serial blood gases.

IV. FURTHER READING

MacKenzie EJ, Morris JA Jr, Smith GS et al. Acute hospital costs of trauma in the United States: implications for regionalized systems of care. *J Trauma* 1990; 29:1096.

Osler T , Hales K, Baack B et al. Trauma in the elderly. *Am J Surg* 1988; 156:537–543.

Scalea TM , Simon HM, Duncan AO et al. Geriatric blunt multiple trauma: improved survival with early invasive monitoring. *J Trauma* 1990; 30:129–136.

Schwab CW, Kauder DR. Trauma in the geriatric patient. *Arch Surg* 1992; 127:701–706.

ANESTHESIA FOR THE TRAUMA PATIENT

I. PREOPERATIVE PREPARATION

A. **INITIAL ASSESSMENT,** evaluation of airway, and physical examination are essential by the anesthesia team.

B. **A DESIGNATED OPERATING ROOM** set up for trauma and readily available with uncross-matched blood (type O, Rh negative) are imperative for unstable trauma patients.

45

C. **STANDARD ANESTHESIA EQUIPMENT.** The standard equipment for a trauma case includes the following:

1. **Anesthesia machine checked and operational**, suction apparatus, and monitors.
2. **Airway equipment**: several sizes of endotracheal tubes.
3. **Laryngoscopy blades** (two sizes) and emergency airway equipment.
4. **Laryngeal mask airways.**
5. **Cricothyroidotomy kit.**
6. **High-flow i.v. fluid infusion devices**, blood warmers (e.g. level I), and automatic transfusers (e.g. cell saver).
7. **Vasoactive medications and anesthetic agents** (drawn up and clearly labeled).
8. **Warming blankets** and a warm trauma room.
9. **Adequate personnel.**

D. **ANESTHETIC DRUGS.**

1. **Induction agents.**
   a. Etomidate (0.2mg/kg).
   b. Ketamine (1–2mg/kg).
   c. Other induction agents may be used if patient is hemodynamically stable and shows no signs of hypovolemia (e.g. sodium thiopental, propofol).

2. **Intubation.**
   a. Succinylcholine (1–2mg/kg).
      1) May cause bradycardia with repeated doses, especially in children.
      2) May cause hyperkalemia and cardiovascular collapse in patients with severe burns, electrolyte imbalance, severe trauma, paraplegia, spinal cord injury, upper motoneuron injury, or muscular dystrophy.
      3) Succinylcholine is contraindicated in patients with genetic disorders of plasma pseudocholinesterases, a family history of malignant hyperthermia, and penetrating eye injuries.
   b. Rocuronium (1mg/kg).
      1) Rapid onset of 60 seconds.
      2) Useful for rapid sequence induction when succinylcholine is contraindicated.

3. **Maintenance agents** – avoid histamine-releasing agents.
a. Rocuronium (0.06–0.6mg/kg).
b. Vecuronium (0.01–0.05mg/kg).
c. Pancuronium (0.01–0.05mg/kg).
4. **Inhalational anesthetic agents.**
a. Carefully titrated.
b. Avoid nitrous oxide to prevent expansion of possible pneumothorax, bowel distension.
5. **Benzodiazepines** – used intraoperatively to prevent recall.
a. Midazolam – 1–4mg i.v. every 1–2 hours.
b. Lorazepam – 1–4mg i.v. every 6–12 hours.
6. **Narcotics** .
a. Carefully titrated.
b. Avoid histamine-releasing agents like morphine.
7. **Resuscitation agents.**
a. Epinephrine – 10–100μg (1.0mg i.v. every 3–5 minutes for cardiac arrest).
b. Sodium bicarbonate – 1mL/kg.
c. Atropine – 0.5–1.0mg i.v.
d. Calcium chloride – 500–1000mg i.v.
e. Lidocaine – 0.5–1.0mg/kg.
f. Ephedrine – 5–10mg i.v.
g. Phenylephrine – 50–100μg i.v.

II. OPERATING ROOM

A. ANESTHETIC TECHNIQUE.

1. **Regional technique** if appropriate for the injury to isolate the limbs and if the patient is hemodynamically stable.
2. **General anesthesia** is required for most trauma patients, especially those with multiple injuries.

B. AIRWAY.

1. **Many hypotensive patients** arrive in the operating room already intubated.
2. **Endotracheal intubation must be reconfirmed** with bilateral breath sounds and evidence of end tidal CO_2 on a capnograph.
3. **All trauma patients should be considered to have a full stomach**.
4. **Awake intubation or rapid sequence induction** should always be performed with cricoid pressure to compress the esophagus and prevent reflux.
5. **Cervical spine stabilization** must be held during intubation if the C-spine has not been cleared by radiography or CT scan.
6. **Airway management can be particularly complex** and requires careful planning in facial, head, and neck trauma.
7. **Consider awake tracheostomy under local anesthesia** if there is uncertainty about the airway.

8. **In emergency situations** the best sequence for intubation is as follows:

a. Give Bicitra 30mL orally and pre-oxygenate with 100% oxygen for 5 minutes.

b. Remove anterior portion of cervical collar and have assistant hold gentle axial traction.

c. Have another assistant apply cricoid pressure starting with induction and continued until endotracheal intubation is confirmed with bilateral breath sounds.

d. Have an experienced laryngoscopist insert endotracheal tube, visualizing the vocal cords with minimal head movement.

e. Confirm endotracheal intubation and replace cervical collar.

C. MAINTENANCE OF ANESTHESIA.

1. **Arterial lines are convenient prior to induction** and are useful for continuous blood pressure monitoring, and serial arterial blood gas and hematocrit determinations.

2. **Use a central venous line or a pulmonary artery catheter** if indicated.

3. **Oxygen, muscle relaxant, and lorazepam** may be the sole anesthetic agents until hypotension and hypovolemia are resolved.

a. Must have good communication between anesthesiologist and surgeons (surgeons may need to pack and allow time for 'catching up').

b. Prevention of hypothermia is important because of myocardial dysfunction, dysrhythmias, coagulopathy, and acidosis that can occur in the cold patient.

   1) Monitor core temperature (esophageal is best).
   2) Warm the room prior to patient arrival.
   3) Warm all i.v. fluids and blood products, use a heated humidifier to warm inhaled gases, use a warming blanket on operating room table, and BAIR™ hugger on upper or lower torso.
   4) Use warm irrigating solutions.

III. FLUID AND BLOOD REPLACEMENT

1. **Ringer's lactate solution or Plasmalyte solution**, along with blood transfusions, are used as necessary for adequate resuscitation.

2. **If a transfusion must be started before a patient's blood type can be determined**, type O Rh negative blood is generally used.

3. **In massive blood transfusions**, dilutional coagulopathy may develop after 1.5 times the patient's blood volume has been transfused.

4. **Fresh-frozen plasma and platelet concentrates** are usually needed after replacement of 1.5 patient blood volumes but should be given based on laboratory data and evidence of 'oozing' or coagulopathy from the surgical field.

5. **In patients with massive continuing hemorrhage:**

a. Keep hematocrit at 30%.

b. Follow labs every 30–60 minutes: hemoglobin, hematocrit, platelet count, PT, PTT, fibrinogen, and electrolytes.
c. Give calcium chloride, 1g, after 1 patient blood volume in packed red blood cells has been given.
d. Infuse platelets after 1.5 patient blood volumes.
e. Infuse fresh-frozen plasma, 2 units, after every 1.5 patient blood volumes.
f. Consider cryoprecipitate after 20 units of packed red blood cells have been given.

IV. ANESTHETIC MANAGEMENT OF THE PREGNANT TRAUMA PATIENT

1. **Surgery is delayed until the 2nd trimester**, if possible.
2. **Regional anesthesia is used**, if possible.
3. **To help relieve anxiety and avoid benzodiazepines** for premedication, the patient is visited before surgery.
4. **Use pentothal for induction, narcotics and inhalational agents for maintenance**: a decreased minimum alveolar concentration for inhalational agents is needed in pregnant patients.
5. **The stomach is emptied** before induction.
6. **Left uterine displacement** is provided.
7. **Premedicate** with Bicitra 30mL, pre-oxygenate, and use rapid sequence induction with cricoid pressure.
8. **Nitrous oxide is avoided**, <50% is used.
9. **Hypotension is treated aggressively** with fluids or ephedrine as the vasopressor of choice to maintain uteroplacental blood flow.
10. **Fetal heart rate is monitored** if the gestational age is >16 weeks.
11. **Uterine activity is recorded** intraoperatively.

V. FURTHER READING

Kirby RR, Brown D. Massive transfusion. In: *Anesthesia for trauma*. Boston: Little, Brown and Co.; 1987:61–71.

Lopez-Viego MA. Anesthesia in trauma. In: *The Parkland trauma handbook*. St Louis: Mosby; 1994:627–630.

Morgan GE, Mikhail MS. Anesthesia for the trauma patient In: *Clinical anesthesiology*, 2nd edn. Norwalk: Appleton and Lange; 1996:683–691.

CARDIOVASCULAR SUPPORT AND MANAGEMENT IN THE INTENSIVE CARE UNIT

I. INTRODUCTION

A. COMMON SYNDROMES. The most common syndromes of cardiac abnormality in the intensive care unit at Parkland Memorial Hospital, following multiple trauma, are:

1. **Primary cardiac dysfunction** (valvular disease or injury, blunt cardiac injury, and myocardial ischemia).
2. **Dysfunction secondary to shock**.
3. **Fluid overload**.
4. **Sepsis**.

B. HYPOVOLEMIC SHOCK.

1. **This is the result of inadequate resuscitation**, third-space losses, or ongoing hemorrhage which occurs soon after injury.
2. **The management** of this problem consists mainly of fluid and blood replacement, as discussed in Chapter 7.

C. CARDIOGENIC SHOCK. This can result from over-aggressive fluid resuscitation, blunt cardiac injury, valvular disease, or injury as well as cardiac dysrhythmias.

II. MEASUREMENTS AND ESTIMATES OF CARDIAC FUNCTION

A. PULMONARY ARTERY WEDGE PRESSURE (PAWP).

1. **Balloon occlusion of the proximal blood flow** in the pulmonary capillaries estimates left atrial pressure and closely approximates left ventricular end diastolic pressure (LVEDP).
2. **The PAWP response to fluid challenge** is a better indicator of volume status than the actual pressure measurement.
3. **The normal range** is 5–10mmHg.

B. CARDIAC OUTPUT.

1. **This is measured as the area under a thermodilution curve**.
2. **This value is the most useful indicator of cardiac function** and is used to determine if a patient is in septic shock or hypovolemic shock.
3. **The normal range** is 5–8L/min.
4. **This value can be indexed to body surface area** and the normal value is 3.5L/min/m^2.

C. RIGHT VENTRICULAR END DIASTOLIC VOLUME (RVEDV).

1. **RVEDV has been shown to be as accurate** and occasionally more accurate than PAWP in estimating volume status.

2. **It is a good estimate of left ventricular function** in patients with normal ventricular wall compliance.
3. **It is measured** with a pulmonary artery catheter and the normal range is 113–225mL or 88mL/m^2.

D. **MIXED VENOUS OXYGEN TENSION.**
1. **Pulmonary artery catheters** equipped with an oximeter at the catheter tip can measure the continuous oxygen tension of mixed venous blood (Smvo$_2$) in the pulmonary artery.
2. **The trend of the Smvo$_2$ is closely monitored** as it may be the first indication of changes in the patient's condition.
3. **Desaturation of Smvo$_2$** may indicate a falling cardiac output, decrease in hemoglobin (hemorrhage), falling SaO$_2$ (hypoxemia), increasing oxygen consumption, or decreased oxygen delivery.
4. **A high Smvo$_2$** may be present in patients with reduced peripheral oxygen consumption, such as septic shock and cyanide poisoning.
5. **The normal value** is 73–80%.

E. **VASCULAR RESISTANCE.**
1. **The systemic vascular resistance index** (SVRI) is a value derived from the equation (MAP–CVP)/CI, where MAP = mean arterial pressure, CVP = central venous pressure, and CI = cardiac index.
2. **The SVRI is used in patients with low CI** to determine the need for vasodilator therapy.
3. **Patients with low CI and high SVRI** will usually benefit from reduction in SVRI, thus improving oxygen delivery to their tissues.
4. **The normal value** is 25L/min/m^2. This value can be multiplied by 80 to convert to dynes/sec.cm^5.

F. **OXYGEN TRANSPORT AND DELIVERY.**
1. **The amount of oxygen delivered to the tissues** (Do$_2$) depends on the cardiac index and the oxygen content of blood: CI × Cao$_2$.
2. **The normal value** is 607mL O$_2$/min/m^2.
3. **Low values can be increased** by increasing CI or determinants of Cao$_2$, such as hemoglobin and arterial oxygen saturation.

G. **OXYGEN CONSUMPTION (Vo$_2$).**
1. **This is the difference between** oxygen delivered by the heart and oxygen returned to the heart: CI × (Cao$_2$ – Cmvo$_2$).
2. **The normal value** is 140mL O$_2$/min/m^2.
3. **Decreases in oxygen consumption** may indicate reduced peripheral oxygen utilization, as in patients with sepsis.

III. HYPOVOLEMIC SHOCK AND RESUSCITATION

1. **Clinical abnormalities** that suggest inadequate resuscitation or ongoing hemorrhage after initial resuscitation (see Chapter 7) include:
a. Hypotension.
b. Oliguria.
c. Metabolic acidosis.
d. Sinus tachycardia.

2. The presence of these findings should prompt re-evaluation and continuous resuscitation while the source of the hemorrhage is identified.
3. Invasive monitoring with a pulmonary artery catheter or central venous line and arterial line should be instituted.
4. Indications for pulmonary artery catheter insertion in the multiply injured patient at Parkland include persistent hemodynamic instability in the setting of:
a. Septic shock.
b. Suspected cardiac injury or myocardial ischemia.
c. Severe pulmonary contusion.

IV. SEPTIC SHOCK

1. Though uncommon in the early postinjury course, septic shock is a common cause of mortality in the intensive care unit.
2. Septic shock usually presents within days to weeks after injury and manifests as a hyperdynamic state (high cardiac outputs 10–15L/min, low SVRI, <1200dynes/sec.cm^5, and increased oxygen consumption) in the presence of signs of sepsis (fever, hypothermia, tachycardia, and cutaneous vasodilatation).
3. Treatment is directed at the causes of sepsis, such as pneumonia, intra-abdominal or severe wound infections, missed injuries, or tissue necrosis.
4. Supportive management of the patient in septic shock can be achieved with norepinephrine or epinephrine (see below) to maintain blood pressure and tissue perfusion, pending removal or definitive treatment of the septic focus.

V. CARDIOGENIC SHOCK

1. The syndrome of low cardiac output and high filling pressures (PAWP, RVEDV, CVP) suggests primary cardiac dysfunction, such as myocardial ischemia or infarction, blunt myocardial injury, pericardial tamponade, or, more commonly, fluid overload from overly aggressive resuscitation.
2. If excessive fluid administration is the source, then diuretics, such as furosemide (40–80mg i.v.) will usually improve end diastolic volumes and allow for optimal contractility.
3. In patients with myocardial ischemia or infarction, treatment with β-blockers, anticoagulants, and thrombolytic agents should be commenced only after consultation with a cardiologist and a trauma surgeon, since these interventions are prone to cause serious complications in the multiply injured patient .
4. Insertion of an intra-aortic balloon for cardiac support is a last resort in patients with primary cardiac dysfunction which is unresponsive to inotropes and vasodilator therapy.

VI. CARDIAC ARRHYTHMIAS

A. PATHOPHYSIOLOGY.

1. **All cardiac dysrhythmias** are caused by either automaticity, or re-entrant current.

2. **The causes of automaticity include**:

a. Hypokalemia.

b. Hypercalcemia.

c. Hypoxia.

d. Increased serum catecholamines.

3. **Re-entrant dysrhythmias** are a result of local tissue conduction delay caused by:

a. Ischemia.

b. Necrosis.

c. Fibrosis.

B. EVALUATION AND MANAGEMENT.

1. **During the care of a patient with an acute dysrhythmia**, it is less important to identify the exact rhythm than to identify what category of dysrhythmia is present.

2. **A 12-lead EKG and serum cardiac enzymes** are routinely obtained at Parkland.

3. **A rapid evaluation needs to be performed** as follows:

a. Is the patient hemodynamically stable?

   1) All hemodynamically unstable patients with acute dysrhythmias should be treated by immediate cardioversion.

   2) The exception to this rule is patients with asystole.

   3) The initial energy level is at least 100J and this can be increased up to a maximum of 400J.

   4) Hemodynamically stable patients can be evaluated depending on the ventricular rate.

b. Is the ventricular rate slow (<60) or fast (>100)?

   1) Slow ventricular rates will usually respond to atropine 0.5mg i.v. This dose can be repeated at 2-minute intervals.

   2) If atropine is unsuccessful, transcutaneous pacing will restore rhythm.

   3) Rapid ventricular rates can be a result of supraventricular tachycardia (SVT), atrial fibrillation, ectopic ventricular foci, or ventricular tachycardia or fibrillation. The first two conditions can be differentiated from the last two by the QRS complex width.

c. Is the QRS complex narrow (<0.08 sec, two small boxes) or wide (>0.08 sec, two small boxes)?

   1) This distinction is important because wide-complex tachycardias require cardioversion and lidocaine

   2) Narrow tachycardias can be safely treated with Verapamil.

d. Narrow-complex tachycardias
   1) Narrow-complex tachycardias are usually supraventricular in origin (sinus tachycardia, paroxysmal supraventricular tachycardia, atrial fibrillation).
   2) They are generally benign compared with the wide-complex arrhythmias.
   3) The exception is a junctional or ventricular ectopic focus, with transmission through aberrant pathways, presenting as a narrow complex tachycardia.
   4) If a narrow-complex rhythm is observed, an attempt should be made to identify the P waves, since the absence of P waves would differentiate atrial fibrillation from paroxysmal SVT.
   5) This differentiation may be difficult to determine in a patient with a heart rate over 160–180 beats per minute.
   6) Occasionally, adenosine 6mg i.v. over 2 seconds is administered at Parkland while obtaining a rhythm strip.
   7) This slows AV conduction enough to identify the different components of the cardiac cycle, such as P waves, and make the diagnosis of atrial fibrillation or SVT with aberrance.
   8) Adenosine may be repeated, 12mg over 2 seconds, at 2-minute intervals to a maximum of 30mg.
   9) Verapamil 1mg/min intravenously can also be used for AV nodal blockade. The profound blockade induces severe vasodilatation, hypotension, and complete heart block, especially in patients with a history of β-blockade.
   10) Verapamil effects are longer in duration and it is used as a second-line drug after adenosine at Parkland.
   11) Atrial fibrillation will also respond to digoxin, propanolol or verapamil.
   12) Sinus tachycardia should prompt evaluation for pain, hemorrhage, fever, infection, and stress. Treatment should be directed towards these causes.
e. Wide-complex tachycardias.
   1) Wide-complex tachycardias are more ominous and portend a poor outcome.
   2) Usually indicate ventricular irritability and require immediate treatment to prevent death.
   3) The most common wide-complex tachycardias are ventricular tachycardia and fibrillation. These will both respond to cardioversion with 100J followed by lidocaine 100mg i.v. to prevent recurrence.

VII. ANTIARRHYTHMIC AGENTS
A. CLASS I – membrane active.
1. Fast sodium channel blockers.

2. Decrease phase 0 depolarization.
3. Prototypes include lidocaine, procainamide, quinidine, and disopyramide.
B. CLASS II – β-blockers.
1. Decrease sympathetic hyperactivity.
2. Propanolol.
C. CLASS III – prolong repolarization and refractory period.
1. Delay phases 2 and 3 of repolarization.
2. Bretylium.
D. CLASS IV – calcium channel blockers.
1. Blocks slow calcium channels but have no effect on fast sodium channels.
2. Verapamil.

VIII. CARDIAC SUPPORT

A. THE PRINCIPAL DETERMINANTS OF CARDIAC OUTPUT are:
1. Preload.
2. Afterload.
3. Contractility.
B. THE PREFERRED FIRST INTERVENTION in a patient with evidence of inadequate tissue perfusion (oliguria, hypotension, tachycardia), is to ensure adequate intravascular volume (preload).
C. PRELOAD MANAGEMENT.
1. A PAWP of 12–15mmHg is considered optimal.
2. High values, >15mmHg, suggest fluid overload and, when combined with evidence of pulmonary edema, warrant diuresis.
3. Low values, <12mmHg, suggest inadequate intravascular volume and are treated by administering crystalloid solutions (lactated Ringer's solution) and observing changes in cardiac output.
a. Increasing the PAWP by 3–5mmHg should increase cardiac output.
b. This response should prompt continuing volume resuscitation until no further response in cardiac output is observed.
4. PAWPs >20–25mmHg are generally associated with pulmonary edema; thus, at Parkland, wedge pressures do not usually increase above 20mmHg.
5. If the CI is still inadequate (<2L/min/m^2), despite adequate preload, the blood pressure and afterload are evaluated at Parkland.
D. AFTERLOAD MANAGEMENT.
1. Calculation of the SVR gives a good estimate of afterload.
2. The normal value is 2000 ± 400dynes/sec.cm^5.
3. Septic shock, autonomic dysfunction, and anaphylactic shock are causes of low SVRI and these causes should be identified and treated appropriately.

4. **Patients with high SVRI and low cardiac output** will usually benefit from afterload reduction with vasodilators.
a. The preferred afterload-reducing agent at Parkland is sodium nitroprusside infusion starting at 0.5μg/kg/min and titrated to obtain the desired effect on cardiac output and SVRI.
   1) This agent has a rapid onset of action that is of short duration.
   2) Disadvantages include thiocyanate toxicity, which is common with infusion rates of >10μg/kg/min for >72 hours.
   3) This can be detected by reduced oxygen consumption manifested as an unexplained increase in $Smvo_2$ or saturation.
   4) Thiocyanate toxicity is managed by i.v. sodium nitrite (10mL of 3% solution) followed by methylene blue (1mg/kg over 5 minutes). If this is unsuccessful, hemodialysis may be instituted.
   5) Profound hypotension is another complication of sodium nitroprusside and can be managed by cessation of the infusion.
b. Other afterload reducing agents include:
   1) Nitroglycerin (5μg/min).
   2) Angiotensin-converting enzyme (ACE) inhibitors, such as enalapril (1.25mg every 6 hours) and trimethaphan camsylate (0.3–3mg/min).
   3) If afterload reduction is unsuccessful in optimizing cardiac output (SVRI <2000dynes/sec.cm^5, CI <2L/min/m^2) the use of inotropes to improve cardiac contractility should be considered.
E. **INOTROPIC SUPPORT.**
1. The preferred inotropic agents at Parkland are dopamine (5–10μg/kg/min) and dobutamine (5–15μg/kg/min).
2. **Dopamine has a dose-dependent action and causes tachycardia.**
a. It also causes significant peripheral vasoconstriction at infusion rates >10–15μg/kg/min, which limits its usefulness at higher doses.
b. At low doses, <5μg/kg/min, it may improve renal perfusion.
3. **Dobutamine is a potent inotropic agent** that has less potential to produce tachycardia and also causes peripheral vasodilatation, especially at doses >20μg/kg/min.
a. This makes it a useful agent in patients with low CI and high SVRI.
b. A significant disadvantage is that it increases myocardial oxygen consumption and subsequent arrhythmogenesis is induced. This limits its usefulness in patients with pre-existing myocardial ischemia.
4. **Other inotropes include:**
a. Epinephrine (0.01mg/kg/min), which is useful for profound hypotension because of its few systemic effects.
b. Norepinephrine, which also increases blood pressure but reduces CI (systemic vasoconstriction).

46

CARDIOVASCULAR SUPPORT AND MANAGEMENT IN THE ICU

5. **Both of these agents are used at Parkland** for cardiac and peripheral vascular support in patients with profound septic shock. However, norepinephrine causes digital necrosis and renal failure from profound vasoconstriction.

6. **When pharmacologic support of the heart is unsuccessful,** intra-aortic balloon counterpulsation (IABP) may be used temporarily until cardiac function improves or is corrected, or as a bridge to cardiac transplantation.

7. **IABP is not a permanent solution to poor cardiac contractility** and the determination that cardiac dysfunction is correctable or reversible should be made before its use.

F. **INTRA-AORTIC BALLOON COUNTERPULSATION.**

1. **The principle of balloon counterpulsation** is maintenance of high diastolic pressure to allow adequate coronary perfusion, as well as diminished myocardial oxygen demand by reduction in afterload.

2. **An intra-aortic balloon is placed through the femoral artery** in the groin and the balloon tip is placed just distal to the origin of the left subclavian artery.

3. **Balloon inflation and deflation are synchronized** with the EKG: inflation occurs during diastole while deflation occurs at the beginning of ventricular systole.

IX. FURTHER READING

Abrams JH, Cerra F, Holcroft JW. Cardiopulmonary monitoring. In: *II, Scientific American Surgery*. New York: Scientific American; 1998:3–23.

Holcroft JW, Shock. ICU management. In: *II, Scientific American Surgery*. New York: Scientific American; 1998:3–17.

Rice CL, Solaro RJ. Support of the failing heart. In: *II, Scientific American Surgery*. New York: Scientific American; 1998:3–11.

PULMONARY DISORDERS

I. PULMONARY PHYSIOLOGY

A. TISSUE OXYGENATION.

1. **The lungs provide oxygen** for use in cellular metabolic needs.
2. **Inability to meet these needs** results in anaerobic metabolism.
3. **The determinants of tissue oxygenation** are:
   a. Oxygen content (Cao_2) is the amount of oxygen in the blood.
      1) Represents the quantity of oxygen in the blood.
      2) This represents the sum of the oxygen bound to hemoglobin (Hb) and dissolved in the blood and is calculated as $Cao_2 = 1.34 \times Hb \times Sao_2 + (0.003 \times Pao_2)$. (The first portion of this equation is derived from the fact that 1g of Hb binds 1.34mL of oxygen.)
      3) Normal value is 20mL O_2/dL.
   b. Oxygen delivery (Do_2) is the delivery of oxygen to tissues.
      1) Represents the quantity of oxygen delivered to tissues.
      2) Calculated by product of Cao_2 and cardiac index (CI): $Do_2 = Cao_2 \times CI$ or $Do_2 = (1.34 \times Hb \times Sao_2 + [0.003 \times Pao_2]) \times CI$.
      3) Therefore, improving Hb amount, saturation, and CI can improve oxygen delivery.
      4) Normal value is 600–1000mL O_2 per minute.
   c. Oxygen consumption (Vo_2) is the utilization of oxygen by tissues.
      1) Represents the amount of oxygen utilized by the body.
      2) Represents the difference between the oxygen content of arterial blood (Cao_2) and the oxygen content of venous blood (Cvo_2).
      3) $Vo_2 = (Cao_2 - Cvo_2) \times CI$ or $= C(a-v)o_2 \times CI$.
      4) Normal value is 110–150mL/m^2 per minute.

B. OXYGEN EXCHANGE.

1. **Alveolar–arterial oxygen gradient.**
   a. The difference between Po_2 in the alveolar gas (Pao_2) and arterial blood (Pao_2) is the alveolar–arterial gradient or A–a gradient.
   b. This gradient provides a measure of oxygen exchange through the alveolar–capillary interface.
   c. It is calculated as follows:
      1) $Pao_2 = Fio_2 [Patm - Ph_2o] - Pao_2$.
      2) Patm = atmospheric pressure = 760mmHg.
      3) Ph_2o = water vapor pressure = 47mmHg.
      4) (A-a) $Do_2 = Pao_2 - Pao_2$.
   d. Normal value is 25–65mmHg on 100% O_2.
   e. The higher the value, the higher the gradient needed for alveolar oxygen to equilibrate with arterial oxygen and therefore the worse the gas exchange.

2. **Shunt fraction (Os/Ot).**
a. Represents the fraction of blood that flows through unventilated pulmonary capillaries.
b. $Os/Ot = (Cco_2 - Cao_2)/(Cco_2 - Cvo_2)$.
   1) Cco_2 = pulmonary artery oxygen content.
   2) This value cannot be directly measured, but can be estimated by placing the patient on 100% oxygen and using Pao_2.
c. Normal value is <10%.
   1) Significant pulmonary dysfunction is indicated by 20–29%.
   2) >30 % is potentially life threatening.

C. **CARBON DIOXIDE REMOVAL (VENTILATION).**

1. **Ventilation is the ability of external air to move into the alveolus.** There are several important determinants.
2. **Minute ventilation (VE).**
a. Minute ventilation is the quantity of air moved into and out of the lungs in a minute.
b. It is a product of tidal volume and respiratory rate.
c. Normal values range between 5 and 8L per minute.
d. Once minute ventilation is >10–12L per minute, it is very difficult for the patient to maintain spontaneous ventilation.
3. **Dead space ventilation.**
a. The 'dead space' is the portion of the respiratory tree that does not participate in gas exchange.
b. It has two components:
   1) Anatomic dead space – the conducting airways (i.e. the trachea).
   2) Physiologic dead space – the ventilated but nonperfused alveoli.
c. The fraction of minute ventilation that does not participate in gas exchange is called the dead space ventilation (Vd).
d. The ratio of dead space ventilation:tidal volume (Vd:Vt) provides another measure of the adequacy of ventilation.
   1) $Vd:Vt = Paco_2 - Petco_2/Paco_2$.
   2) $Petco_2$ = end tidal CO_2 tension.
e. Normal values are 0.2–0.3.
f. Values of 0.6–0.7 represent severe cases of acute respiratory failure.
4. **Compliance.**
a. Defined as the ratio of change of volume over pressure or $\Delta V:\Delta P$.
b. Estimates the distensibility or 'stiffness' of the lungs and the chest wall.
c. Static compliance (Cstat).
   1) Compliance measured at the end of air flow.
   2) $Cstat = Vt/plateau$ pressure – PEEP(positive end expiratory pressure).
   3) Normal value is 70–160mL/cm H_2O.
   4) Difficult to maintain spontaneous ventilation with values <40mL/cmH_2O.

d. Dynamic compliance (Cdyn).
1) Measures compliance of the lung during air movement.
2) Cdyn = Vt/peak inspiratory pressure - PEEP.
3) Normal value is 50–80mL/cmH$_2$O.

5. Inspiratory force.

a. Maximum inspiratory force (MIF) or negative inspiratory force (NIF).

b. Provides an estimate of ventilatory muscle 'power'.

c. The minimum negative force to support spontaneous ventilation is 25cmH$_2$O.

6. Vital capacity.

a. Is the volume of air generated by maximum expiration after maximal inspiration.

b. Normal values are 65–75mL/kg.

c. Minimally adequate values are between 10 and 15mL/kg.

7. Pulmonary circulation.

a. Relationship between pulmonary blood flow and alveolar pressure divides the lung into three zones (i.e. West Zones).
1) Zone I – alveolar pressure > pulmonary artery pressure > pulmonary venous pressure; no blood flow therefore no gas exchange occurs.
2) Zone II – pulmonary arterial pressure > pulmonary alveolar pressure > pulmonary venous pressure; flow is intermittent and varies with respiratory cycle.
3) Zone III – pulmonary arterial pressure > pulmonary venous pressure > pulmonary alveolar pressure; continuous blood flow.

b. Zones change with changes in patient position; therefore changes in patient position (i.e. supine to sitting position) will change ventilation and perfusion relationships.

8. Lung volumes.

a. Tidal volume is the volume of air inspired or expired in a normal breath.

b. Inspiratory reserve volume (IRV) is the volume of air that can be inspired after normal inspiration.

c. Expiratory reserve volume (ERV) is the volume of air that can be expired after normal expiration.

d. Residual volume (RV) is the volume of air remaining after maximal expiration.

e. Total lung capacity (TLC) is the amount of air in the lung after maximal inspiration (TLC = VC + RV).

f. Inspiratory capacity (IC) is the maximum amount of air that can be inspired after normal expiration (IC = IRV + VT).

g. Vital capacity (VC) is the maximum amount of air that can be expired after maximal inspiration (VC = IRV + ERV + VT).

h. Functional residual capacity (FRC) is the amount of air in the lungs after normal expiration (FRC = ERV + RV).

II. RESPIRATORY FAILURE

A. **DEFINITION.** Respiratory failure is defined as functional lung impairment that does not allow the alveoli to perform gas exchange and is characterized by hypoxemia and hypercapnia. There are two major causes.

B. **VENTILATION AND PERFUSION MISMATCH.**

1. **In normal lungs,** ventilation and perfusion are closely matched for a V:Q ratio close to 1.

2. **Two manifestations of ventilation and perfusion abnormalities** are shunt and dead space ventilation.

a. Shunt:

   1) When a perfused alveoli is not ventilated (V:Q = 0).
   2) Venous blood travels back into the arterial circulation and results in arterial hypoxemia.
   3) Hypercapnia is often not seen, however, because chemoreceptors increase VE to maintain normal $Paco_2$.
   4) Can be estimated using alveolar gas equation, P:F ratio, or shunt fraction.
   5) When the shunt fraction is >50%, Pao_2 is not improved with increased Fio_2.

b. Dead space ventilation:

   1) Ventilated alveoli that are not perfused.
   2) These alveoli do not contribute to gas exchange (V:Q = infinity).
   3) This produces both hypoxemia and hypercapnia.

C. **ALVEOLAR HYPOVENTILATION.**

1. **This is defined as a decrease in alveolar ventilation** for a given carbon dioxide production.

2. **It is usually secondary** to a decrease in VE.

3. **The A–a gradient remains the same** but Pao_2 decreases and $Paco_2$ increases.

D. **DIAGNOSIS.**

1. **Relies on arterial blood gases to confirm clinical signs of hypoxemia.**

2. **Symptoms include:**

a. Tachypnea.

b. Dyspnea.

c. Mental status changes (confusion).

3. **Cyanosis** is a key sign.

4. **Hypercapnia** may lead to lethargy and coma.

5. **The parameters for the diagnosis of acute respiratory failure** are listed in Table 47.1.

III. MANAGEMENT OF RESPIRATORY FAILURE

A. **FOUR COMPONENTS.**

1. **Airway management** – if patent airway cannot be maintained, endotracheal intubation or tracheostomy must be performed.

TABLE 47.1	
ACUTE RESPIRATORY FAILURE	
Parameter	
Vital capacity	<10mL/kg
Functional residual capacity (mL/kg)	<60% predicted
Vd:Vt	0.6
Static compliance	35–45mL/cmH$_2$O
Inspiratory force	20cmH$_2$O
Shunt (Qs/Qt)	20–29%
Room air Pao$_2$	<60mmHg
Paco$_2$	60mmHg
Respiration rate	>35 breaths per minute
Work of breathing	Excessively increased

2. Ventilation.
3. Oxygenation.
4. Treatment of underlying disease.
B. **VENTILATION.**
1. **Types.**
a. Volume
   1) Volume-controlled mechanical support.
   2) Each mechanical breath may be terminated after a selected time (time cycled) or volume (volume cycled) is delivered.
b. Pressure – each mechanical breath may be terminated after selected interval (time cycled) or when flow declines to selected level (flow cycled).
2. **Modes.** (Note: control implies the ventilator controls all phases of the respiratory cycle.)
a. Continuous mandatory ventilation (CMV).
   1) Machine delivers breaths based on time cycle.
   2) Preset Vt and rate is selected.
   3) All aspects of respiratory phase are controlled by machine, independent of patient respiratory drive.
   4) The patient is unable to initiate breath and this mode is poorly tolerated by the awake patient.
b. Assist controlled (AC).
   1) This mode relies on spontaneous breath to trigger ventilator.
   2) With each patient respiratory effort, the ventilator responds with a full preset Vt.
   3) If the patient is apneic, a 'backup' (control) mode is triggered and the ventilator provides all aspects of ventilator support (essentially CMV).

       4) The disadvantages is that it does not allow spontaneous respiratory support between breaths.

       5) May be poorly tolerated by awake patients, and may lead to 'breath stacking' and respiratory alkalosis.

c. Intermittent mandatory ventilation (IMV).

       1) Ventilator delivers preset Vt and preset rate.

       2) Flow is also provided between the machine breaths for the patient's spontaneous respiratory efforts.

       3) If the ventilator breaths are synchronized so that it commences with a spontaneous respiratory effort, the mode is called SIMV.

       4) SIMV avoids breath stacking.

       5) (S)IMV is a versatile mode that can offer 0–100% of respiratory support.

d. Pressure support ventilation (PSV).

       1) Patient's spontaneous breath triggers the machine to deliver the gas mixture until a preselected pressure is achieved, after which flow ceases.

       2) Patient controls Vt and respiratory rate.

       3) Pressure support is used to augment patient's spontaneous Vt.

       4) This mode can be used to offset the work imposed by an endotracheal tube.

       5) The circuit of the machine requires an intact respiratory drive.

       6) This mode can be used by itself or in combination with another mode of ventilation (e.g. SIMV).

e. Pressure control ventilation (PCV).

       1) Gas is delivered at a preset pressure, but the machine controls all aspects of the respiratory cycle.

       2) Vt is determined by inspiratory flow, pulmonary compliance, and inspiratory time.

       3) Advantages include highest flow and therefore largest portion of Vt delivered at the beginning of breath, resulting in an increased mean airway pressure and improved oxygenation.

       4) Other advantages include limited airway pressures.

f. Inverse ratio ventilation.

       1) In spontaneous breaths the normal inspiratory:expiratory ratio is 1:2 or 1:3.

       2) Inverse ratio ventilation reverses the normal ratio, spending more time in inspiration and thus achieves relatively high mean airway pressures and improving oxygenation.

       3) Problems include excessive gas trapping and 'autoPEEP' can develop, owing to shortened expiratory time.

       4) This mode is unnatural and requires paralysis and sedation.

g. Mandatory minute ventilation (MMV).

       1) VE is programmed and machine adjusts the pressure support to ensure adequate spontaneous Vt is reached.

2) If the patient's spontaneous ventilation is greater than or equal to predetermined VE, the patient receives no support.

3) If the patient becomes apneic, the machine provides all support (i.e. the preset VE).

C. WEANING FROM THE VENTILATOR.

1. **Basic considerations.**

a. >70% of patients requiring respiratory support are able to be extubated within 72 hours with little difficulty.

b. Consider these general principles prior to extubation:

1) Cardiovascular stability – adequate oxygen supply to muscle, particularly respiratory muscle, is essential for adequate respiratory function.

2) Nutrition – malnutrition has many adverse effects on the respiratory system, including changes in respiratory muscle mass and contractility.

3) Metabolic abnormalities – electrolyte abnormalities, such as phosphate, calcium, and magnesium, may adversely affect respiratory functions.

2. **Specific weaning criteria** attempt to predict the outcome of weaning.

a. Measurements of oxygenation.

1) Pao_2 >70mmHg or Fio_2 40%.

2) Arterial saturation >90%.

3) A–a oxygen gradient <300–350.

4) Shunt fraction <15%.

5) Pao_2:Fio_2 >200.

b. Measurements of ventilation and respiratory muscle.

1) $Paco_2$ <50mmHg.

2) Arterial pH >7.25.

3) Respiratory rate <24 breaths per minute.

4) Vt = 5–8mL/kg.

5) VE <10L per minute.

6) NIF >–200cmH$_2$O.

7) Dead space to Vt ratio <0.6.

3. **Methods of weaning from the ventilator.**

a. Overall concept is gradually to increase stress on respiratory muscles to increase endurance and strength and therefore enable spontaneous ventilation.

b. T-bar.

1) 'T-bar' or 'T-piece' attaches to the endotracheal tube so that oxygen-rich gas flows by the patient and prevents inhalation of exhaled gas.

2) Patients are given spontaneous breathing trials and are first started with brief periods (e.g. 15 minutes) off the ventilator on the T-piece.

47

PULMONARY DISORDERS

  3) When the patient is on the T-piece, their respiratory rate, heart rate, and breathing pattern should be closely observed.
  4) Tachypnea (respiratory rate >35), tachycardia (heart rate >125), or an abnormal breathing pattern imply intolerance of ventilator wean and the trial should be halted.
  5) The periods off the ventilator are gradually increased.
  6) If a patient has required intubation for a short period of time prior to T-piece trial, a successful 2-hour T-bar trial can be followed by extubation.
  7) Patients intubated for a longer time, however, should tolerate 24 hours off the ventilator (on the T-bar) prior to extubation.
c. IMV.
  1) Mode of ventilation delivers set rate of Vt machine breaths.
  2) Between these breaths, the patient is free to breathe spontaneously.
  3) The patient is weaned by gradual decrease in machine delivered breaths, usually in increments of 1–2 breaths.
  4) The number of breaths is gradually decreased to zero.
  5) The rate of tapering breaths is extremely variable and depends on the patient's condition.

IV. SPECIFIC CAUSES OF RESPIRATORY FAILURE

A. ACUTE RESPIRATORY DISTRESS SYNDROME (ARDS).

1. **Characterized** by severe hypoxia, decreased lung compliance, decreased FRC, and characteristic (but nonspecific) chest radiograph findings and a definable event or risk factor.
2. **ARDS is seen with many conditions** (e.g. fat emboli, Gram-negative sepsis, aspiration, shock, and pancreatitis).
3. **All of these processes** commonly cause the systemic inflammatory response syndrome (SIRS); therefore, ARDS may represent a localized pulmonary manifestation of a systemic disease.
4. **Pathophysiology.**
a. Alveolar epithelial cells and pulmonary capillary endothelial cells both rest on a thin basement membrane and are separated by an interstitial space.
b. This alveolar–capillary interface allows for gas exchange.
c. After injury, capillary permeability is increased and fluid and protein extravasates from the endothelium to the interstitium. This fluid is usually drained by pulmonary lymphatics, but once the lymphatics are overwhelmed, edema fluid accumulates.
d. Alveolar type I cells are most fragile and are destroyed.
e. These cells are sloughed and the alveolar basement membrane is quickly denuded.

f. Alveolar type II cells then proliferate in an attempt to cover the basement membrane.
g. Plasma proteins, fibrin, and sloughed cells lie on the alveolar surface forming characteristic hyaline membranes.
h. The loss of surfactant, as well as surfactant inactivation, leads to widespread microatelectasis, loss of lung compliance (stiff lungs), intrapulmonary shunting, and hypoxemia.

5. Clinical manifestations.
a. Initial manifestations include tachypnea, dyspnea, and tachycardia.
b. Eventually, severe tachypnea and dyspnea, progressive hypoxemia (Pao_2:Fio_2 <200), and decreased lung compliance develop and respiratory failure requiring mechanical ventilation ensues.
c. A characteristic, but nonspecific, pattern of diffuse interstitial infiltrates develop on chest radiography.
d. Initially, it may be difficult to distinguish ARDS from cardiogenic pulmonary edema, although the former will lack cardiomegaly or pleural effusions.
e. Eventually, a pattern of diffuse interstitial fibrosis may ensue, characterized by a patchy, nodular pattern on chest radiography.

6. Management.
a. Overall management is supportive.
b. The basic tenet is the use of mechanical ventilation with PEEP to maintain the FRC by stabilizing collapsing alveoli.
   1) PEEP is titrated to keep Pao_2 >60mmHg and Fio_2 <50%.
   2) High Fio_2 is avoided to prevent oxygen toxicity.
   3) Using high levels of PEEP (>15cmH$_2$O) can lead to hemodynamic compromise and barotrauma.
   4) At levels >12cmH$_2$O, use of a pulmonary artery catheter is suggested to assess the hemodynamic status.
   5) Peak inspiratory pressures should be kept below 40cmH$_2$O.
   6) Initially the volume control mode is used, but increasing peak pressures can be limited by the pressure control mode.
   7) Progressive hypoxemia can be counteracted with inverse ratio ventilation.
   8) Disadvantages of inverse ratio ventilation include excessive gas trapping and autoPEEP as well as decreased carbon dioxide elimination.
   9) Patients receiving inverse ratio ventilation often require paralysis and sedation.
   10) No increased survival has been demonstrated with the use of pressure control.

47

PULMONARY DISORDERS

B. **PULMONARY EMBOLISM.**
1. **Basic considerations.**
a. Annually there are 500,000 cases of which 200,000 result in death.
b. Of adult patients who undergo major operative procedures, 0.1–0.5% die of pulmonary embolism (PE) in the postoperative period.
c. Most emboli originate from the lower extremity pelvic deep venous thrombosis (DVT).
2. **Risk factors** include:
a. Immobilization.
b. Cardiac disease.
c. Age >40 years.
d. Malignancy.
e. Trauma.
f. Pregnancy.
g. Use of oral contraceptives.
h. Previous DVT or PE.
i. Hypercoaguability states.
3. **Preventive measures.**
a. Nonpharmacologic
   1) Early postoperative ambulation.
   2) Intermittent compression boots may work through decreasing stasis as well as activation of the endogenous fibrinolytic system.
   3) Graduated compression stockings.
b. Pharmacologic
   1) Low dose heparin dosage – 5000 units s.c. 2–3 times daily.
   2) Low molecular weight heparin (LMWH) dosage – 30mg subcutaneously twice daily.
   3) Warfarin.
C. **PULMONARY ASPIRATION SYNDROME.**
1. **The signs and symptoms** depend on the quality and quantity of the aspirate.
2. **Particulate aspiration** can lead to airway obstruction while chemical (gastric acid) may produce local injury as well as a systemic inflammatory response.
3. **This may produce a spectrum of clinical responses** ranging from mild respiratory distress to ARDS.
4. **The magnitude of injury** is determined by the pH of the aspirated fluid.
5. **Risk factors for aspiration.**
a. Perioperative state.
b. Decreased level of consciousness.
c. Laryngeal incompetence.
d. Nasogastric feedings.
e. Artificial airways.

f. Gastroesophageal reflux disease.
g. Obesity.
h. Pregnancy.
6. Clinical presentation comprises four stages.
a. Mechanical effects of obstruction.
    1) Immediate.
    2) Unconscious patients may present with airway obstruction.
b. Chemical burn of airway.
    1) Occurs within hours of aspiration.
    2) Dyspnea and wheezing occur.
    3) Severe irritation of airway, broncho-obstruction, and bronchorrhea may be present.
    4) Damage to cilia decrease the clearance of particles.
c. Lung inflammatory response.
    1) Occurs 1–2 days after injury.
    2) Neutrophils and platelets infiltrate the pulmonary microvasculature and release vasoactive compounds.
    3) This leads to an increase in pulmonary vascular permeability.
    4) Subsequent alveolar flooding leads to decreased and altered surfactant with subsequent alveolar collapse, atelectasis, and hypoxemia.
d. Infectious complications.
    1) Occurs 4–5 days after injury.
    2) This represents the potential complication of secondary bacterial infection.
    3) Can lead to bacterial pneumonia and lung abscess.
    4) Mortality is 50% in the presence of infection.

7. Diagnosis.
a. Maintain high index of suspicion for high-risk patients.
b. Patients often develop acute onset of wheezing, tachypnea, and cyanosis.
c. Chest radiography.
    1) Severe aspiration can cause diffuse bilateral pulmonary infiltrates.
    2) Radiographic findings often lag behind clinical symptoms by 1–2 days.
d. The right mainstem bronchus is the most direct pathway to the lungs, therefore, the right lower lobe is most frequently affected.
e. The left lower lobe is the second most frequently involved.

8. Initial treatment.
a. Suction airway.
b. Administer supplemental oxygen.

9. Management.
a. Supportive treatment.
    1) Often supplemental oxygen is all that is needed.

       2) Progressive hypoxemia may require mechanical ventilation.

       3) Bronchospasm can be treated with aerosolized bronchodilators.

       4) Surfactant replacement and steroids are of no value.

       5) Antibiotics should be withheld until clinical evidence of infection is present.

       6) Clues to developing infection include new and worsening infiltrates; cavitation on chest radiograph; purulent sputum; leukocytosis; and persistent fever.

       7) Antibiotic coverage should include anaerobic bacteria.

  b. Prevent further aspiration.

       1) Maintain head of bed at 45° angle.

       2) Antacids, H_2 blockers, or omeprazole.

       3) Promote gastric bacterial growth by increasing gastric pH with sulcralfate.

DISORDERS OF TEMPERATURE REGULATION IN THE INTENSIVE CARE UNIT

I. TEMPERATURE HOMEOSTASIS

A. **CORE TEMPERATURE** is normally 36.7–37.6°C with typical variations of ± 1.5°C.

B. **CHILDREN <2 YEARS OF AGE** lack stable homeostatic mechanisms and can experience wide fluctuations in body temperature when they are subjected to extreme temperatures.

C. **THE ELDERLY** (persons >70 years of age) likewise may be less able to compensate for unusual ranges of temperature.

D. **RECTAL TEMPERATURES** are the most accurate noninvasive means of measurement.

E. **MECHANISMS OF HEAT TRANSFER.**

1. **Conduction** – transfer of heat between two masses that are in contact with each other. (Lying on a cold, wet surface is one of the fastest ways to lose body heat.)

2. **Convection** – transfer of heat through the flow of liquids or gases over a surface. (Significant heat loss can occur during transport or in a cold room with high air flow.)

3. **Radiation** – transfer of radiant heat which is the result of electromagnetic transmission. This type of heat transfer occurs between the body and its surroundings.

4. **Evaporation** – loss of heat by evaporation of water from the surface of the body.

a. Heat loss occurs from the open abdomen.

b. Heat loss can be reduced by placing intestines in dry towels or plastic bags rather than using cold, wet towels.

II. HYPOTHERMIA

A. **ETIOLOGY.**

1. **Accidental environmental exposure** is the usual etiology of primary hypothermia.

2. **Secondary hypothermia** in the general surgical or trauma patient may arise from any single factor or a combination of several:

a. Long intra-abdominal operations.

b. Cardiopulmonary bypass.

c. Sepsis.

d. Multiple metabolic abnormalities such as hypoglycemia, hypopituitarism, hypothyroidism, and hypothalamic dysfunction can contribute to or cause hypothermia.

3. **Chemicals,** such as ethanol, barbiturates, phenothiazines, and anesthetics.

B. **PATHOPHYSIOLOGY.**

1. **Secondary hypothermia is more common** than primary hypothermia and carries a more lethal prognosis.

2. **The alterations in homeostasis** produced by even mild degrees of hypothermia are poorly tolerated when superimposed on patients with shock, hemorrhage, or major tissue injury.

3. **Hypothermia in the surgical or trauma patient** is usually in the range 32–35°C.

a. These temperatures are not associated with a significant risk of problems, such as ventricular fibrillation, altered pH regulation, cold-induced diuresis, respiratory depression, rewarming shock, or core afterdrop.

b. The primary problems in this setting are alterations in oxygen supply and demand and coagulopathy.

4. **Increase in oxygen consumption.**

a. At rest, average oxygen concentration (Vo_2) is approximately 210mL/min in an adult, which produces 64kcal/hour of heat.

b. In a patient with limited cardiopulmonary reserves, hypothermia may worsen any imbalance between oxygen supply and demand leading to anaerobic metabolism and lactic acidosis.

c. With shivering, Vo_2 can increase to as much as 500% of normal.

d. Patient energy expenditure to overcome or simply to maintain hypothermia is detrimental.

e. The thermoneutral temperature (28°C) is the ambient temperature at which the basal rate of thermogenesis is sufficient to offset ongoing heat losses.

f. Maintaining normothermia, when the temperature around the body drops below the thermoneutral zone, requires an increase in heat production.

g. Because humans produce heat by combustion, extra oxygen is needed as substrate.

C. **BLOOD AND COAGULATION.**

1. **Hypothermia can prolong coagulation** and cause severe clotting-factor deficiencies.

2. **Because the PT and PTT are temperature-standardized tests,** the extent of the hypothermia-induced coagulopathy is often underestimated.

3. **Hypothermia also affects platelet function.**

a. Platelets sequester in the portal circulation during hypothermia and, at temperatures <20°C, they are nearly absent from the peripheral circulation.

b. Platelets liberate thromboxane A_2, a potent vasoconstrictor necessary for platelet aggregation.

c. The production of thromboxane A_2 is temperature dependent, and bleeding time is significantly prolonged in hypothermia secondary to a defect in the platelet's ability to produce this prostaglandin at the bleeding site.

d. This problem is reversed with rewarming.

4. **Transfusions of fresh-frozen plasma and platelets** may not correct coagulopathic bleeding if the dysfunction is temperature related.

5. **Blood viscosity is increased during hypothermia**, and thrombotic complications are seen with severe hypothermia.

D. **CARDIOVASCULAR.**

1. **Initially, the cardiovascular response is tachycardia**, followed by progressive bradycardia beginning at about 34°C and resulting in a 50% decrease in heart rate at 28°C.

2. **Although stroke volume is relatively well preserved**, a decline in cardiac output occurs secondary to the effect of hypothermia on heart rate.

3. **On the EKG,** the PR, then the QRS, and finally the QT interval become progressively prolonged.

4. **An Osborne wave, or J-wave** (hypothermic hump), is sometimes seen at the junction of the QRS and ST segments in leads II and V6.

5. **Below 32°C**, atrial and then predominantly ventricular dysrhythmias occur.

6. **At 28°C**, the risk of dysrhythmias increases significantly.

7. **Below 28°C**, the body behaves in a cold-blooded fashion, and below 25°C, virtually all patients will be asystolic.

8. **Generally, 'freezing to death' has implied ventricular fibrillation**, but asystole may be the primary fatal rhythm.

E. **RESPIRATORY.**

1. **During the early stages of hypothermia**, respiratory drive is increased, but progressive respiratory depression occurs at temperatures <33°C.

2. **This results in a decline in minute ventilation.**

3. **Noncardiogenic pulmonary edema** is also reported after prolonged hypothermia.

F. **CENTRAL NERVOUS SYSTEM.**

1. **As the core temperature falls, progressive confusion**, slurred speech, and incoordination occur.

2. **At temperatures <32°C**, patients are often amnestic.

3. **Below 31°C**, most patients lose consciousness; shivering and deep tendon reflexes are lost as well.

4. **At temperatures <30°C**, the pupils become dilated with slow or absent light response, and the patient has a flaccid appearance.

5. **Below 26°C**, the pupils dilate and loss of cerebral autoregulation occurs.

6. **Below 33°C**, the electroencephalogram (EEG) becomes abnormal; and below 20°C it is silent.

G. RENAL.

1. **Decreases in blood pressure and cardiac output** cause a concomitant decrease in the glomerular filtration rate.

2. **Urine output is maintained** because of an impairment in renal tubular Na^+ reabsorption (cold diuresis).

3. **The initial vasoconstriction which occurs in response to hypothermia** also causes an increase in central blood volume that prompts a diuresis.

H. GASTROINTESTINAL.

1. **Hypothermia causes decreased gastrointestinal motility** and results in gastric dilatation, ileus, and colonic distention.

2. **Hepatic dysfunction occurs** as well, secondary to a decrease in splanchnic blood flow.

3. **Gastric mucosal erosions are also common.**

I. ENDOCRINE.

1. **Insulin release and insulin uptake are inhibited** at receptor sites.

2. **Hyperglycemia is common,** especially at temperatures <30°C.

J. DIAGNOSIS.

1. **Hypothermia is a core temperature <35°C.**

2. **Hypothermia has been divided in ranges** based on physiologic changes that occur at each level.

a. Mild hypothermia – 32–35°C.

b. Moderate hypothermia – 28–32°C.

c. Severe hypothermia – 20–28°C.

d. Profound hypothermia – 14–20°C.

e. Deep hypothermia – <14°C.

III. TREATMENT

A. AGGRESSIVE REWARMING of trauma patients lowers mortality rates, and decreases blood loss, fluid requirements, episodes of organ failure, and length of intensive care unit (ICU) stay.

B. DEMANDS ON BODY RESERVES for extra energy, and the accelerated rate of nitrogen loss and consequent increase in oxygen utilization, can be attenuated by controlling environmental factors that lead to heat loss.

C. PASSIVE EXTERNAL REWARMING.

1. **This is used for patients with temperatures >30°C** who have intact homeostasis mechanisms (i.e. they are shivering).

2. **In these patients,** 100% oxygen is administered, external heat is applied, and i.v. fluids and inspired air are warmed.

3. **Attempts are made to achieve a temperature of 35°C** by raising the body temperature by 1–1.5°C per hour.

D. ACTIVE EXTERNAL REWARMING.

1. **Because skin temperature may be 10–15°C cooler then the core temperature** in hypothermic patients, external rewarming techniques

cannot transfer heat to the core until the temperature of the skin is raised to at least the level of the core.

2. **During the time that skin rewarming is occurring**, the core temperature can continue to decrease by a phenomenon called afterdrop.

3. **When using a heating blanket**, the blanket should be placed above the patient rather than below to prevent burns and to trap heat between the blanket and the mattress.

4. **Convective warmers serve to prevent most heat loss**, but do very little in terms of rewarming the patient.

5. **Attempting to prevent or to treat hypothermia by increasing the operating room temperature** has very little effect except in pediatric or burn patients.

6. **Warm water immersion** is the only external rewarming technique that transfers a significant amount of heat, but this method is associated with a high rate of cardiovascular collapse secondary to vasodilatation.

7. **Covering the head with reflective material is helpful**. Scalp vessels do not undergo vasoconstriction, and 50% of radiant heat loss occurs above the neck.

E. **ACTIVE CORE REWARMING.**

1. **Typically used for temperature <30ºC** or when regulatory mechanisms are impaired. This includes airway rewarming, heated peritoneal or pleural lavage, warm i.v. fluids, and extracorporeal circulation.

2. **Heated gastric, bladder, or colonic lavage** uses too small a surface area for effective heat transfer.

3. **Airway rewarming** has little effect on core temperature.

4. **Pleural or peritoneal lavage result in significant heat transfer** and are roughly equivalent although fluid return may be better with pleural lavage.

5. **The pleural cavity may be preferred in a patient with arrhythmias** because the heart may be rewarmed faster than with peritoneal lavage.

6. **Two ipsilateral chest tubes are used for pleural lavage** to enable a continuous flow of water.

7. **A two-tube method is preferred for peritoneal lavage.**

a. The liver is more likely to be warmed with peritoneal lavage, thereby restoring its synthetic and metabolic properties more quickly.

b. This method is not feasible in patients who have undergone celiotomy.

8. **When lavaging body cavities**, a temperature of <44ºC is acceptable in patients who are not in hemodynamic collapse. In the setting of cardiac arrest or severely diminished blood flow, bowel necrosis can occur with lavage fluid at a high temperature.

9. **Since cold i.v. fluid administration is the fastest way to induce hypothermia**, giving warm i.v. fluids is critical in preventing it as well as in its treatment.

a. Blood products should be warmed as well.

b. A bolus of cold i.v. fluid can increase cardiac irritability by directly affecting the conducting system.

48

DISORDERS OF TEMPERATURE REGULATION IN THE INTENSIVE CARE UNIT

c. The use of warm i.v. fluids will help reduce the incidence of intraoperative cardiac arrest, coagulopathy, and acidosis.

d. Warm i.v. fluids also provide the simplest means of transferring significant amounts of heat to patients requiring massive fluid resuscitation.

10. **Cardiopulmonary bypass is the most efficient warming technique** and should be used for the rewarming of fibrillating patients with primary accidental hypothermia.

a. Rewarming surgical patients does not require cardiac pump assistance or membrane oxygenation.

b. Continuous arteriovenous rewarming (CAVR) is an effective method that does not require a mechanical pump or heparin.

11. **Patients who are aggressively rewarmed** suffer fewer consequences of hypothermia.

12. **Rapidly rewarmed patients** require fewer blood products and less volume resuscitation; they have better pulmonary function, fewer organ failures, and shorter ICU stays.

13. **The mortality is reduced** in hypothermic trauma patients by rapid rewarming.

IV. OTHER CONSIDERATIONS

A. **OXYGEN CONSUMPTION.**

1. **By preventing shivering,** anesthetics and neuromuscular blocking agents can attenuate the increase in Vo_2 associated with hypothermia.

2. **During anesthesia, aggressive rewarming should be pursued** so that emergence from anesthesia does not overly stress the patient from a cardiovascular standpoint.

3. **Even in the absence of shivering,** the catecholamine response to hypothermia causes an increase in metabolic rate, making prevention and treatment of importance.

B. **CARDIOVASCULAR.**

1. **Weak, bradycardic pulses in hypothermic patients** may be difficult to palpate; hence the presence of an organized rhythm is taken as a sign of life which contraindicates cardiopulmonary resuscitation (CPR).

2. **If the patient does not have an organized rhythm** and field conditions are such that CPR cannot be instituted, rewarming should not be undertaken until CPR can be instituted.

3. **There are reports of patients with hypothermic cardiac arrest** who have been successfully resuscitated after many hours of CPR.

4. **Rewarming will generally reverse the bradycardia and mild hypotension** that may occur with hypothermia.

5. **Vasoconstrictors should be used with extreme caution** in cases of refractory hypotension because they may be arrhythmogenic, may deleteriously affect frostbitten tissues, and may decrease the effectiveness of external rewarming.

C. RESPIRATORY.
1. Arterial blood gases (ABGs) should be assessed at 37°C without temperature correction.
2. The pH of blood increases by 0.015 pH units for every 1.0°C decrease in temperature
3. Hypothermia shifts the oxyhemoglobin dissociation curve to the left, but has very little effect on arterial saturation.
D. ENDOCRINE. Do not treat hyperglycemia at temperatures <30°C because of rebound hypoglycemia during rewarming.
E. COMPLICATIONS. Rewarming can lead to sudden decreases in peripheral vascular resistance which can lead to hypotension or lactic acidosis.

V. HYPERTHERMIA SYNDROMES: FEVER
A. PATHOPHYSIOLOGY AND ETIOLOGY.
1. The febrile response is secondary to endogenous pyrogens including the cytokines (IL-1, IL-2, IL-6, TNF, IFN-α, IFN-β, and IFN-γ) and prostaglandins which increase the hypothalamic thermal set point.
2. IL-1 elicits fever by altering the activity of temperate-sensitive neurons in the anterior hypothalamus.
3. Exogenous pyrogens may also cause fever indirectly by stimulating the production of endogenous pyrogens; an example is lipopolysaccharide (LPS) which stimulates production and release of TNF and IL-1.
4. For every degree of fever, oxygen consumption increases 7%, cardiac work is increased, and the seizure threshold of the brain is lowered.
5. Negative feedback mechanisms usually maintain temperatures <41°C.
6. Any temperature >38°C is considered a fever and should warrant evaluation; however, fever, especially in the early postoperative period, is a poor predictor of infection.
a. Temperature elevations (>37.5°C) should not be ignored and may be an early sign of some abnormal condition.
b. Minimal temperature elevations warrant close observation but do not require an aggressive workup.
7. Most fevers due to infections in surgical patients begin on or after the third postoperative day.
8. Intermittent fever, in which body temperature returns to normal each day, is characteristic of pyogenic infections.
9. Remittent fever, in which the temperature falls but not to normal, is considered the most common febrile response to diseases.
10. Common sources of fever in surgical and trauma patients include:
a. Infections (bacterial, viral, and fungal involving lungs, wounds, salivary glands, prostate, colon, decubitus ulcers, perirectal area, urine, i.v. sites, sinuses, etc.).

b. Pancreatitis.

c. Thromboembolism.

d. Drugs (up to 30% of hospitalized patients experience some type of adverse drug reaction).

e. Blood transfusions.

f. *Clostridium difficile* colitis.

g. Overwhelming postsplenectomy infection (OPSI).

h. Myocardial infarction.

i. Direct tissue trauma.

j. Alcoholic hepatitis.

k. Crush syndrome.

l. Alcohol and drug withdrawal.

11. Less common causes of fever include:

a. Antigen–antibody complexes.

b. Neoplasms.

c. Central nervous system disorders.

d. Connective tissue and immunologic disorders.

e. Metabolic and endocrine disorders (thyroid storm, gout, porphyria, adrenocortical insufficiency, pheochromocytoma).

f. Tetanus.

g. Malignant hyperthermia.

B. EVALUATION OF THE FEBRILE RESPONSE.

1. Assess the patient for any underlying cause of fever.

2. The first febrile episode should be evaluated with a careful history and physical examination.

3. If the physical examination fails to identify the source of fever, no further work-up is necessary unless the patient is immunocompromised or has a high probability of bacteremia.

4. For a second febrile episode, aggressive pulmonary toilet, ambulation, and diagnostic tests should be pursued.

a. Urinalysis, chest radiograph, and sputum Gram stain will yield the quickest results.

b. Blood, sputum, and urine can be cultured as well as central line tips.

5. For persistently elevated temperatures after intra-abdominal procedures, abdominal computed tomography (CT) may be helpful as early as postoperative day 7.

C. PHYSICAL EXAMINATION CHARACTERISTICS.

1. Temperature.

a. Normal oral temperature is 37.0°C.

b. Diurnal variation is 1.3°C (greatest from 16.00 to 20.00 hours).

c. Core temperature is 0.5°C higher than oral.

d. Fever is a temperature >38.0°C.

2. Hemodynamic status.

a. Heart rate increase is approximately 5–10 beats per minute/°C.

b. Hypotension may be associated with advanced sepsis and systemic inflammatory response syndrome (SIRS).
c. Tachypnea manifests as a respiratory rate >20.

3. **Neurologic.**
a. Decreased level of consciousness.
b. Focal neurologic deficit.

4. **Head, eye, ear, nose, and throat (HEENT).**
a. Facial tenderness.
b. Nuchal rigidity.
c. Nasal and sinus drainage.

5. **Lungs** – abnormal breath sounds.

6. **Cardiac.**
a. Murmur
b. Pericardial friction rub.
c. Sternal instability (postcardiac surgery).

7. **Abdomen.**
a. Abdominal tenderness.
b. Mass.
c. Distension.
d. Rectal.
e. Perirectal mass and tenderness.

8. **Skin and soft tissue.**
a. Erythema.
b. Tenderness.
c. Swelling.
d. Heat.

9. **Intravascular catheter sites.**

D. LABORATORY AND RADIOGRAPHIC EVALUATION.

1. **Hematology (CBC).**
a. White blood cells increased; may be decreased with overwhelming infection.
b. Thrombocytopenia is sometimes associated with sepsis.

2. **Blood culture.**
a. Obtain two sets of peripheral blood cultures.
b. Obtain a central line blood culture if catheter infection is suspected.

3. **Urinalysis.**
a. Obtain a urinalysis looking for white blood cells, nitrite, and leukocyte esterase.
b. Obtain a urine culture.

4. **Chest radiography.**
a. Infiltrate with signs of infection is suggestive of pneumonic process.
b. Effusion (parapneumonic, sympathetic).
c. Air–fluid level is suspicious for lung abscess.
d. Subdiaphragmatic air is a sensitive indicator of hollow visceral perforation, but normal variant in postceliotomy period.

5. **CT** is suspicious for intra-abdominal process and abscess.

48

DISORDERS OF TEMPERATURE REGULATION IN THE INTENSIVE CARE UNIT

VI. HYPERTHERMIA SYNDROMES: SPECIAL CONCERNS

A. RESPIRATORY.

1. Pneumonia is one of the most common hospital-acquired infections and may lead to death in 10–20% of ventilated patients.

2. If a patient has been intubated >48 hours, tracheal colonization has already occurred.

3. Operative procedures lasting >2 hours increase the risk of development of pneumonia.

4. With aspiration pneumonia, the initial injury is chemical and results in bronchospasm, hypoxemia, and fever.

5. 15–30% of patients intubated with cuffed endotracheal tubes or tracheostomy tubes will aspirate significantly.

6. In the first 24 hours postoperation, atelectasis is often the cause of fever, but it is rarely the cause of temperatures >39.5°C.

7. Atelectasis is probably the most common cause of postoperative, noninfectious fever.

B. NEUROLOGIC.

1. Meningitis is an uncommon cause of fever in surgical ICUs but should be considered in any critical patient with altered mental status and high fever.

2. Meningitis usually results from bacteria in contiguous sites of colonization or infection, but may rarely be secondary to hematogenous spread from a distant site of infection.

3. Meningitis following head or spinal cord injury appears to be uncommon, but bacterial meningitis develops in about 1% of patients with closed head injuries after blunt trauma.

4. Patients at risk are those with basilar skull fractures with a dural tear that creates a communication between the subarachnoid space and the nasal cavity, paranasal sinuses, or the ear canal.

5. Infecting organisms are almost always enteric Gram-negative bacilli.

C. DRUG REACTION.

1. Fever may be the first sign of the two most serious types of allergic drug reactions: anaphylaxis and serum sickness.

2. Anaphylactic reactions are rare, but potentially fatal with a maximum allergic response within 5–30 minutes.

3. These types of reactions are type I, IgE-mediated reactions with associated itching, urticaria, angio-edema, dyspnea, peripheral eosinophilia, joint pain, and abdominal pain.

4. In the ICU, early symptoms may go unrecognized until bronchospasm and hypotension occur.

5. Drugs associated with fatal anaphylactic reactions include penicillins, opiates, aspirin, heparin, cephalosporins, and insulin.

6. Serum sickness is a type III or immune complex reaction which develops 6–21 days after drug administration.

7. **The symptoms** include:
a. Fever.
b. Rash.
c. Lymphadenopathy.
d. Arthralgias or arthritis.
e. Edema.
f. Neuritis.
8. **Avoid the injudicious use of atropine or other parasympathomimetic drugs** that interfere with sweating.

D. **WOUND INFECTIONS.**
1. **Although wound infections and problems typically appear** on postoperative days 5–7, any fever should warrant a look at the wound even in the first few hours after surgery or trauma.
2. **High fevers may be secondary** to occult evisceration, or virulent gas-forming or necrotizing organisms such as *Escherichia coli*, group A streptococcus, and clostridia.
3. **The crush injury syndrome** and occasionally tetanus can cause fever in the postoperative trauma patient.

E. **OTHER INFECTIONS.**
1. **Infections induce an inflammatory response** in the host tissue that consists of vascular endothelial injury, edema, and neutrophil and macrophage infiltration.
2. **Sepsis** is manifested by fluid sequestration, hypotension, organ dysfunction, and ultimately death.
3. **In 2% of all abdominal operations,** reoperation or percutaneous drainage for a deep infectious complication is requires within 30 days of the original procedure.
4. **Mortality for intra-abdominal infection** is 15–50%.
5. **A leaking bowel anastomosis or missed bowel injury** is a potential cause of early life-threatening postoperative infection and fever.
6. **Toxic shock syndrome** secondary to *Staphylococcus aureus* infection is a rare, but severe, cause of fever and wound infection that occurs within 48 hours after operation.
a. Symptoms include fever, vomiting, watery diarrhea, erythroderma, and hypotension.
b. Usually, the wound initially appears normal.
c. Treatment is drainage of the wound and systemic antistaphylococcal antibiotics.

F. **TRANSFUSION.**
1. **90% of blood transfusion reactions** are allergic or febrile.
2. **If a patient has received blood products** within 3 weeks prior to the fever, transfusion-associated viral infections should be considered.

48

DISORDERS OF TEMPERATURE REGULATION IN THE INTENSIVE CARE UNIT

3. **The most common etiology** is hepatitis C followed by hepatitis B.
4. **Cytomegalovirus (CMV) has also been recognized as a cause of post-transfusion infection** and is most commonly associated with cardiac surgery; it may also be more common in postsplenectomy patients.

G. **TREATMENT PRINCIPLES.**

1. **For temperature elevations without an increased white blood count**, consider hyperpyrexia.
2. **Obvious sources of infection should be cultured** (if possible) and then treated with antibiotics.
3. **Symptomatic treatment of fever** is warranted for myalgias and cardiovascular stress.
4. **Nonsteroidals or acetaminophen** may be used.
5. **Sharp reductions in temperature can be avoided** by administering antipyretics at least every 3 hours around the clock rather than prescribing these agents only for temperature elevations above certain levels.
6. Cooling blankets do not decrease fever and actually increase metabolic demand unless the hypothalamus is blocked by sedation or paralysis.

H. **COMPLICATIONS OF PERSISTENT FEVER.**

1. **Febrile seizures** are rare after 6 years of age.
2. **Fever is a serious problem for patients with limited cardiovascular reserve** because of increased oxygen consumption and decreased systemic vascular resistance.

VII. MISCELLANEOUS SYNDROMES

A. **MALIGNANT HYPERTHERMIA.**

1. **Fulminant in 1/250,000 anesthetics.**
2. **Secondary to increased exothermic metabolic activity.**
3. **Usually precipitated by volatile anesthesia** (halothane, enflurane, isoflurane, and depolarizing muscarinic relaxants, such as succinylcholine).
4. **Malignant hyperthermia is caused by a genetic myopathy** involving skeletal muscle.
5. **Intracellular calcium is increased** which leads to intense metabolic activity and muscular contracture with a resultant increase in lactic acid.
6. **The reaction may occur on induction of anesthesia** or within 24 hours.
7. **Temperature may rise 1°C every 5 minute**s. (Barbiturates, ketamine, vecuronium, atracurium, pancuronium, opioids, benzodiazepines, and local anesthetics are considered safe.)
8. **Even with dantrolene therapy**, mortality rates are no less than 10%.
9. **Diagnosis.**
a. Signs include: tachycardia, metabolic acidosis, hypoxemia, hypercarbia,

hyperkalemia, hypernatremia, anxiety, skin mottling, cyanosis, hypertension or unstable blood pressure, masseter rigidity (initial event in 50% of patients), and temperatures as high as 43°C.

b. Early symptoms may be confused with thyrotoxicosis, undiagnosed pheochromocytoma, or neuroleptic malignant syndrome.

c. Ultimately, metabolic exhaustion occurs with edema, disseminated intramuscular coagulation, and multiple system organ failure.

d. For definitive diagnosis, caffeine and halothane contracture tests can be given.

e. Muscle biopsy is the gold standard.

10. Treatment.

a. Stop the anesthetic agent. (For neuroleptic malignant syndrome, 5–7 days may be needed for return to baseline.)

b. Hyperventilate the patient with 100% oxygen.

c. Give dantrolene 2.5mg/kg i.v. immediately and every 5 minutes up to a dose of 10mg/kg. (Dantrolene inhibits calcium release from the sarcoplasmic reticulum.)

d. Treat ventricular arrhythmias with procaine or procainamide.

e. Maintain urine output with hydration and mannitol (12.5g i.v.) to prevent myoglobinuria.

f. Some authors advocate giving sodium bicarbonate at 2–4 mEq/kg and titrate to maintain normal acid–base balance.

g. Obtain a creatine phosphokinase (CPK) level and check for disseminated intravascular coagulation.

h. Use surface cooling for temperatures >39°C.

i. Dantrolene 2.5mg/kg can be given 10–30 minutes before anesthetic induction or 3mg/kg daily for 2 days preoperatively as pretreatment.

11. Complications.

a. Similar to those of heat stroke (see below).

b. Complications may be more severe because temperature elevations are more extreme.

c. Disseminated intravascular coagulation is more common.

B. NEUROLEPTIC MALIGNANT SYNDROME.

1. **Administration of certain neuroleptic drugs** may cause a reaction similar to malignant hyperthermia, although the elevation of core temperature is usually less.

2. **Physiologic heat-dissipating mechanisms and hypothalamic regulation of temperature** may be impaired.

3. **Profound muscular rigidity occurs.**

4. **Hypothalamic temperature set-point regulation may be affected** by drug-induced dopamine-receptor blockade. Associated drugs include phenothiazines, butyrophenones, thioxanthenes, dibenzoxepines, dopamine-depleting drugs, and dopamine agonist withdrawal.

5. Diagnosis.
a. Suspect in patients given any neuroleptic drug who develop muscular rigidity, dystonia, or unexplained catatonic behavior along with hyperpyrexia.
b. Diaphoresis, tachycardia, hypertension or hypotension, and tachypnea may also be present.
6. **Treatment** – see above (under malignant hyperthermia).
7. Complications.
a. Similar to heat stoke (see below).
b. May also be at increased risk for aspiration pneumonia secondary to dystonia and impaired ability to handle secretions.
C. HEAT STROKE.
1. **Heat-related illness** with body temperatures $\geq 41°C$.
2. **Temperatures $\geq 40.6°C$**, anhydrosis, and altered mental status also qualifies as heat stroke.
3. **Irritability or irrationality** may precede either form of heat stroke.
4. **Creatine kinase is always elevated**, and some consider this to be necessary for the diagnosis.
5. **Disseminated intravascular coagulation is rare**, but is a poor prognostic marker if present.
6. **ABG, $Paco_2$, and Pao_2 will be falsely low** and the pH falsely high unless the gas is corrected for temperature.
7. **70% mortality** if untreated.
8. **Classified as exertional or nonexertional** (classic).
9. **Exertional heat stroke.**
a. Typically occurs in young, healthy adults who overexert themselves at times of high ambient temperatures or in an environment to which they are not acclimatized.
b. Thermoregulatory mechanisms are intact, at least initially, but endogenous heat production outstrips heat-dissipating mechanisms.
c. Usually there is little clinical warning.
d. Body temperature climbs rapidly, and patients can quickly lapse into coma with high core temperatures.
e. Cardiac muscle damage and infarction occur frequently and are related to the toxic effects of heat on myocytes and to coronary artery hypoperfusion in the face of hypovolemia.
10. Nonexertional heat stroke.
a. Affects elderly and debilitated persons with chronic medical illnesses during times of increased ambient temperatures.
b. Thermoregulatory mechanisms are impaired from the outset.
c. Advancing age decreases the ability to produce sweat and impairs perception of changes in ambient or body temperatures.

d. Drugs which may be associated with nonexertional heat stroke include alcohol, diuretics, phenothiazines, antiparkinsonians, anticholinergics, β-blockers, tricyclic antidepressants, amphetamines, hallucinogens, and butyrophenones).

11. Treatment of heat stroke.

a. Survival is inversely related to the intensity and duration of hyperpyrexia.

b. Effective lowering of the core temperature is usually possible with external techniques, such as immersion in an ice water bath, wetting the skin with tepid water or alcohol, and using fans to help with heat dissipation and evaporation.

c. Gastric or peritoneal lavage with iced saline is rarely needed.

d. Vigorous skin massage should accompany immersion cooling to prevent dermal stasis of cooled blood in vasoconstricted skin.

e. Once the patient's temperature approaches 39°C, cooling efforts should be terminated.

f. Intravenous chlorpromazine (10–50mg every 6 hours) may help prevent shivering and associated thermogenesis.

g. Dantrolene may decrease the time required to cool patients with heat stroke.

h. Isoproterenol is the traditional inotropic drug of choice for heat stroke with myocardial dysfunction and inadequate cardiac output because it has very little agonist affect on peripheral α-receptors.

12. Complications associated with heat stroke.

a. Myocardial pump failure.

b. Dysrhythmias.

c. Myocardial infarction.

d. Acute renal failure (multifactorial).

e. Rhabdomyolysis (exertional). Severe hypocalcemia often develops in these patients, but exogenous calcium should be avoided unless the patient develops serious ventricular ectopy secondary to hyperkalemia because calcium may worsen the rhabdomyolysis.

f. Seizures.

g. Cerebral edema.

h. Petechial hemorrhages.

i. Marked depression of mental status.

j. Hepatic failure which is reversible.

k. Cholestasis and centrolobular necrosis elevate the bilirubin and serum transaminases.

l. Acute respiratory distress syndrome (ARDS).

m. Heat enhances plasma fibrinolytic activity, directly activates platelets, and may specifically trigger disseminated intravascular coagulation.

48

DISORDERS OF TEMPERATURE REGULATION IN THE INTENSIVE CARE UNIT

D. ACUTE ADRENOCORTICAL INSUFFICIENCY.

1. Occurs in patients who are being weaned from steroids and suddenly develop increased temperature and hypotension.

2. In elective surgical cases, acute adrenal insufficiency usually develops within the first 72 hours after operation.

3. The severe metabolic stress resulting from systemic sepsis or multiple organ dysfunction (MOD) may produce acute adrenal insufficiency.

4. Treatment.

a. If the diagnosis is suspected, the patient should be treated immediately.

b. Hydrocortisone (200mg) is given i.v., followed by 50–100mg every 6 hours, unless there is a question of underlying sepsis or multiple system organ failure.

c. For these patients, higher steroid doses may be necessary.

d. Dramatic clinical improvement may be expected within minutes of steroid administration when adrenocortical insufficiency is the cause of fever and hypotension.

e. For any temperature >40°C, a cooling blanket is used until the temperature reaches 39°C.

I. ANATOMY OF BODY FLUIDS

A. **WATER** constitutes 50–70% of total body weight.

B. **FAT CONTAINS LITTLE WATER,** therefore lean patients have a greater percent of total body water.

C. **INTRACELLULAR FLUID.**

1. Makes up two-thirds of total body water.
2. Major cations are potassium (K^+) and magnesium (Mg^{2+}).
3. Major anions are phosphates and proteins.

D. **EXTRACELLULAR FLUID.**

1. Makes up one-third of total body water.
2. Two major subdivisions: interstitial fluid and plasma.
   a. Interstitial fluid is 75% of the extracellular fluid.
   b. Plasma is 25% of the extracellular fluid.
3. Major cation of extracellular fluid is sodium (Na^+).
4. Major anion of extracellular fluid is chloride (Cl^-).
5. The third space is nonfunctional fluid formed from internal losses of the extracellular fluid.
6. Third-space losses can be significant following major trauma or burns.

II. DAILY FLUID AND ELECTROLYTE REQUIREMENTS AND MAINTENANCE

A. **WATER REQUIREMENTS** in the hemodynamically stable patient:

1. Adults require 35mL/kg per 24 hours.
2. The following formula can be used for children and to a lesser degree for adults over a 24 hour period:
   a. First 10kg multiply by 100mL/kg.
   b. Second 10kg multiply by 50mL/kg and add 1000mL (from the first 10kg).
   c. Each additional kg multiply by 20mL/kg and add 1500mL (from the first 20 kg).
   d. This formula can be simplified on an hourly basis to:
      1) 4mL/kg per hour for the first 10 kg.
      2) 2mL/kg per hour for the next 10kg.
      3) 1mL/kg per hour for each additional kg.
3. Fever increases basal requirements by 15% for each degree over 37°C.
4. Tachypnea increases requirements by 50% for each doubling of rate.

B. **ELECTROLYTE REQUIREMENTS:**
1. **Sodium** – 1–2mEq/kg per day for adults or 1mEq/kg per day for children.
2. **Chloride** – 1–2mEq/kg per day for adults or 1mEq/kg per day for children.
3. **Potassium** – 1mEq/kg per day.

III. EVALUATION

A. **EXTRACELLULAR FLUID DEPLETION.** The signs and symptoms of volume deficit.
1. **Mild volume deficit** (4–6% of total body weight):
a. Agitation.
b. Increased heart rate, or asymptomatic.
2. **Moderate volume deficit** (6–8% of total body weight):
a. Orthostatic hypotension.
b. Tachycardia.
c. Collapsed veins.
d. Apathy.
e. Anorexia.
f. Drowsiness.
g. Decreased skin turgor.
h. Oliguria.
3. **Severe volume deficit** (8–10% of total body weight):
a. Hypotension.
b. Stupor.
c. Coma.
d. Atonic muscles.
e. Sunken eyes.
f. Marked decrease of body temperature.
g. Anuria.
B. **EXTRACELLULAR FLUID VOLUME EXCESS.** The signs and symptoms include:
1. **Distended jugular veins.**
2. **Rales.**
3. **Anasarca.**
C. **CAREFUL MONITORING** of intake and output as well as daily weights is crucial for fluid balance calculations.
D. **VOLUME, CONCENTRATION, AND COMPOSITION STATUS.** The volume status, concentration status (serum sodium), and composition status (potassium, calcium, trace elements, acid–base and other parameters that make up the composition of fluids) should be evaluated daily for all patients receiving i.v. fluids.
1. **Volume assessment** is accomplished by evaluating the patient clinically at the bedside using the parameters described above.

2. **Patients may not need labs every day** if their condition remains stable.
3. **Critically ill patients may require evaluation more frequently,** depending on the rate of change occurring with their fluid and electrolyte needs.

IV. REPLACEMENT OF FLUID LOSSES

A. **DEFICIT CALCULATION.** The deficit is calculated by considering the following:
1. **Extracellular fluid losses** average 750 –800mL per hour during celiotomy.
2. **Quantify measurable losses,** such as nasogastric output, fistulae, drains, vomiting, and diarrhea.
B. **MAINTENANCE FLUID REQUIREMENTS.**
1. **Insensible losses** (600–900mL per day), which may increase with tachypnea or fever.
2. **Replacement of urine output,** which averages 1000mL per day.
C. **FLUID LOSSES.** These should be replaced with a solution of similar electrolyte composition.
1. **Extracellular fluid losses** are replaced with a balanced salt solution, such as Ringer's lactate.
2. **This includes most measurable losses,** such as nasogastric output, vomitus, diarrhea, and fistula drainage, whether biliary or enteric.
3. **Fluid losses due to a gastric outlet obstruction** (at the pylorus) are replaced with normal saline.
4. **Maintenance fluids** (insensible and urine output) are generally given as half-normal saline, but in the absence of a salt-wasting nephropathy can be supplied as D5W.
D. **MONITORING FLUID REPLACEMENT.** Urine output and clinical evaluation are usually sufficient to monitor fluid replacement.
1. **Central venous monitoring** is used in patients with cardiovascular disease and complex fluid and electrolyte problems.
2. **A physician must be present to monitor patients who are receiving fluids** in excess of 1L per hour.

V. ELECTROLYTE DISORDERS

A. **HYPERNATREMIA.**
1. **The signs and symptoms include:**
a. Lethargy.
b. Muscular tremor.
c. Rigidity.
d. Coma.
e. Convulsions.
2. **Acute hypernatremia can lead to intracranial hemorrhage** from brain shrinkage and avulsion of the meningeal vessels.

49

DISORDERS OF ACID–BASE, FLUIDS, AND ELECTROLYTES

3. **Common causes of hypernatremia** in the trauma setting are excessive sodium administration or diabetes insipidus (DI).
4. **The etiology** can be determined with the help of a patient history, physical examination, evaluation of patient data for fluid status, urine osmolality, and urine sodium.
5. **DI can be diagnosed** with a urine osmolality <200mOsm; serum osmolality >290mOsm, and a normal glomerular filtration rate.
6. **Correction of hypernatremia** depends on the length of time the patient has been hypernatremic and needs to be well monitored in order to prevent sudden uncompensated fluid shifts in the brain which may cause swelling.
7. **Acute changes within 24 hours**, occurring in the absence of neurologic symptoms, can be more leisurely corrected.
8. **Sodium abnormalities are related to volume changes;** therefore correct treatment of hypernatremia depends on the patient's volume status and correction of those deficits.
9. **Hypovolemic hypernatremia** is treated by first correcting the fluid deficit. The following formula may be used:
   a. Water deficit = $0.6 \times$ body weight $\times (1 - 140/\text{serum Na})$.
   b. Intravascular volume is first repleted using isotonic fluids.
   c. Thereafter hypotonic fluids such as D5W may be used to correct the free-water deficit.
   d. Maintenance fluids are continued throughout this process.
10. **Euvolemic hypernatremia** is treated with free water enterally or D5W parenterally.
11. **Hypervolemic hypernatremia** is treated by removing fluid excess with loop diuretics (furosemide) and the use of D5W. If renal failure occurs, dialysis is necessary.
12. **DI is often seen in head injury patients** and is characterized by excretion of large quantities of dilute urine.
   a. Treatment requires intravenous fluids which may necessitate replacement of urine output with 1ml D5W (5% dextrose in water) per ml of urine every hour.
   b. Desmopressin is given 2–4μg intranasally twice a day.
   c. Severe cases can be treated with vasopressin 5–10 units s.c. every 4–6 hours.
B. **HYPONATREMIA.**
1. **The signs and symptoms include:**
   a. Muscle cramps.
   b. Weakness.
   c. Fatigue.
   d. Seizures.
   e. Coma.
2. **Evaluation** includes history, physical examination, assessment of fluid status, serum osmolality, urine osmolality, and urine sodium.

3. **Dilutional hyponatremia and syndrome of inappropriate ADH secretion** (SIADH) are frequent causes of this abnormality in the trauma patient.

4. **Other causes of hyponatremia** can be classified according to osmolality.

5. **SIADH also presents with low serum and high urine osmolalities** yet the urine sodium is >30mEq/L (30mmol/L).

a. The patient may have a history of head trauma.

b. Physical examination may be consistent with euvolemia.

c. Treatment for SIADH is fluid restriction.

6. **Hyponatremia is seen in burn patients** and is usually due to a reset osmostat. Treatment requires strict fluid restriction.

7. **Hypervolemic hyponatremia** can be treated with fluid restriction and diuresis.

8. **Severe hyponatremia** (<120mEq/L; <120mmol/L) or symptomatic hyponatremia can be treated with 3% sodium chloride.

a. This is administered slowly and with caution so as not to cause central pontine myelinolysis.

b. One half of the calculated deficit is given and then the patient re-evaluated.

c. Once sodium is >120mEq/L (>120mmol/L), hypertonic saline should be stopped.

C. **HYPERKALEMIA.**

1. **Intracellular potassium** is released into the extracellular space after trauma, acidosis, and catabolic states

2. **Renal failure or myoglobinuria** may cause rapid increases in serum potassium.

3. **The signs of hyperkalemia include:**

a. Nausea.

b. Vomiting.

c. Diarrhea.

4. **EKG changes include:**

a. High-peaked T-waves.

b. Widened QRS complexes.

c. Depressed ST segments.

d. Disappearance of T-waves, heart block, or cardiac arrest with increasing potassium levels.

5. **Treatment** is aimed at identifying and eliminating the cause of the hyperkalemia.

a. Potassium chloride supplementation is stopped and a potassium level is measured in nonhemolyzed blood.

b. Renal failure patients are dialyzed.

c. For potassium levels between 6.0–6.5mEq/L (6.0–6.5mmol/L), and in the absence of EKG changes, furosemide or sodium polystyrene sulfonate (kayexalate 15g orally 1–4 times per day) may be given.

   d. Peaked T-waves or a potassium >6.5mEq/L requires EKG monitoring, furosemide, and sodium polystyrene sulfonate.
      1) It may be necessary to give the patient insulin, 10 units i.v. in 50mL of D50W.
      2) Dialysis may be necessary if the patient is in renal failure.
   e. If EKG changes progress, calcium gluconate (90mg of elemental calcium in a 10mL ampule given over 2 minutes) or bicarbonate (50mEq/50mL over 5 minutes) is given.

D. HYPOKALEMIA.

1. The causes include:
a. Gastrointestinal losses.
b. Inappropriate supplementation.
c. Excessive renal excretion.
d. Movement of potassium into cells.
e. Alkalosis may cause hypokalemia due to excretion of potassium rather than hydrogen by the kidney.

2. Hypokalemia can cause alkalosis by renal tubular excretion of hydrogen due to the lack of potassium.

3. The signs include:
a. Weakness.
b. Paralysis.
c. Absent tendon reflexes.
d. Ileus.
e. Propensity for digoxin toxicity.
f. Flattening of ST segments on EKG.

4. The treatment consists of:
a. Oral, or i.v. administration of no more than 10mEq/L potassium per hour of potassium chloride in 100mL of saline given through a peripheral line.
b. >10mEq/L potassium per hour may be given through a central line with EKG monitoring and frequent potassium determinations.

E. CALCIUM METABOLISM.

1. Normal values – 8.5–10.5mg/dL.

2. Total serum calcium must be corrected for albumin level.

F. HYPERCALCEMIA.

1. Uncommon in trauma patients.

2. The causes include:
a. Iatrogenic.
b. Use of diuretics.
c. Thyrotoxicosis.
d. Granulomatous disease.
e. Renal disease.
f. Hyperparathyroidism.
g. Hypophosphatemia.

3. The signs and symptoms include:
a. Fatigue.
b. Lethargy.
c. Confusion.
d. Anorexia.
e. Nausea.
f. Constipation.
f. Polydipsia.
g. Polyuria.
h. Bradycardia.
i. Heart block.
4. **Treatment** is a combination of oral phosphate (if phosphate level is low), hydration, and furosemide.
G. HYPOCALCEMIA.
1. **Massive transfusions** can cause calcium depletion by citrate binding.
2. **Ionized calcium should be monitored** frequently and kept >3.8mg/dL or 1mmol/L.
3. **Other causes of hypocalcemia include:**
a. Alkalosis.
b. Acute pancreatitis.
c. Renal failure.
d. Fistulae.
e. Rhabdomyolysis.
f. Sepsis.
4. **The signs and symptoms include:**
a. Numbness and tingling of lips or fingers.
b. Hyperactive tendon reflexes.
c. Chvostek's sign.
d. Trousseaus' sign.
e. Tetany.
f. Prolongation of QT interval.
g. Reduction of cardiac contractility.
h. Ventricular fibrillation.
5. **Treatment.**
a. Bolus therapy of calcium chloride (1g over 10–30 minutes) or calcium gluconate (1g over 10–30 minutes).
b. Calcium chloride has a larger elemental calcium load.
H. MAGNESIUM METABOLISM.
1. **Magnesium is crucial** as a cofactor to multiple enzymes of metabolism.
2. **It is important** for neuromuscular transmission and muscle contraction.
3. **The normal serum level** is 1.6–2.4mg/dL.

4. **Physiologically active magnesium** is in an ionized form which is difficult to measure.

I. HYPERMAGNESEMIA.

1. **This is a rare condition.**
2. **Etiology.**
a. Impaired renal function.
b. Excessive magnesium administration.
c. Acidosis.
3. **The signs include:**
a. Lethargy.
b. Loss of deep tendon reflexes.
c. EKG changes with increased PR interval, widened QRS complex, and elevated T-waves leading to cardiac arrest.
4. **Treatment.**
a. Calcium may help control symptoms.
b. Some patients may need dialysis.

J. HYPOMAGNESEMIA.

1. **Magnesium deficiency can present with:**
a. Hyperactive tendon reflexes.
b. Muscle tremors.
c. Tetany and positive Chvostek's sign with progression to delirium and convulsions.
2. **Serum levels may be normal** with a magnesium deficiency.
3. **Potassium levels cannot be repleted with a magnesium deficiency.** This occurs because magnesium depletion can result in renal potassium wasting, and magnesium is required for potassium to enter cells.
4. **Treatment consists of 2g of magnesium sulfate** i.v. over several minutes. A maximum of 10g can be given in a 24 hour period.

K. PHOSPHORUS METABOLISM.

1. **Normal serum phosphate** is 2.5–4.5 mg/dL.
2. **Hyperphosphatemia.**
a. Most common cause is renal failure.
b. Treatment
   1) Aluminum hydroxide (i.e. Amphojel) as an oral phosphorus-binding agent.
   2) Furosemide or acetazolamide.
   3) Dialysis may be necessary.
3. **Hypophosphatemia.**
a. Causes include:
   1) Redistribution between intracellular and extracellular space.
   2) Gastrointestinal losses.
   3) Renal losses.
   4) Use of phosphorus-binding antacids.

b. Severe deficits can be treated with i.v. sodium phosphate or potassium phosphate.

c. Mild deficits can be treated with oral Neutraphos or Fleet's Phosphosoda.

VI. ACID–BASE DISTURBANCES

A. ACID–BASE REGULATION is important for homeostasis including enzyme function, coagulation factors, oxygen delivery, cardiovascular function, and other cellular processes.

B. ARTERIAL BLOOD GAS VALUES.

1. pH 7.36–7.44.

2. $Paco_2$ 35–45mmHg.

3. Pao_2 80–100mmHg.

4. Base excess –-3–3mEq/L.

C. ARTERIAL BLOOD GASES are used to monitor patient's ventilation, confirm acid–base disturbances, and evaluate therapeutic maneuvers.

D. SHOCK, blood component therapy, and over or under resuscitation are common causes for acid–base disorders in the trauma patient.

E. RESPIRATORY DISTURBANCES.

1. Respiratory acidosis.

a. Arises from poor ventilation, such as respiratory distress, oversedation, head injury, intoxication, or agonal states.

b. The pH will decrease by 0.08 for each 10mmHg rise in the $Paco_2$.

c. The degree of metabolic compensation is important to estimate so a mixed acid–base disturbance, which is common in trauma patients, is not missed.

d. Bicarbonate (HCO_3) will increase by 1mmol for each 10mmHg increase of $Paco_2$ above 40mmHg in patients with acute hypercapnia.

e. Bicarbonate will increase by 4mmol for each 10mmHg increase of $Paco_2$ above 40mmHg in patients with chronic hypercapnia.

f. Treatment.

   1) Correction of underlying cause.

   2) If this cannot be done quickly mechanical ventilation is instituted.

2. Respiratory alkalosis.

a. Hyperventilation is the most common cause in the trauma patient.

b. For each 10mmHg decrease of the $Paco_2$ the pH will increase 0.08.

c. Metabolic compensation can be estimated by:

   1) Acute hypocapnia in which the bicarbonate decreases 2mmol/L for each 10mmHg decrease of $Paco_2$ below 40mmHg

   2) Chronic hypocapnia in which the bicarbonate decreases 5–7mmol/L for each decrease of $Paco_2$ below 40mmHg.

49

DISORDERS OF ACID–BASE, FLUIDS, AND ELECTROLYTES

    d. Treatment.
       1) Ventilatory control.
       2) Possible mechanical ventilation.

F. METABOLIC DISTURBANCES.

1. Metabolic acidosis.

a. Anion gap = $Na - (Cl + HCO_3)$.
    1) Normal is 8–14.
    2) Bicarbonate is commonly decreased as a result of diarrhea, fistulae, and renal tubular acidosis.
    3) Causes of an elevated anion gap (>14) include lactic acidosis, keto-acidosis, overingestion of aspirin, ingestion of ethylene glycol, methylene glycol, or paraldehyde, and chronic renal insufficiency. The most common cause in trauma is fluid under-resuscitation or shock.

b. Base excess can be a helpful measure of fluid resuscitation.
    1) It is an index of nonrespiratory acid–base balance and a measure of total serum buffer anions (including proteins and red blood cells).
    2) Calculation is made from measurements of pH, $Paco_2$, and hematocrit and plotted on a nomogram.

c. Hyperventilation causes respiratory compensation and inappropriate compensation may reveal a mixed disorder.

d. Treatment.
    1) Correct the underlying cause.
    2) Adequate fluid resuscitation.

e. A pH <7.2 may require bicarbonate administration.
    1) Bicarbonate administration may worsen the acidosis if the patient cannot ventilate the excess CO_2.
    2) Bicarbonate may be administered using the bicarbonate deficit formula: $0.4 \times$ body weight (kg) $\times$ (HCO_3 desired – HCO_3 calculated). One-half of this amount should be given over 8 hours with frequent monitoring of arterial blood gases.

f. If the patient is in renal failure dialysis is indicated.

2. Metabolic alkalosis.

a. Classified as chloride responsive or chloride resistant.

b. Chloride responsive.
    1) Nasogastric suction.
    2) Use of diuretics.
    3) Volume contraction.

c. Chloride resistant
    1) Bicarbonate administration.
    2) Hyperaldosteronism.
    3) Cushing's syndrome.

d. Spot urine chloride <10–20mEq/L indicates a chloride-responsive alkalosis; >10–20mEq/L usually represents a chloride-resistant alkalosis.
e. Respiratory compensation: 5–7mmHg increase of $Paco_2$ for each 10mmol/L increase of HCO_3.
f. Treatment of chloride-responsive alkalosis:
    1) Appropriate chloride-containing fluids such as normal saline.
    2) Acetazolamide 250–500mg i.v. may be used.
g. Treatment of chloride-resistant alkalosis:
    1) Correction of underlying cause.
    2) Discontinue steroid or bicarbonate use.

VII. ACUTE RENAL FAILURE
A. CLASSIFICATION.
1. **Oliguric acute renal failure** – urine output <400mL per 24 hours.
2. **Nonoliguric acute renal failure** – urine output >400mL per 24 hours. Mortality is one-half that of oliguric acute renal failure.
B. ETIOLOGY.
1. **Prerenal.**
a. Decrease in intravascular volume is common in trauma patients after hemorrhage, third-space fluid loss, or fluid drainage.
b. Impaired cardiac function.
c. Renal vascular obstruction.
2. **Renal.**
a. Prolonged prerenal or postrenal states.
b. Parenchymal lesions of the glomerulus or tubules due to nephrotoxins, such as aminoglycosides, amphotericin B, acetaminophen, and radiologic contrast agents.
    1) Acute renal failure is more likely to occur after the administration of radiologic contrast agents if the patient is diabetic or has pre-existing chronic renal insufficiency, decreased intravascular volume, hypertension, peripheral vascular disease, or is of increased age, or if other nephrotoxic drugs are being used concomitantly.
    2) Myoglobin precipitates in the renal tubules causing obstruction.
c. Nonsteroidal anti-inflammatory drugs may increase renal vasoconstriction in patients with pre-existing prerenal conditions.
3. **Postrenal** – anatomic obstruction of the urinary tract.
C. DIAGNOSIS OF ACUTE RENAL FAILURE.
1. **Acute renal failure can be assessed** by an accurate history and physical examination focusing on prerenal, renal, or postrenal etiologic factors.
2. **Laboratory assessment.**
a. Blood urea nitrogen and creatinine will rise with decreased renal function.

49

DISORDERS OF ACID–BASE, FLUIDS, AND ELECTROLYTES

   b. Urine chemistries should be determined before diuretics are used.

   c. Fraction excretion of Na (FENa) is a measure of the kidneys' concentrating ability.

     1) Calculation: (urine Na × serum creatinine/serum Na × urine creatinine) × 100%.

     2) In prerenal patients the FENa is <1%.

     3) In renal parenchymal injury the FENa is >3%.

   d. Prerenal patients will have unremarkable urinalysis.

     1) Urine osmolality >350mOsm.

     2) Urine Na <10mEq/L.

   e. Patients with intrinsic renal failure may have:

     1) Proteinuria.

     2) Pyuria.

     3) Casts (protein, white blood cells, or epithelial) in their urine.

     4) Urine osmolality will equal plasma osmolality.

     5) Urine Na will be >10mEq/L.

   f. Patients with postrenal failure will have:

     1) An unremarkable urinalysis.

     2) Unremarkable urine electrolytes.

     3) A need for imaging studies to confirm the diagnosis.

   g. Patients with rhabdomyolysis will have a positive urine dip for blood, but no microscopic red blood cells.

D. TREATMENT.

1. Prerenal.

   a. Restoration of intravascular volume.

   b. Correction of cardiac output.

   c. Correction of renal vascular perfusion.

   d. Swan–Ganz catheter may be necessary for hemodynamic monitoring.

   e. Establish urine output.

2. Renal.

   a. Withhold nephrotoxic agents.

   b. Myoglobinuria will require vigorous fluid administration until urine is free of myoglobin.

     1) Mannitol (25g) is given for an osmotic diuresis.

     2) Urine alkalization is achieved with bicarbonate (50mEq/50mL vial).

3. Postrenal – urinary obstruction should be corrected.

E. MANAGEMENT.

1. Establish urine output (0.5–1mL/kg per hour).

2. Optimize intravascular volume and hemodynamic status for appropriate renal perfusion.

3. Use osmotic or loop diuretics to increase urine output for fluid management.

4. Use all precautions to prevent hyperkalemia.
5. **Low-dose dopamine**:
a. Increases renal blood flow and glomerular filtration rate.
b. Dose 0.5–2.5µg/kg per minute.
c. Complications: tachyarrhythmias, pulmonary shunting.
6. **Dialysis** – common indications include:
a. Volume overload.
b. Hyperkalemia (electrolyte abnormalities).
c. Metabolic acidosis.
d. Signs and symptoms of severe uremia.
7. **Peritoneal dialysis.**
a. Advantages
   1) Technically easy.
   2) Less associated hypotension.
   3) No need for anticoagulation.
b. Disadvantages
   1) Risk of peritonitis.
   2) Inappropriate after recent celiotomy.
8. **Intermittent hemodialysis** is the standard therapy for acute renal failure.
9. **Continuous venovenous (CVVH) and arteriovenous hemodialysis** (CAVH) have benefits over intermittent hemodialysis:
a. Advantages.
   1) Precise fluid and metabolic control.
   2) Less accidental hypotension.
   3) Ability to administer nutritional support.
b. Disadvantages.
   1) Need for prolonged anticoagulation.
   2) Constant sophisticated surveillance.

VIII. FURTHER READING

Carrico CJ, Mileski WJ, Kaplan HS. Transfusion, autotransfusion, and blood substitutes. In: Feliciano DV, Moore EE, Mattox KL (eds.) *Trauma*, 3rd edn. Stamford: Appleton and Lange; 1996:181–191.

Lyerly HK, Gaynor JW (eds.) *The handbook of surgical intensive care,* 3rd edn. St Louis: Mosby Year Book; 1992.

Shires GT III, Shires GT. Fluid and electrolyte management of the surgical patient. In: Sabiston DC, ed. *Textbook of surgery: the biological basis of modern surgical practice,* 15th edn. Philadelphia: WB Saunders; 1997:92–111.

Thadhani R, Pascual M, Bonventre JV. Acute renal failure. *N Engl J Med* 1996; 334:1448–1460.

DISORDERS OF ACID–BASE, FLUIDS, AND ELECTROLYTES

49

INFECTION IN THE SURGICAL INTENSIVE CARE UNIT

50

I. STATISTICS

1. **Infection and inflammation** are among the most common causes of admission and extended length of stay in the surgical intensive care unit (ICU).
2. **There are an estimated 250,000–500,000 cases of sepsis** in the United States yearly associated with a mortality of 20–30%.
3. **Early recognition and institution of therapy** are paramount in decreasing the morbidity and cost associated with this disease process.

II. DEFINITIONS OF INFECTION AND INFLAMMATION

A. **INFECTION.** This is a microbiologic diagnosis.

B. **SYSTEMIC INFLAMMATORY RESPONSE SYNDROME (SIRS).**

1. **Fever + elevated white blood count (WBC) = SIRS.**
2. **Two or more of the following criteria:**
   a. Temperature >38ºC or temperature <36ºC.
   b. Heart rate >90 beats per minute.
   c. Respiratory rate >20 or Pao_2 <32mmHg.
   d. WBC >12 or WBC <4 or immature forms >10%.

C. **SEPSIS.**

1. **SIRS + infection = sepsis.**
2. **Hypermetabolic response** associated with increased oxygen demand.
3. **Systemic inflammation** in response to infection.

D. **SEPTIC SHOCK.**

1. **Sepsis + hypotension = septic shock.**
2. **Associated with decreased tissue oxygen extraction and oxygen debt.**

E. **MULTIPLE ORGAN DYSFUNCTION.**

1. **Predisposing factors** include sepsis and systemic inflammatory response syndrome (SIRS).
2. **Functional abnormality** of more than one organ system.
3. **Pathophysiology related to overwhelmed host defense.**

III. HOST DEFENSE AND INFLAMMATORY RESPONSE

A. **ACUTE INFLAMMATORY RESPONSE.**

B. **CELLULAR.**

1. **Tissue injury** leads to polymorphonuclear leukocyte chemotaxis and adhesion.
2. **Neutrophil degranulation and phagocytosis** effect bacterial killing.
3. **Stimulated macrophages** produce cytokines in response to bacteria and lipopolysaccharide (LPS).

C. **CYTOKINES.**

1. **These are factors released in response to injury** which potentiate inflammatory response.

2. **Their controlled production** attempts to reinstate homeostasis, but overproduction is potentially deleterious.

D. IMMUNOLOGIC.

1. **Humoral immunity** is mediated by B lymphocytes.
2. **Cellular immunity** is mediated by T lymphocytes.

IV. EVALUATION OF THE FEBRILE RESPONSE
See Chapter 48.

V. ETIOLOGY OF HYPERTHERMIA

A. INFECTION AND INFLAMMATION.

B. DEEP VENOUS THROMBOSIS (DVT) and pulmonary embolus (PE) (see Chapter 33).

C. TRANSFUSION.

D. DRUGS.

1. **Antibiotics** (e.g. penicillins, cephalosporins, rifampin, vancomycin).
2. **Antifungals** (e.g. amphotericin B).
3. **Antiarrhythmics** (e.g. procainamide, quinidine).
4. **Thrombolytics** (e.g. streptokinase).
5. **Anticonvulsants** (e.g. dilantin, carbamazepine).

E. HYPOTHALAMIC DYSFUNCTION – preoptic nucleus of the anterior hypothalamus.

F. TRAUMA.

G. MALIGNANCY.

H. INFARCTION (e.g. cerebrovascular accident).

I. HEMORRHAGE (e.g. hypertension).

J. ENDOCRINE AND METABOLIC.

1. **Thyroid storm** is the extreme manifestation of thyrotoxicosis associated with fever, disproportionate tachycardia relative to fever, and central nervous system (CNS) aberrations.
a. Inciting factors include thyroid manipulation, infection, trauma, diabetic keto-acidosis, myocardial infarction, and drugs.
b. Diagnosis is based on thyroid function tests.
c. Treatment is aimed at the minimization of thyroid hormone and the acute control of the hemodynamic effects of thyroid hormone excess by β-blockade.

2. **Adrenal insufficiency**
a. The pathophysiology is related to adrenocortical dysfunction with a decreased production of glucocorticoids.
b. The primary causes are adrenal in origin and include trauma, hemorrhage, infarction, and malignancy.
c. Secondary causes are associated with the suppression of the hypothalamic–pituitary–adrenal axis by exogenous steroids.
d. The signs may include hyperthermia and refractory hypotension.

e. Diagnosis is based on an ACTH stimulation test to document the cortisol production in response to exogenous hormone administration.

f. A CT head scan may be useful to exclude a CNS abnormality.

g. Treatment is i.v. steroid and supportive measures, including the possible necessity for inotropic support.

3. Gout.

a. Manifests by increased serum urate in conjunction with arthritis, most common at first metatarsophalangeal joints.

b. Treatment is supportive.

4. Cardiac – acute myocardial infarction.

5. Drug withdrawal (e.g. ethanol).

6. Sympathetic response associated with hypertension, tachycardia, and mental status changes (e.g. narcotic).

K. IATROGENIC.

1. Warming blanket.

2. Infusion devices and blood warmers.

3. Ventilator circuit warming.

L. MISCELLANEOUS.

1. Malignant hyperthermia.

a. Hyperthermia is usually associated with general anesthetics (e.g. halothane, enflurane, isoflurane) and depolarizing neuromuscular blockade (e.g. succinylcholine).

b. Malignant hyperthermia occurs in 1 in 16,000 administration of general anesthetics; also 1 in 50,000 adults have a genetic predisposition to malignant hyperthermia.

c. Mortality of untreated cases is 80% and treated cases 10%.

d. May occur intraoperatively or within 24 hours postoperatively.

e. Etiology is the excess release of calcium by the sarcoplasmic reticulum of skeletal muscle associated with sustained contraction.

f. Symptoms include temperature >104ºC, mental status changes, and muscular rigidity.

g. Laboratory findings are consistent with coagulopathy, metabolic acidosis, and progressive renal insufficiency associated with rhabdomyolysis.

h. Treatment is discontinuation of anesthetic followed by a dantrolene 2mg/kg bolus subsequently followed every 10 minutes by 2mg/kg to a total dose of 10mg/kg.

i. Hemodynamic or ventilatory support may be needed.

2. Neuroleptic malignant syndrome.

a. Presentation is similar to malignant hyperthermia.

b. Associated with neuroleptic therapy, most commonly haloperidol (commonly used in ICU settings).

c. Originates centrally and presynaptically.

d. Treatment is the same as for malignant hyperthermia.

1. **Risk factors** include:
a. Prolonged site utilization.
b. Catheter manipulation.
c. Occlusive dressings.
d. Poor sterile technique on insertion.
2. **Signs and symptoms.**
a. Fever.
b. Local erythema.
c. Pain and tenderness.
3. **Diagnostic evaluation.**
a. Complete blood count.
b. Blood cultures: two peripheral and one through the central line.
c. Central line culture.
4. **Diagnostic criteria.**
a. Colonization:
   1) Line with >15 colony-forming units (CFU).
   2) Cultures negative.
b. Infection:
   1) Line with >15CFU.
   2) Cultures positive with same organism.
5. **Treatment.**
a. Catheter removal.
b. Antistaphylococcal therapy (e.g. nafcillin, first-generation cephalosporin).
c. Elevation and comfort measures.
d. Phlebectomy required for suppurative thrombophlebitis.
B. **WOUND AND SOFT TISSUE.**
1. **Superficial.**
a. Signs and symptoms.
   1) Fever.
   2) Pain.
   3) Erythema.
   4) Tenderness.
   5) Rubor.
   6) Lymphangitis.
b. Diagnostic evaluation.
   1) CBC.
   2) Clinical evaluation.
c. Treatment.
   1) Antibiotics directed against most likely Gram-positive pathogens (e.g. nafcillin).
   2) Incision and drainage (I&D) superficial abscess.

2.   **Invasive.**
a.   Risk factors include:
   1)   Immunosuppression.
   2)   Diabetes.
   3)   Advanced age.
   4)   Malnutrition.
   5)   Exogenous steroids.
   6)   Radiation.
   7)   Chemotherapy.
b.   Types of infection.
   1)   Polymicrobial.
   2)   Clostridial – produces progressive myonecrosis.
   3)   Streptococcal – exotoxin and lytic enzymes which cleave prefascial tissue planes associated with rapidly advancing infection.
c.   Signs and symptoms.
   1)   Fever.
   2)   Pain.
   3)   Symptoms of shock.
   4)   Tenderness.
   5)   Erythema.
   6)   Skin discoloration and bullae.
   7)   Crepitus.
   8)   Clostridia associated with characteristic 'dishwater colored' effluent.

VII.   DIAGNOSIS AND TREATMENT
A.   **GENERAL PRINCIPLES.**
1.   **Diagnostic evaluation.**
a.   No special diagnostic studies.
b.   Therapy is based on clinical judgment.
2.   **Treatment.**
a.   Surgical emergency: hallmark of therapy is the wide débridement of nonviable tissue.
b.   Broad-spectrum antibiotic therapy is instituted, including a high-dose penicillin (against clostridia and streptococci).
B.   **TETANUS.**
1.   **May be heralded by:**
a.   Trismus.
b.   Dysphagia.
c.   Fever.
2.   **The interval between the first symptom and the first severe spasms** may be from 24 hours to >10 days.

3. **In severe cases**, muscular spasms are superimposed on the baseline muscular hypertonicity, leading to crush fractures of vertebrae and death from respiratory failure.

4. **Any wound may be a nidus for tetanus** although deep penetrating injuries with a necrotic focus create the highest risk.

5. **The toxin attacks nerve synapses.**

6. **Treatment.**

a. Passive immunization with human tetanus immune globulin.

b. Active immunization with tetanus toxoid.

c. Penicillin.

d. Débridement and drainage of wounds.

e. Supportive care with mechanical ventilation and complete muscle paralysis may be necessary for 6–8 weeks.

7. **Recovery is complete in survivors.**

8. **The diagnosis is completely clinical** because cultures are rarely positive.

C. **MELENEY'S ULCER.**

1. **A rare synergistic infection** usually due to a microaerophilic streptococcus and hemolytic *Staphylococcus aureus*.

2. **It is a tender lesion** with a central area of purple-appearing necrosis surrounded by cellulitis.

3. **It can occur** around surgical drains, sutures, and stomas after 1–2 weeks.

4. **The lesion progressively enlarges**, but seldom involves underlying fascia.

5. **Treatment.**

a. Antistaphylococcal drug.

b. Minor débridement.

D. **PULMONARY AND THORACIC.**

1. **Pneumonia.**

a. Predisposing conditions include:

    1) Endotracheal airway with loss of mucociliary clearance.

    2) Nasogastric intubation.

    3) H2 blocker therapy.

    4) Prolonged recumbency.

b. Signs and symptoms.

    1) Fever.

    2) Dyspnea.

    3) Cough.

    4) Chest pain.

    5) Abnormal breath sounds.

    6) Hypoxia.

c. Diagnostic evaluation.

    1) Chest radiography to exclude infiltrate.

2) Sputum culture.
3) Broncho-alveolar lavage and culture (10^4 organisms per mL has 70–100% sensitivity for pneumonia).

d. Treatment.
1) Chest physiotherapy.
2) May require ventilatory support.
3) Antimicrobial agents directed by culture results (*Pseudomonas* species require double synergistic coverage).

2. **Empyema.**
a. Risk factors include:
1) Penetrating thoracic trauma.
2) Retained hemothorax.
3) Tube thoracostomy.
4) Parapneumonic effusion.
b. Signs and symptoms.
1) Fever.
2) Chest pain.
3) Dyspnea.
c. Diagnostic evaluation.
1) Chest radiography to evaluate for gross pathology.
2) Chest CT scan.
d. Treatment.
1) Antimicrobial agent directed at source of contamination: endogenous (broad spectrum); exogenous (Gram-positive coverage).
2) Tube thoracostomy drainage.
3) Thoracoscopy or thoracotomy with decortication reserved for conservative-treatment failures.

3. **Mediastinitis.**
a. Posterior mediastinitis is usually related to inflammatory esophageal pathology and perforation.
b. Anterior mediastinitis is associated with poststernotomy procedures.
c. Signs and symptoms.
1) Fever.
2) Chest pain.
3) Dyspnea.
4) May present with signs of shock, especially posterior mediastinitis.
5) May have sternal instability (anterior mediastinitis).
d. Diagnostic evaluation.
1) Chest radiography may show left basilar effusion consistent with esophageal perforation or pneumomediastinum.
2) Cineradiographic evaluation if esophageal perforation is suspected.

e. Treatment.
  1) Anterior mediastinitis: Gram-positive coverage (e.g. vancomycin).
  2) Surgical débridement with pectoralis major flap coverage.
  3) Posterior mediastinitis: broad-spectrum coverage.
  4) Esophageal repair or exclusion.

4. Pericarditis.
a. Generally associated with poststernotomy procedures, uremia, or viruses.
b. Signs and symptoms.
  1) Fever.
  2) Chest pain.
c. Diagnostic evaluation.
  1) Chest radiography.
  2) Echocardiography if suspicious of significant effusion.
d. Treatment.
  1) Supportive.
  2) Anti-inflammatory drugs.
  3) Percutaneous or open subxiphoid drainage for suspected purulent pericarditis or tamponade.

E. URINARY TRACT.
1. Microorganism migration along indwelling catheter.
2. Accounts for 35–40% of nosocomial infections.
3. Gram-negative organisms predominate.
4. Signs and symptoms.
a. Fever.
b. Dysuria.
c. Flank and suprapubic tenderness.
5. Diagnostic evaluation.
a. Urinalysis
  1) WBC.
  2) Leukocyte esterase, nitrite.
b. Urine culture.
6. Treatment.
a. Removal of Foley catheter.
b. Antimicrobial therapy directed at Gram-negative organisms (e.g. combination penicillin and β-lactamase inhibitor).
F. INTRA-ABDOMINAL ABSCESS.
1. Predisposing conditions include:
a. Perforated ulcer, diverticulitis, appendicitis, or gallbladder.
b. Postceliotomy.
c. Missed traumatic injury.
2. Signs and symptoms.
a. Fever.

b. Abdominal pain.

c. Nausea.

d. Vomiting.

e. Abdominal tenderness (local tenderness and diffuse peritonitis).

f. Abdominal mass.

3. Diagnostic evaluation.

a. Chest radiography may demonstrate free air or a sympathetic effusion.

b. Kidney, ureter, and bladder radiography (KUB) obtained to rule out obstruction or free air.

c. CT of the abdomen is the single best diagnostic test as it is highly sensitive and specific.

4. Treatment.

a. Broad-spectrum antibiotics to cover, especially, Gram-negative organisms and anaerobes.

b. Percutaneous CT-guided drainage.

c. Surgical drainage.

G. CHOLECYSTITIS (ACALCULOUS).

1. Predisposing factors.

a. Burns.

b. Trauma.

c. Ischemia.

d. Biliary stasis.

e. Cystic duct obstruction.

2. Signs and symptoms.

a. Fever.

b. Abdominal pain.

c. Nausea.

d. Vomiting.

e. Right upper quadrant abdominal tenderness.

3. Diagnostic evaluation – right upper quadrant ultrasound for gallbladder distension and sludge, pericholecystic fluid, or wall thickening.

4. Treatment.

a. Gram-negative antibiotic coverage, with or without anaerobe coverage.

b. Cholecystectomy.

c. Unstable patients may be temporized by ultrasonic or CT-guided percutaneous cholecystostomy.

H. CHOLANGITIS.

1. Associated with:

a. Common bile duct obstruction.

b. Biliary stasis.

c. Transendothelial migration of bacteria.

2. Signs and symptoms – Charcot's triad.

a. Fever.

b. Jaundice.

c. Right upper quadrant abdominal pain.

3. Diagnostic evaluation – right upper quadrant ultrasound to evaluate biliary system.

4. Treatment.

a. Gram-negative antimicrobial agents.

b. Endoscopic retrograde cholangiopancreatography (ERCP) with sphincterotomy.

c. Open or CT-guided cholecystostomy in patients who are not ERCP candidates.

d. Percutaneous transhepatic drainage.

I. PANCREATITIS.

1. Associated factors include:

a. Ductal obstruction.

b. Alcohol use.

c. Trauma.

d. Ischemia.

e. Drugs and antibiotics.

2. Signs and symptoms.

a. Epigastric abdominal pain.

b. Nausea.

c. Vomiting.

d. Fever.

e. Epigastric abdominal tenderness.

f. Signs of shock consistent with necrotizing infection or abscess.

3. Diagnostic evaluation.

a. Amylase.

b. Lipase.

c. Liver function tests.

d. Right upper quadrant ultrasound to exclude common bile duct obstruction or cholelithiasis.

e. CT of the abdomen to evaluate for phlegmon and abscess.

4. Treatment.

a. Broad-spectrum antibiotics.

b. Surgical drainage and debridement for necrotizing infection or abscess.

c. Supportive measures, may require vigorous volume support.

J. ENTERIC.

1. Pseudomembranous enterocolitis.

a. Enteric overgrowth of *Clostridium difficile* with production of mucosal pseudomembrane and enterotoxin.

b. Predisposing factor is related to antecedent antibiotic therapy.

c. Associated with increased risk of toxic megacolon.

2. Signs and symptoms.

a. Fever.

b. Abdominal pain.
c. Diarrhea.
d. Abdominal tenderness.
3. **Diagnostic evaluation.**
a. Stool analysis:
   1) Difficile toxin.
   2) Fecal white blood cells.
b. KUB to exclude colonic distension (toxic megacolon).
c. Lower endoscopy.
   1) Pseudomembrane visualization.
   2) Culture and biopsy.
4. **Treatment.**
a. Parenteral or enteral metronidazole are first line of therapy.
b. Enteral vancomycin is reserved for refractory illness.
c. Toxic megacolon may require surgical intervention.

K. **SINUSITIS.**
1. **Predisposing factors** include:
a. Paranasal sinus fracture.
b. Prolonged nasogastric or nasotracheal intubation or nasal packing.
2. **Signs and symptoms.**
a. Fever.
b. Headache.
c. Facial pain.
d. Maxillary or frontal tenderness, nasal discharge.
3. **Diagnostic evaluation.**
a. Radiographs (facial series).
b. CT of face including paranasal sinuses.
c. Sinus aspiration ($>10^3$ organisms per mL is indicative of infection).
4. **Treatment.**
a. Antibiotics.
b. Aspiration or open sinus drainage (Caldwell Luc approach).

L. **MENINGITIS.**
1. **Associated with:**
a. Hematogenous spread.
b. Trauma.
c. Postcraniospinal surgery.
2. **Signs and symptoms.**
a. Fever.
b. Headache.
c. Obtundation.
d. Nuchal rigidity.
3. **Diagnostic evaluation.**
a. CT of head to rule out mass lesion.

b. Lumbar puncture.

4. **Treatment** – antibiotics, which must cross the blood–brain barrier.

M. MISCELLANEOUS.

1. **Toxic shock syndrome (TSS).**

a. Mucocutaneous colonization and infection with exotoxin-producing *S. aureus*.

b. Predisposing factors include:
   1) Retained tampons.
   2) Nasal packs, etc.

2. **Signs and symptoms.**

a. Fever.

b. Headache.

c. Diarrhea.

d. Diffuse erythematous rash.

3. **Diagnostic evaluation** – culture of the affected tissue.

4. **Treatment.**

a. Mainly supportive.

b. Use of antibiotics is variable (blood cultures usually sterile).

VIII. THERAPY OF INFECTION AND INFLAMMATION

A. VOLUME RESUSCITATION.

1. **Isotonic fluid resuscitation** (lactated Ringer's, 0.9% NaCl) is instituted to restore intravascular volume.

2. **Ongoing evaluation of volume status** by monitoring hemodynamic status and urine output.

B. INVASIVE PHYSIOLOGIC MONITORING. The criteria influencing the decision to place a pulmonary artery catheter include:

1. **High fluid volume support.**

2. **High ventilatory support** (PEEP >10).

3. **Cardiac disease** (e.g. congestive heart failure, coronary artery disease, etc.).

4. **Pulmonary disease** (e.g. COPD, pulmonary contusion, pulmonary hypertension, etc.).

5. **Age** >65 years.

C. SEPSIS AND SIRS.

1. **Early phase** is characterized by elevated cardiac output and decreased systemic vascular resistance.

2. **Cardiac output** below normal in late phases; precedes cardiac failure.

D. INOTROPIC SUPPORT.

1. **The goal** is to optimize oxygen consumption and delivery.

2. **Dopamine.**

a. 2–5µg/kg body weight/minute exerts renal effect via dopaminergic receptors.

b. 5–10µg/kg body weight/minute mainly affects the heart rate via β receptors.

c. Doses over 10μg/kg body weight/minute are associated with vasoconstriction via β-receptor binding.

3. Dobutamine.

a. Initial dose 2–5μg/kg body weight/minute.

b. Selective β effect produces inotropy and decreased systemic vascular resistance.

c. Is associated with improved cardiac output.

d. May cause hypotension in the hypovolemic patient.

4. Norepinephrine.

a. Pure agonist; used sparingly.

b. Produces vasoconstriction and increases afterload which may impair cardiac output and oxygen delivery in the face of increased metabolic demand.

5. Epinephrine (Levophed).

a. Both α and β effects.

b. Stimulates the epinephrine response.

c. Useful for unstable patients and those refractory to dopamine therapy.

d. Complications include myocardial and visceral ischemia.

E. SURGICAL CONTROL OF INFECTION AND INFLAMMATION.

1. Control source.

2. Débridement.

3. Drainage.

F. ANTIBIOTIC THERAPY.

1. General principles.

a. Bacteriostatic.

    1) Action of the antibiotic inhibits bacterial cell growth and division.

    2) Bacteria subsequently cleared by host defenses.

b. Bacteriocidal.

    1) Antibiotic which exerts direct effect on organism to effect cell killing.

    2) Crucial form of therapy in the immunocompromised host.

c. Synergy – combinations of antibiotics which act by different mechanisms.

d. Resistance – antibiotic associated, penicillins and cephalosporins are especially susceptible, owing to bacterial mutations conferring increased β-lactamase activity.

e. Complications.

    1) Allergy and hypersensitivity.

    2) Fever.

    3) Nephrotoxicity (e.g. aminoglycosides).

    4) Seizures (e.g. imipenem).

    5) Bone marrow toxicity.

f. Empiric therapy.

      1) Azole antifungal or broad-spectrum antibiotic therapy.
      2) Indications include unstable or deteriorating patients with clinical sepsis or SIRS.
      3) Useful for suspected candidiasis associated with fever of unknown origin.
  g. Prophylactic therapy.
      1) Institution of antibiotic therapy prior to surgical procedures to minimize postoperative wound infection.
      2) Antibiotics given 30–60 minutes preoperatively are associated with adequate tissue levels at the time of surgical incision.
  h. Wound morbidity is associated with the class of procedure.
      1) Clean (e.g. hernia, thoracotomy): 1–2%.
      2) Clean–contaminated (e.g. biliary, esophageal, gastric): 2–5%.
      3) Contaminated (e.g. unprepared colon): 5–30%.
      4) Infected (e.g. intra-abdominal abscess): >30%.

2. Aminoglycosides.
a. Spectrum – Gram-negative aerobes and facultative anaerobes.
b. Effect bacterial killing by inhibition of protein synthesis.
c. Single daily dose based on nomogram.
d. Indications.
      1) Urinary tract infection.
      2) Synergistic therapy.

3. Antianaerobes.
a. Spectrum – anaerobe and Gram-positive.
b. Indications.
      1) Intra-abdominal abscess.
      2) Oral or dental abscess.
      3) Aspiration pneumonia.

4. Lactams.
a. Penicillins.
b. Inhibit bacterial cell wall synthesis.
c. Spectrum – Gram-positive cocci and bacilli.
d. Indications.
      1) Clostridial myonecrosis.
      2) Streptococcal soft tissue infection.
      3) Streptococcal pneumonia.

5. Cephalosporins.
a. General.
      1) Mechanism – inhibition of cell wall synthesis.
      2) Bacteriocidal.
b. First generation.
      1) Spectrum – Gram positive.

      2) Indications – superficial soft tissue infection and prophylactic therapy for clean operative cases.

c. Second generation.

      1) Spectrum – moderate Gram positive, moderate Gram negative.

      2) Indications – prophylactic therapy for enteric surgical procedures; perioperative prophylaxis for suspected clean–contaminated and contaminated cases; ERCP prophylaxis; and combination therapy for intra-abdominal sepsis.

d. Third generation.

      1) Spectrum – broad spectrum Gram negative.

      2) Indications – community-acquired pneumonia; pseudomonas coverage, should be used in synergy with another agent.

e. Fourth generation.

      1) Spectrum – excellent Gram-negative coverage.

      2) Indications – resistant organisms; and nosocomial pneumonia.

6. Monobactams (e.g. aztreonam).

a. Spectrum – Gram-negative aerobe, including *Pseudomonas* species.

b. Indications.

      1) Synergistic antipseudomonal therapy.

      2) Gram-negative coverage in patients with contraindications to aminoglycosides.

7. Carbapenems (e.g. imipenem).

a. Spectrum – most broad-coverage penicillin.

b. Indications.

      1) Intra-abdominal sepsis.

      2) Resistant pneumonia.

      3) Synergistic antipseudomonal coverage.

8. Glycopeptides (e.g. vancomycin).

a. Spectrum – Gram-positive, including *Staphylococcus epidermidis*, methicillin resistant *Staphylococcus aureus* (MRSA), and enterococcus.

b. Indications.

      1) Pseudomembranous enterocolitis (third-line choice).

      2) Sternal wound infection and postcoronary artery bypass (CAB) mediastinitis.

      3) MRSA.

      4) Coagulase negative staphylococcus.

      5) Ampicillin resistant enterococcus.

      6) Selective indications to prevent emergence of vancomycin-resistant *Enterococcus* species.

9. Quinolones.

a. Spectrum – broad Gram-negative coverage, including *Pseudomonas* species.

  b. Gram-positive coverage intermediate.
  c. Indications.
      1) Nosocomial pneumonia.
      2) Intra-abdominal sepsis.
      3) Urinary tract infection.

10. Macrolides.
  a. Spectrum – Gram-positive organisms.
  b. Bacteriostatic at low concentrations and bacteriocidal at high concentrations.
  c. Indications.
      1) Pre-operative prophylaxis for elective colonic operations.
      2) Synergistic combination against resistant Gram-positive organisms.

11. Sulfa drugs.
  a. Spectrum – Gram-negative rods.
  b. Indications.
      1) Urinary tract infection.
      2) *Pneumocystitis carinii* infection.

12. Antifungal therapy.
  a. Amphotericin B.
      1) Indications – hematogenous fungal infection and disseminated fungal infection.
      2) Risk factors for disseminated fungal infection include: immunosuppression; trauma and burns; and broad-spectrum antibiotics.
      3) Treatment is with initial 1mg test dose and, if no hypersensitivity, daily dosing is based according to renal function.
  b. Fluconazole.
      1) Indications – nonhematogenous and nondisseminated *Candida albicans* infection; limited role for treatment of invasive *C. albicans* infection (e.g. patients with hypersensitivity to amphotericin B); and empiric therapy for inflammatory process of unknown origin in high-risk population (e.g. immunosuppression, burn, trauma, broad-spectrum antibiotics).
      2) Many *Candida* species are resistant.
  c. Nystatin.
      1) Treatment of mucocutaneous candidiasis and oral thrush.
      2) Topical application 10mL three times daily.

13. Antiviral therapy.
  a. Acyclovir.
      1) Herpes simplex virus.
      2) Post-transplant.
      3) HIV.
      4) Epstein–Barr virus.

b. Gancyclovir.
   1) Cytomegalovirus (CMV).
   2) Post-transplant.
   3) HIV.
c. Interferon.
   1) Immunomodulator.
   2) Potentially useful against hepatitides (HCV >HBV).
d. Nucleoside analogs.
   1) Inhibit reverse transcription HIV virus.
   2) Limits retroviral replication and protein synthesis.
e. Ribavirin.
   1) Respiratory syncytial virus.
   2) Viral hepatitis.

METABOLISM AND NUTRITION

I. INTRODUCTION

After the initial resuscitation, stabilization, and correction of anatomic and physiologic insults, the next obstacle facing the critically injured patient is the maintenance of nutritional support.

II. METABOLISM

A. **STARVATION VS POST-TRAUMATIC HYPERMETABOLIC STATE.**
Knowledge of the metabolic response to starvation and its comparison to the stressed patient provides insight and understanding for the basis of nutritional support (Table 51.1).

B. **MEDIATORS OF STRESS RESPONSE.**

1. **Catecholamine and sympathetic nervous system.**
   a. Increase heart rate and contractility.
   b. Increase in vascular tone.
   c. Increase in minute ventilation.
   d. Increase in oxygen consumption.
   e. Increase in glycogenolysis and gluconeogenesis.
   f. Increase in lipolysis.

2. **Hormonal mediators.**
   a. ADH (vasopressin)
      1) Acts on renal tubules to increase reabsorption of free water by the peritubular vessels.
      2) Vasoconstriction (especially splanchnic).
      3) Increases glycogenolysis and gluconeogenesis.

TABLE 51.1		
METABOLIC COMPARISION CHART		
Metabolic parameter	**Starvation**	**Hypermetabolic state**
Resting energy expenditure (REE)	Increased	Increased
Respiratory quotient (RQ)	0.8–0.7 (fat fuel source)	>0.8 (protein fuel source)
Glucose metabolism	Normo or hypoglycemia	Hyperglycemia
Protein metabolism	Minimal protein loss	Negative nitrogen balance
Fat metabolism	FFA primary fuel source	Increased lipolysis and oxidation of ϭ-6-fatty acids

FFA, free fatty acids.

   b. Cortisol.
      1) Increase in blood glucose through gluconeogenesis.
      2) Increase in lipolysis; decrease lipogenesis.
      3) Increase in proteolysis.
      4) Potentiates actions of glucagon and catecholamine.
   c. Glucagon.
      1) Opposes insulin effects.
      2) Increases gluconeogenesis.
      3) Promotes amino acid uptake by the liver.
      4) Increases hepatic ketogenesis.
      5) Increase in lipolysis.
   d. Insulin.
      1) Initial suppression of insulin during first few hours of injury.
      2) Insulin levels rise after initial suppression.
      3) Decrease in the insulin:glucose ratio (physiologic suppression).
   e. Growth hormone.
      1) Increase in lipolysis.
      2) Promotes protein conservation.
      3) Increases hepatic ketogenesis.
      4) Decreases plasma insulin levels.
      5) Promotes release of insulin-like growth factor (IGF)-1 and IGF-2.
      6) IGF-1 secretion decreases: levels have been shown to correlate with nitrogen balance and recombinant infusions in traumatized patients may attenuate nitrogen loss.

3. Cytokines.
   a. TNF, IL-6.
   b. Increase resting energy expenditure.
   c. Synergistic effects on proteolysis.
   d. Inhibit lipoprotein lipase in adipose tissue reducing triglyceride clearance.
   e. Induce liver production of acute-phase reactants and downregulates production of nonacute-phase proteins (albumin and transferrin).

III. NUTRITIONAL SUPPORT

A. WHO SHOULD BE PLACED ON NUTRITIONAL SUPPORT?
1. Trauma patients who were malnourished prior to traumatic event.
2. Patients with severe traumatic injury who will not take adequate oral intake for 5–7 days.

B. GOALS OF NUTRITIONAL SUPPORT.
1. Maintenance of organ structure and function.
2. Treatment of malnutrition.
3. Prevention of nutrient deficiencies.

C. WHEN TO INITIATE NUTRITIONAL SUPPORT. Support should begin after the initial resuscitation.

D. **ESTIMATION OF ENERGY REQUIREMENTS.**

1. **Harris-Benedict equation** – an estimation of basal energy expenditure (BEE) in the fasted, resting, nonstressed state.

a. Men – BEE (kcal per day) = 66 + (13.7 × weight (kg)) + (5 × height (cm)) – (6.8 × age (years)).

b. Women – BEE (kcal per day) = 665 + (9.6 × weight (kg)) + (1.7 × height (cm)) – (4.7 × age (years)).

c. Trauma patients, especially burn patients, require a stress factor applied to the above equations. Current stress factors range from 1.2 to 1.6.

2. **Metabolic cart.**

a. Many intensive care units are now equipped with metabolic carts which can compute the REE for a given patient using the equation: REE = $5.083(V_{O_2})$ – $0.138(V_{CO_2})$ – $0.128(NM)$; where V_{O_2} is oxygen consumption, V_{CO_2} is carbon dioxide production, and NM is derived from urine urea nitrogen.

b. Although indirect calorimetry is accurate; it is somewhat cumbersome, expensive, and provides only a snapshot (20–30 minutes) of the patient's REE. It may be useful in the troublesome hypermetabolic patient who is difficult to wean from the ventilator.

E. **NUTRITIONAL MANAGEMENT.**

1. **At Parkland Memorial Hospital, 25–30kcal/kg per day are provided** as non protein calories, depending on injury severity.

a. This is provided in the form of glucose at 2–4g/kg per day since the body is unable to oxidize glucose at a faster rate.

b. The total daily administration of glucose never exceeds 5g/kg per day at Parkland.

2. **Approximately 7% of total calories** should be given to prevent essential fatty acid (FA) deficiency.

a. Providing excess FAs, especially in the form of ϖ-6-FA has been associated with immune dysfunction as well as perhaps accentuating the eicosanoid inflammatory response.

b. Parenteral FAs are given as a separate infusion twice weekly and contain 50% ϖ-6-FA.

3. **Protein is provided** at a rate of 1.5–2.0g/kg per day or 1g of nitrogen per 100–150 nonprotein kcal in the trauma patient.

a. In the severely stressed patient this ratio may decrease to 1gN:80kcal or lower.

b. 1g of nitrogen = 6.25g of protein.

4. **Assessment of nitrogen balance** is accomplished by obtaining a 24-hour measurement of urinary nitrogen excretion.

a. An estimation of total urinary nitrogen (TUN) excretion is the urinary urea nitrogen (UUN). This is easily obtained by collecting a 24-hour urine sample.

b. Urea accounts for about 80% of TUN; therefore TUN can be estimated by the formula, UUN + 20% UUN + 2g (nitrogen from skin and stool losses).

c. Nitrogen balance can then be determined by: (protein intake(g)/6.25) − UUN − 20% UUN − 2.

5. **Patients undergoing total parenteral nutrition (TPN)** should have daily measurements of electrolytes with changes incorporated into TPN formulations.

a. It is important to keep in mind that these changes will not be administered until the next bag of TPN formula is prepared (usually ~6–12 hours).

b. Acute changes need correction by supplemental i.v. repletion.

6. **Vitamins and trace elements.**

a. Daily requirements should be administered as per the AMA Nutritional Advisory Group guidelines.

b. Most enteral nutrition formulas contain the recommended daily allowances.

c. Intravenous multivitamin preparations can be prepared with the daily parenteral formula.

d. Deficiencies in copper and zinc may occur from excessive gastrointestinal (GI) losses.

F. ENTERAL VS PARENTERAL NUTRITION.

1. **Current consensus is to utilize the GI tract** for nutritional support whenever feasible.

2. **Experimental evidence has demonstrated** that total enteral nutrition when compared with TPN, prevents gut mucosal atrophy, attenuates the stress injury response, maintains immunocompetence, and preserves normal gut flora.

3. **Maintaining the gut mucosa** in the severely injured patient is thought to preserve the normal immune barrier to bacteria, thus preventing the adverse effects of bacterial translocation.

G. ENTERAL NUTRITION.

1. **Contraindications.**

a. Free perforation.

b. Peritonitis or intra-abdominal infection.

c. Complete mechanical bowel obstruction.

2. **Route of administration.**

a. Nasogastric feedings

   1) Easiest way to obtain access.

   2) Owing to possible gastric atony (gastric motility may be the last portion of GI tract to resolve from an ileus), the patient may not be able to tolerate feedings.

   3) May also predispose to aspiration pneumonia.

b. Naso-enteric feedings.
   1) Tubes are made of silastic rubber, 108–110cm in length, usually weighted, and have a wire stylet to aid in placement.
   2) The tube is placed past the pylorus and placement confirmed by obtaining a plain abdominal radiograph.
   3) Greater success with tube placement has been described with fluoroscopic or endoscopic guidance.
c. Surgical placement of feeding tubes.
   1) A naso-enteric or oro-enteric feeding tube can be positioned at the time of celiotomy, especially if the duodenum has been mobilized.
   2) Gastrostomy or jejunostomy tubes should be placed if the patient is expected to require long-term tube feedings >3 weeks.
   3) Tubes that contain a proximal gastric port for gastric decompression and a distal postpyloric port for enteral feedings have been used with good success.
   4) Placement of a postpyloric tube ensures that early feeding may begin even in the presence of a postoperative ileus.

3. **Feeding regimen.**
a. Initial continuous infusion rates should be between 20 and 30mL per hour.
b. Advance to a calculated goal rate that will administer 25–30kcal/kg per day.
c. Residuals should be checked and tube feeds held for 1–2 hours when >200–300mL.
d. At Parkland, a hydrolysate lactose-free formula is administered that contains 1kcal/mL, 300mOsm/kg of water, and a nonprotein kcal:g of nitrogen ratio of 125:1, is administered.
e. When initially starting tube feeds, a hyperosmolar formula (i.e. >400mOsm/kg of water) should be avoided because this may cause some intolerance to tube feeds (i.e. diarrhea).
f. Commercially available special enteric formulas containing arginine, fish-oils, and various other supplements are not used at Parkland.
g. Certain formulas are useful for patients with specific organ dysfunction that require adjustments to their nutritional supplements including:
   1) Liver failure – formulations that are high in branched-chain amino acids and low in aromatic amino acids may improve hepatic encephalopathy.
   2) Renal failure – these formulations contain essential amino acids and low protein which may diminish the increase in blood urea nitrogen. Furthermore the amount of calories administered per mL of fluid is often greater than that in standard formulas, thus

diminishing excess fluid administration. They also contain low or balanced electrolytes in order to prevent serum electrolyte abnormalities.

   3) Pulmonary failure – these formulas contain low carbohydrate and high fat thus reducing CO_2 production. The lowering of the respiratory quotient may diminish minute ventilation and thus reduce the need for ventilatory support. These formulas may cause steatorrhea due to fat malabsorption.

4. Complications of enteral feedings.

a. Aspiration.

   1) Aspiration from gastric vs postpyloric tube feeds continues to be an area of debate, with studies showing both no difference as well as an increased risk with gastric feeding.

   2) Parkland's policy is to start tube feeds and attempt to place a postpyloric tube.

   3) Tube feeds are usually started with a nasogastric tube and if postpyloric placement has not been achieved then gastric feedings are continued.

   4) Precautions, such as elevating the head to 30°, checking gastric residual volumes, and placing food coloring in the feedings, may help prevent aspiration.

b. Diarrhea.

   1) Can occur with high rates of administration of hyperosmolar solutions.

   2) This can be avoided by using solutions with lower osmolality administered at a low rate as outlined above. The rate can then be increased to goal rate.

   3) The avoidance of hyperosmolar solutions in the small intestine will also aid in the prevention of diarrhea.

   4) Hyperosmolar solutions tend to be handled better when administered via the stomach.

   5) The utilization of formulas with increased fiber may also help.

   6) The use of agents which decrease gut motility can be used cautiously once all other possible causes of diarrhea have been evaluated (i.e. malabsorption syndromes, infectious etiologies, lactase deficiencies, etc.).

c. Clogged feeding tubes.

   1) May create a problem, especially in surgically positioned tubes that cannot be easily replaced.

   2) Prevention can be achieved by precluding the administration of medications through the tube, using low-residue tube feeds, and flushing the tube periodically.

   3) Once clogged, numerous agents can be used to relieve the blockage (e.g. meat tenderizer, cola, cranberry juice, vinegar).

H. PARENTERAL NUTRITION.

1. **Total parenteral nutrition** is associated with more complications than enteral nutrition.

2. **Despite the inability to nutritionally support patients via enteral feeding**, Parkland attempts to provide at least 20–30% of nutritional needs via the GI tract as this will maintain the mucosal barrier through its trophic effects on the gut mucosa.

3. **Composition of parenteral nutrition**

a. Carbohydrates.
   1) Administered in the form of dextrose solutions ranging from 10 to 70%.
   2) Solutions are hyperosmolar and, as a result, most must be infused through a large central vein.
   3) Each dextrose solution is presented as mg/dL; thus a 10% dextrose solution will contain 100g of dextrose in 1L of solution. The amount of calories per liter of solution can then be easily determined since there are 3.4kcal/g of dextrose (Table 51.2).

b. Protein.
   1) Given in the form of single amino acid mixtures.
   2) Peptides cannot be utilized when given i.v.
   3) Amino acid solutions contain essential and nonessential amino acids.

c. Fat.
   1) Supplied as emulsions derived from safflower oil or soybean oil.
   2) Unlike dextrose and amino acid solutions, these emulsions are isosmolar to plasma and can be given through peripheral i.v. infusions.
   3) The commercially available emulsions contain 1–2kcal/mL.
   4) At Parkland, the standard TPN order supplies most, if not all, of the nonprotein calories as carbohydrate.
   5) Fat emulsions are primarily administered to provide linoleic acid and prevent essential fatty acid deficiency.

TABLE 51.2

CALORIFIC VALUE DETERMINATION CHART – DEXTROSE SOLUTIONS

Dextrose concentration (%)	Dextrose (g/dL)	Calories (kcal/L)
7	70	238
10	100	340
20	200	680
25	250	850
50	500	1700
70	700	2380

51

METABOLISM AND NUTRITION

6) The administration of fat as a primary fuel source may be indicated in patients that are glucose intolerant.

d. Electrolytes, vitamins, and minerals.

1) Supplied as standard additives to the TPN solution.
2) Standard electrolyte mixtures contain sodium, potassium, chloride, acetate, phosphorus, calcium, and magnesium.
3) The standard daily electrolyte and trace element additives used at Parkland are listed in Table 51.3.
4) A multivitamin commercial packet is also added to each day's TPN mixture.
5) Most patients' daily requirements will be met with the above standard additives.
6) Patients with electrolyte disturbances will need to have their additives tailored to meet their needs.
7) TPN orders should be written only after reviewing the patient's daily electrolyte profile.
8) It must be kept in mind that any changes made in the TPN formula will not be instituted until the new formula is administered (~6–12 hours later).

4. Practical guidelines for administering and ordering TPN

a. Route of administration – central venous access must be used for hyperosmolar solutions.

b. The lipid emulsions discussed above can be administered peripherally.

c. Administration of hyperosmolar solutions of amino acids can cause thrombophlebitis.

TABLE 51.3

STANDARD DAILY ELECTROLYTE AND TRACE ELEMENT ADDITIVES

Electrolyte/trace element	Amount (per day)
Sodium	103mEq
Zinc	1000µg
Potassium	60mEq
Copper	400µg
Chloride	90mEq
Manganese	100µg
Acetate	90mEq
Chromium	4µg
Phosphorus	21mEq
Selenium	20µg
Calcium	15mEq
Magnesium	15mEq

1) Use of more dilute solutions of amino acids can cause volume overload.
2) The current recommendation is that the peripheral route be reserved for patients who do not have accessible central venous sites and for patients who require only supplementation.

d. Writing TPN orders.

1) Daily TPN orders should begin with a clinical assessment of the patient including pulmonary, cardiovascular, and renal status, as well as ongoing infections, wounds, and daily electrolytes.
2) The energy requirements for most patients can be achieved by supplying 25–30kcal/kg per day supplied as nonprotein calories. In an 80kg patient, 2000 nonprotein kilocalories should be administered daily in the form of a 25% dextrose solution. Each liter of D25 will contain 850kcal (see above), thus this patient will need 2350mL of D25 per day.
3) Daily protein requirements should be 1–2g/kg per day. An 80kg patient will require 120g of protein per day or 19g of nitrogen per day.
4) An 80kg patient will require a final TPN solution consisting of 25% dextrose and 5% amino acids administered at a rate of 100mL per hour. Conversely, this can be determined by figuring out the amount of daily nitrogen (protein) requirement and multiplying that number by 100 to determine the amount of daily nonprotein calories required.
5) TPN is started at 50–70% of the computed rate, owing to possible glucose intolerance. If the patient is able to tolerate this rate, the rate is advanced to the goal on the subsequent day.
6) The patient's electrolytes should be checked daily and the TPN formula tailored to meet each patient's requirements.
7) Other additives include multivitamins, trace elements, and H2 antagonists for patients at risk for stress gastritis.
8) Each patient's blood glucose is checked every 4 hours after initiation of TPN. Patients should be placed on a regular insulin sliding scale to keep their blood glucose between 100 and 200mg/dL. If the patient's daily insulin requirement is relatively stable, then insulin can be added to each day's TPN formula.

5. **Complications of parenteral nutrition.**

a. Technical complications.

1) Pneumothorax.
2) Hemothorax.
3) Hydrothorax.
4) Air embolism.
5) Guide wire or catheter embolism.
6) Subclavian or carotid artery injury.

       7) Nerve injury.
       8) Thoracic duct injury.
       9) Erosion of catheter into right atrium.
      10) Subclavian thrombosis.
      11) Thrombophlebitis.
      12) Catheter sepsis.
      13) Cardiac arrhythmias.
  b. Electrolyte and other substance abnormalities.
      1) Trace metal deficiencies (e.g. zinc, copper, chromium, selenium).
      2) Essential fatty acid deficiency.
      3) Hyperglycemia.
      4) Hypoglycemia.
      5) Hepatic steatosis.

I. NUTRITION MODIFICATION AND IMMUNOMODULATION .

1. Fatty acid modification.

  a. The use of medium-chain triglycerides as opposed to long-chain triglycerides may improve nitrogen balance when used as an alternate fuel source in parenteral nutrition.

  b. The enteral administration of short-chain triglycerides may have trophic effects on bowel mucosa.

2. Growth hormone.

  a. Growth hormone levels are depressed in severely injured patients.

  b. Growth hormone has been shown to attenuate proteolysis, promote lipolysis, and improve immune function.

  c. Although still experimental, exogenous administration of growth hormone has been shown to improve negative nitrogen balance and diminish muscle protein catabolism in trauma and burn patients.

3. Immunomodulation.

  a. Dietary supplementation with ϖ-3-polyunsaturated fatty acids may have beneficial anti-inflammatory effects.

  b. Antioxidants (α-tocopherol and ascorbic acid) may also have immunomodulatory effects and have been shown to improve neutrophil function when given to blunt-trauma patients.

IV. PEARLS AND PITFALLS

1. **Nutritional support should be initiated for trauma patients** who are unable to maintain adequate oral nutrition for 5–7 days.

2. **Do not overfeed** – most trauma patients will require 25–30kcal/kg per day.

3. **Glucose administration** should not exceed 5g/kg per day.

4. **If the GI tract works use it!** (Ileus does not preclude some form of enteral nutrition.)

5. **Postpyloric tube feeds may be tolerated better than gastric feedings**; however, postpyloric placement is not essential to the administration of enteral nutrition.

6. **Initiate tube feeds at a low rate**, 20–30 mL per hour, and then advance to goal rate as tolerated.
7. **Hyperosmolar solutions** may not be well tolerated and can cause diarrhea.
8. **Total parenteral nutrition** is associated with a higher morbidity than enteral nutrition.
9. **Providing 20–30% of nutritional needs via the GI tract** may prevent gut mucosal atrophy and maintain mucosal barrier.
10. **Dressings on central venous lines** should be changed daily and monitored for signs of infection.
11. **Patients' blood glucose** should be checked every 4–6 hours and they should be placed on an insulin sliding scale.
12. **Every effort should be made to avoid aspiration** (e.g. by elevating head of bed, placing food coloring in tube feeds).

V. FURTHER READING

Cerra FB. Metabolic and nutritional support. In: Feliciano DV, Moore EE, Mattox KL (eds.) *Trauma,* 3rd edn. Stanford: Appleton and Lange; 1996:1155.

Endres S, Ghorbani R, Kelley VE et al. The effects of dietary supplementation with n-3 polyunsaturated fatty acids on the synthesis of interleukin-1 and tumor necrosis factor by mononuclear cells. *N Engl J Med* 1989; 320(5):265–271.

Fischer JE. Metabolism in surgical patients. In: Sabiston DC (ed.) *Textbook of surgery: the biologic basis of modern surgical practice,* 15th edn. Philadelphia: WB Saunders; 1997:137–175.

Herskowitz K, Souba WW. Intestinal glutamine metabolism during critical illness: a surgical perspective. *Nutrition* 1990; 6(3):199–206.

Jiang Z, Zhang S, Wang X et al. A comparison of medium-chain and long-chain triglycerides in surgical patients. *Ann Surg* 1993; 217(2):175–184.

Kudsk KA, Croce MA, Fabian TC et al. Enteral vs parenteral feeding: effects on septic morbidity after blunt and penetrating abdominal trauma. *Ann Surg* 1991; 215(5):503–511.

Moore FA, Feliciano DV, Andrassy RJ, et al. Early enteral feeding, compared with parenteral, reduces postoperative complications. *Ann Surg* 1991; 216(2):172–183.

Rombeau JL, Kripke SA. Metabolic and intestinal effects of short-chain fatty acids. *JPEN* 1990; 14(5)S:181S–184S.

Strong RM, Condon SC, Solinger MR et al. Equal aspiration rates from postpylorus and intragastric-placed small-bore naso-enteric feeding tubes: a randomized, prospective study. *JPEN* 1992; 16:59–63.

Zaloga GP. Bedside method for placing small bowel feeding tubes in critically ill patients: a prospective study. *Chest* 1991; 100:1643–1646

51

METABOLISM AND NUTRITION

MANAGEMENT OF THE ORGAN DONOR

52

I. INTRODUCTION

1. **Major advances have been made** in the areas of organ preservation, operative techniques, and immunosuppression that have significantly improved outcomes in organ transplantation.
2. **The limiting factor** continues to be the shortage of donors.
3. **As severe head injury is the leading cause of death in organ donors**, it is important for the trauma surgeon to recognize patients as potential donors, and to refer them to the appropriate organ procurement agency.

II. DONOR CRITERIA

1. **The preferred candidate for organ donation** is an otherwise healthy patient who has sustained irreversible brain injury due to:
   a. Head trauma.
   b. Subarachnoid hemorrhage.
   c. Drug overdose.
   d. Primary brain tumor.
   e. Cerebral ischemia.
2. **Age is no longer considered an absolute exclusion criteria**, and each case should be reviewed on an individual basis.
3. **Contraindications to donation** include:
   a. Malignancies other than primary brain or localized skin cancers.
   b. Sepsis.
   c. History of tuberculosis or syphilis.
   d. Acute viral infections, including hepatitis, HIV, cytomegalovirus, systemic herpes, or viral encephalitis.
   e. The donor should not have a history of chronic unstable hypertension or diabetes, have undergone prolonged hypotension or asystole, or have required high-dose vasoactive drugs.
   f. There should be no evidence of infection, trauma, or a chronic disease involving the specific organs considered for donation.
   g. A recent history of i.v. drug use.
4. **Should a patient fail to meet the criteria for organ donation** or die from cardiac arrest, consideration should be given for tissue donation (i.e. corneas, whole eyes, skin, tendon, bone, or heart valves).
5. **If questions arise as to whether a donor is eligible**, these specific issues should be addressed by the organ procurement agency or transplant team.

III. ESTABLISHING BRAIN DEATH

A. LEGAL DEFINITION.

1. **A person is considered legally dead** if there is irreversible cessation of spontaneous respiratory and circulatory functions.
2. **If artificial means of support are utilized,** a person is declared dead if there is irreversible cessation of all spontaneous brain and brain-stem function. Death is then pronounced before artificial means of support are terminated.

B. GENERALIZED CRITERIA FOR BRAIN DEATH.

1. **Etiology of coma** must be defined.
2. **No major abnormalities** in acid–base, serum electrolytes, or glucose metabolism.
3. **Correction of hypotension, hypothermia** (<32ºC), and hypoxia.
4. **Absence of central nervous system depressants, neuromuscular blocking agents, and toxins.**
5. **Absence of spontaneous movements,** including posturing.
6. **Absent brain-stem reflexes:** pupillary, corneal, gag, oculocephalic, and oculovestibular.
7. **Apnea test.**
   a. The patient is removed from the ventilator while oxygen is administered at 6–8L per minute by cannula via the endotracheal tube.
   b. An arterial blood gas is drawn in 5 minutes to document no spontaneous respirations in the presence of hypercarbia (Pco_2 >60).
   c. The test is discontinued for evidence of bradycardia, hypotension, or hypoxia, and an arterial blood gas is immediately drawn.
   d. Spinal reflexes may be present during this test, but do not exclude brain death.
8. **The period of observation** may range from 2 to 24 hours, depending on clinical circumstances.
9. **Confirmatory tests** – in the presence of confounding factors, such as certain drugs, the absence of cerebral circulation can be confirmed by cerebral angiography, radionuclide imaging, cerebral blood flow scans, or electrocerebral silence on electroencephalogram (EEG).

IV. CONSENT FOR DONATION

1. **The Uniform Anatomical Gift Act** allows adults to donate all or parts of their body for research, education, or transplantation. It also establishes a hierarchy for next of kin from whom to obtain consent:
   a. Spouse.
   b. Adult son or daughter.
   c. Either parent.
   d. Guardian.
   e. Other authorized person.
2. **Should a discrepancy exist between the donor's and the family's**

wishes, this can frequently be resolved with help from the organ bank and the hospital chaplain's office. In reality, the family's wishes are frequently honored over the donor's.

3. **Permission must also be granted by the medical examiner's office** when appropriate.

4. **The family should not be approached** about organ donation until brain death has been declared, and they have been allowed sufficient time to accept this reality. The topic may be discussed earlier if it is brought up by the family.

5. **Attempts by organ bank personnel to obtain consent** are frequently more successful than those by physicians, and they are available to assist in this matter.

6. **It is important to be able to answer questions** that the family may have, and to assure them that funeral proceedings, body presentation, and financial costs incurred will not be altered by the decision to donate.

7. **Many families may lessen their grief** by realizing their loved one has helped to sustain the lives of others.

V. MEDICAL MANAGEMENT OF THE DONOR

A. **THE GOALS** of medical therapy for the organ donor are to maintain tissue oxygenation and perfusion.

B. **HEMODYNAMICS.**

1. **Restore and maintain circulation volume.**

2. **Infuse lactated Ringer's solution, colloid, or blood products** as needed to maintain a cardiovascular pressure of 8–15 and systolic blood pressure >100mmHg.

3. **If a vasopressor or inotrope is required**, dopamine is recommended. Use the lowest dose possible, preferably <10µg/kg body weight/minute.

4. **Avoid receptor agonists**, such as norepinephrine.

5. **Match urine output with lactated Ringer's solution**, roughly mL for mL, plus an additional 50mL per hour for maintenance.

6. **Utilize nitroprusside infusion for hypertension**: systolic blood pressure >170mmHg, diastolic blood pressure >110mmHg.

7. **Resuscitate as required.** Bradyarrhythmias are common, and may not respond to atropine.

8. **Maintain normothermia** (>35°C).

C. **OXYGENATION AND VENTILATION.**

1. **Monitor arterial blood gases frequently**, every 4 hours.

2. **Normalize Pco_2 to** maintain a normal or slightly alkalotic pH.

3. **Regulate Fio_2 to** maintain Po_2 >100. PEEP may be added as needed.

4. **Maintain adequate hemoglobin** to optimize oxygen-carrying capacity.

5. **Use aggressive pulmonary toilet** to minimize pulmonary complications.

D. RENAL SYSTEM.
1. **Maintain urine output** at >75mL per hour, or >1mL/kg per hour, replacing losses with lactated Ringer's.
2. **Colloids may be added** as needed.
3. **If the central venous pressure is adequate,** furosemide may be used to maintain diuresis.
4. **If poor response to furosemide** (up to 120mg), mannitol may be used, starting with a 12.5g dose.
5. **Monitor serum electrolytes frequently,** every 4 hours.
6. **Diabetes insipidus.**
   a. Treat if urine output >300mL per hour for 2 consecutive hours.
   b. Replace urine output mL for mL if normotensive.
   c. Desmopressin:
      1) Administer 0.5–2g i.v. to produce ADH effect for 8–12 hours.
      2) Repeat dose in 2 hours if poor response initially.
   d. Pitressin drip may also be used (50 units in 500mL normal saline) at 0.5–2 units per hour, or for urine output 75–250mL per hour.
7. **Check urine for glucose,** treat hyperglycemia with insulin.

VI. FURTHER READING

Guidelines to donor management. Dallas: Southwest Organ Bank.

Organ and tissue procurement procedure. In: *Dallas County Hospital District Administrative Manual*.

INDEX